We live in a world where psychiatric diagnoses, like autism, are treated differently than any other medical condition. Once a psychiatric diagnosis is made, there is no consideration of the biochemistry involved in a diagnosis or that changing the biochemistry can change outcomes. Marcia Hind's book, *I Know You're in There*, serves as a reminder that autism is a neurologic condition with causes and solutions. It shows parents and physicians that when a child gets proper medical intervention recovery becomes possible. I have witnessed firsthand my autism patients regain their health. Ryan's story is a beacon of hope for all families with children on the spectrum."

—James Neuenschwander, MD, director of the Bio Energy Medical Center

Parents need to read *I Know You're in There*. This motivating and encouraging story proves that optimal outcomes are possible for children with autism when families look positively to the future by embracing cutting-edge medical treatment combined with standard-of-care rehabilitation."

—Richard Frye, PhD, MD, chief of the Division of Neurodevelopmental Disorders, Phoenix Children's Hospital neurologist and autism expert

After reading Ryan's story, parents will realize there is hope and recovery is possible. This book shows the medical treatment is different and individual for every child. *I Know You're in There* helps the reader understand that medicine alone is not enough. We must use a child's interests and strengths to help them overcome autism."

—Sidney McDonald Baker, MD, founder of Autism360.org

There is an urgent need for the worldwide autism paradigm to change: children with the diagnostic label of autism are medically ill and need help. With proper medical intervention, they can recover or significantly improve in health and function. Every child deserves that chance. Marcia Hinds' book, *I Know You're in There*, encourages parents, therapists, and others to give these precious children this opportunity. Marcia wants all children to have what her recovered son now has; she can't leave the other kids behind."

—Ed and Teri Arranga, president and executive director, AutismOne

ADVANCE PRAISE

"Ryan's recovery was not miraculous. It was the result of having h
illness treated. His family persisted in looking for answers until th
doctor who would do just that. Maybe that was the miracle."

—Bruce L. Ri

"This book is a MUST read for any family struggling with autism. As
nologist, my intuition said my son's dysfunctional immune system
core of his illness. Marcia's experience correcting Ryan's immune s
recovering the whole child is shared openly and honestly in this
Hinds family could have taken the easy path, walked away from A
moved on with their life. Instead of letting others figure it out for
Ryan's story will inspire and inform crucial medical and educationa
This unique book offers the hope and tenacity parents need to find
for their children in the midst of a journey that is turbulent and
Hope is contagious. Now that we know what is possible, we must ne
on recovery."

—Melinda Borrello Sharma, PhD, director of Autism Spectrum

"*I Know You're in There* shows that autism is not a hardwired i
stamped into the brain by the child's genes and destined to remain fi
as we're often told. Instead, it is the TOTAL LOAD of challenges
whole system that overloads the brain and causes the behaviors asso
autism. Even a few treatments that reduce the load and increase su
make a huge difference. Ryan's recovery is a testimony to this appro

—Martha Herbert, PhD, MD
The Autism Revolution: Whole-Body Strategies for Making Life Al
Harvard Medical School neurologist, researcher, ar

"Ryan's story of diagnosis and recovery illustrates that there is a medical basis for most, if not all, cases of autism. Today, powerful technologies are available which can help doctors make a more accurate and timely diagnosis of this medical basis. If there is one message in this book it is *Never give up trying!*"

—Rosario Trifiletti, MD, PhD, pediatric neurologist, PANDAS/PANS Institute

"A compelling story of a courageous mom who helped her son overcome the challenges faced by Autism. She inspires all parents to never give up and how important it is to not overlook the biomedical component. A must read for ALL parents!"

—Alisa Wolf, Med-SPED, executive director/founder, Actors for Autism

"*I Know You're in There* is an inspiring true story of one mother's fight to help her son overcome autism. Ryan's recovery involved a combination of approaches, including biomedical therapies, behavioral interventions, as well as love and determination. It is a very personal story about the challenges their family faced, and how they overcame them. It shows what can happen for some children, and we hope for many more as we learn more about effective treatments for autism."

—James B. Adams, PhD, Autism/Asperger's Research Program Arizona State University

"*I Know You're in There* should be given to every family when they receive an autism diagnosis. This book will help parents understand the importance of digging deep to identify possible underlying immune dysfunction rather than just accepting therapy alone as the only option for improving development. More importantly Ryan's story should serve as a source of encouragement to families struggling to manage daily life as they navigate the challenges of this complex disease process. The title is perfect. If you know your child is IN THERE, use this book to inspire you in the hardest of times to never, ever give up hope that you can find a path to recovery."

—Victoria L. Falcone, DO, Falcone Center for Functional, Cosmetic and Integrative Medicine

"Marcia Hinds provides a detailed case history of how her child responded to various treatment interventions, many of which are not yet considered evidenced-based by the scientific community. I truly hope this book will inspire researchers worldwide to study these interventions. Once validated, these treatments will likely become accepted by the autism and medical communities and covered by health insurance companies."

—Steve Edelson, PhD, executive director, Autism Research Institute

"*I Know You're in There* presents a wonderful example for families dealing with autism. With knowledge, flexibility, patience and creativeness on the part of both parents and health care providers, it becomes possible to address the root medical causes of autism. Ryan's story provides hope. With perseverance and proper treatment, children with autism can improve. Some who might have unnecessarily drifted through life with limited abilities and untapped potential can even achieve 'normalcy'."

—Morton M. Teich, MD, Pediatric Allergy and Immunology, former president of the American Academy of Environmental Medicine

"Too many parents of children diagnosed with autism are told that recovery is not possible. In *I Know You're in There*, Marcia Hinds courageously retells the story of her son's journey out of autism and provides hope and inspiration for the millions of families affected by the tidal wave of chronic childhood illnesses sweeping through our world. While everyone's route to recovery will be different, Ryan's story reinforces what we know to be true: Children can get better!"

—Beth Lambert, author of *A Compromised Generation*, executive producer of the Canary Kids Project, executive director, Epidemic Answers

"Families must realize that successful individuals with autism are no longer a 'fluke.' It takes educating yourself, tough decisions, and perseverance. *I Know You're in There* offers real life solutions to families. Ryan triumphed because his family educated themselves and combined multiple approaches for his success. Exciting!"

—Ann Millan, author of *Autism—Believe in the Future*

"*I Know You're in There* is a compelling read that helps parents realize they are not alone while facing the challenges, along the autism road so many of us travel. In this inspiring story told so well by Marcia, we all share a renewed hope for the future of our children."

—Karen Simmons, founder and CEO of Autism Today,
co-author of *Chicken Soup for the Soul, Children with Special Needs*

"Ryan's success demonstrates the effectiveness of the UCLA (Lovaas) Model of Applied Behavior Analysis. ABA was in its infancy when Ryan's program began twenty years ago. Now, even more empirical research and data are in and show that what happened for Ryan is possible for others with autism. I hope that Ryan's success story, as described in *I Know You're in There*, will inspire others to take this challenging but worthwhile path toward recovery."

—Scott Wright, president and CEO of Lovaas Institute
and LIFE Midwest, Inc.

"The combination of hard work on the part of the parents, teachers, therapists, and medical care specifically for the treatment of autism can make children improve dramatically. But in Ryan's case it resulted in complete recovery. This book gives us all hope for the future."

— Katherine E. Robertson, RN, MSN, LTC (ret.) U.S. Army, founder of the
Northern New York Autism Foundation

"When I first met Ryan around age five, he was disengaged and had significant social and communication problems. While Ryan's deficits were extensive, he made remarkable progress after we implemented the Applied Behavior Analysis program designed specifically to meet his needs. I feel fortunate and proud to have been a part of his amazing success and continue to be inspired by him and his family's relentless dedication that lead to his recovery."

— Mindi Fisher Pohlenz, BCBA, MSc SLT,
director of the Behavior Intervention Group

"*I Know You're in There* is an important book for families dealing with autism. This heartfelt story destroys many of the myths associated with the diagnosis. Readers will come to understand how autism can be treatable and surmountable when children receive proper interventions for their medical needs. We want to thank Ryan and his family for bravely sharing their story because in doing so they will undoubtedly help other families looking for answers."

—Treating Autism nonprofit, United Kingdom
(Treating Autism provides support to families affected by autism)

I Know You're in There

Winning Our War Against Autism

MARCIA HINDS

FOREWORD BY DR. JAMES B. ADAMS

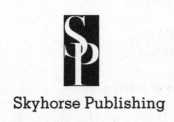

Skyhorse Publishing

Skyhorse Publishing books may be purchased in bulk at special discounts for sales promotion, corporate gifts, fund-raising, or educational purposes. Special editions can also be created to specifications. For details, contact the Special Sales Department, Skyhorse Publishing, 307 West 36th Street, 11th Floor, New York, NY 10018 or info@skyhorsepublishing.com.

Skyhorse® and Skyhorse Publishing® are registered trademarks of Skyhorse Publishing, Inc.®, a Delaware corporation.

Visit our website at www.skyhorsepublishing.com.

10 9 8 7 6 5 4 3 2 1

Library of Congress Cataloging-in-Publication Data is available on file.

Cover design by Paul Qualcom
Cover image credit: Getty Images

Print ISBN: 978-1-5107-4825-5
Ebook ISBN: 978-1-5107-4826-2

Printed in the United States of America

This book is dedicated to the army of people who climbed into the trenches with us. You helped Ryan win the battle of his life and our war against autism.

To Aunt Debbie, Uncle Dean, Grandma, and Auntie Two Shoes: You loved Ryan unconditionally. Your acceptance helped him more than you'll ever know.

To my husband, Frank, and my daughter, Megan: Ryan recovered because of your hard work and sacrifice. Our family made it through the dark side. We are better and stronger because of your efforts.

And, most of all, to my son, Ryan: No one taught me more about what is important in life. You defied the odds and conquered autism, sometimes in spite of your overprotective mother. You continue to be my personal hero.

Some people think we should just accept autism. And that if a child is treated, it changes who that kid is. I am still the same person I was, only now I'm happy and can enjoy life. It is hard to understand that children are not receiving proper medical treatment because some people think we should celebrate autism. When doctors believe the medical issues associated with autism are just part of a "developmental disorder," children are not treated for the same medical conditions as every other kid. Is that really okay?

—Ryan Hinds, My Son

AUTHOR'S NOTE

Some of the names in this book were changed to protect people's privacy. Others were changed because I wanted to write an honest account of our story and not worry about being sued. I am an expert at only one thing and that is being Ryan's mom. Even so, I made a lot of mistakes along the way. I fought doctors when they were right. I went along with snake oil salesmen when I shouldn't have. The thing I did right is that I never gave up. Please do not take this book as a blueprint for what you should do for your child, medically or otherwise. When it comes to the treatment of autism, one size doesn't fit all. You must find your own path and follow it. And God help anyone who gets in your way.

The information contained herein is meant to be of a general nature and should not be construed as medical or any other type of professional advice. Any intervention must be decided upon on an individual basis and administered by professionals skilled in their respective discipline. Please do not do anything stated or implied in this book without proper supervision.

TABLE OF CONTENTS

PREFACE BY MY SON, RYAN HINDS

While we try to teach our children all about life, our children teach us
what life is all about.

—Angela Schwindt

MY MOM ASKED me to read the book to make sure I was okay with the
things she wrote. That was hard to do. I learned about events I didn't remember
and things that were just embarrassing. I know I shouldn't be concerned about
the weird things I did back then, because I was ill. But I am embarrassed by
them and would rather keep them in my past forever. I wish I could forget all
the horrible things that happened and everything to do with autism.

While I want to provide hope and encouragement to others, I still have
mixed feelings about telling my story. Who really wants every detail of their
childhood out there for the world to see? I don't want the first thing people
know about me to be that I was once severely affected by autism. But more than
that, I don't want anyone to question the things my mom said in this book.
Some will say I never really had autism or maybe that I was only mildly affected.
I wish that were true.

Our story has a happy ending, but how many parents are still told there is no
hope for their children? And how many kids will not get better proper medical
care or get better as a result? My family never gave up on me because, like the
title of this book, they knew I was in there. When experts told them I would
never be okay and would probably end up in a group home, they still didn't give
up. As a result, I was able to leave my autism label behind.

As much as I don't want to admit to anything autistic, I know my story is important to help others realize autism is medical, treatable, and surmountable. I was lucky to have a family who fought back and never gave up on me. They were always there, no matter how difficult I made things for them.

FOREWORD

I KNOW YOU'RE in There is an inspiring true story of one family's fight to help their son overcome autism. Ryan's recovery involved a combination of approaches, including biomedical therapies, behavioral interventions, as well as love and determination. It is a very personal story about the challenges Marcia's family faced, and how they overcame them. It shows what is possible for some children, and we hope it will be possible for many more as we continue to learn about effective treatments for autism.

I'm writing this foreword from multiple viewpoints, based on my experience as a father of an adult daughter with autism, an autism researcher with over forty publications focused on biomedical causes of autism and treatments for it, as the president of the Autism Society of Greater Phoenix for nineteen years, as the president of the Autism Nutrition Research Center, as the co-leader of the scientific advisory board of the Autism Research Institute, and as the co-founder of the Neurological Health Foundation.

I think one of the most important messages in Marcia's story is the love she has for her son. We all seem to have a similar beginning. When my daughter Kim was diagnosed with autism and a severe intellectual disability at age two and a half in 1994, my wife and I were devastated. Like many parents, we were told that autism was incurable and that eventually our daughter would need institutionalization. The expert multi-disciplinary team who diagnosed her said they did not know how to treat her and advised us to go to the local Autism

Society of America group to learn more. There, we met other parents and realized how little was known about the causes of autism or how to help our children. Eventually that led us to another parent, Dr. Bernard Rimland, founder of the Autism Research Institute, who helped us understand that autism is a medical condition and treatable.

Autism is simply the label given to children who have a certain set of symptoms in early childhood, including major impairments in communication, social interaction, and restricted, repetitive behaviors. In reality, what we call autism is a complex medical condition, and so it makes sense to first evaluate the most common medical problems and to develop treatments for them. The bottom line is that "autism" is very heterogeneous, and different children have different genetic and/or environmental causes of autism. This means that the family and their physician need to work together to identify what particular medical conditions the child has, and to try to identify treatments for them. Ryan's story is a great example of the complexities of autism. Each child has unique medical problems that must be treated. Our challenge as parents is to identify our children's medical problems and try to find the treatment that will address the root causes.

It is up to each family to work with a knowledgeable physician to test for different medical conditions and treat them appropriately. Ryan's story shows how his family kept looking until they found the medical answers that helped him. It is important to remember what works for one child may not be the right treatment for another due to the differences in underlying biochemistry and physiology. Sadly, most physicians today are still focused on using standard psychiatric medications for treating behavior symptoms, instead of identifying and treating the root causes of autism.

There is already a large amount of research which demonstrates that these children often have many medical abnormalities, such as impaired methylation (which effects gene expression), low glutathione (an important anti-oxidant and defense against toxic metals), low sulfate (which affects neurotransmitter deactivation and lubrication of the gastrointestinal tract), abnormal gut bacteria (which can cause constipation and/or diarrhea), reduced melatonin (causing sleep problems), cerebral folate deficiency (leading to impaired mental function), impaired mitochondrial function (leading to low energy for the body and brain), low lactase (needed to digest lactose, the sugar in milk), and more. However, although many children with autism do have one or more of these conditions, there is no one medical condition common to all children with autism. I suspect that further research will reveal that low levels of essential vitamins, minerals, and other nutrients may also contribute to autism, and proper nutrition is an active part of our research. For more discussion about preventing autism and other medical disorders during pregnancy, see the "Healthy Child Guide" by the Neurological Health Foundation (www.neurologicalhealth.org)

But there is still much hope for the future of our children. The answers and treatments are coming. My research team is currently doing trials for Microbiota Transfer Therapy (MTT) in both adults and children. The initial results have shown 44 percent of participants with "severe" autism no longer qualified for an ASD diagnosis two years later. The Food and Drug Administration is fast-tracking our studies, which helps with faster review and we hope will eventually lead to approval by the FDA. That means once they are approved, any doctor will be able to prescribe this treatment for any individual on the spectrum. You can find more info about these trials at http://autism.asu.edu.

Currently behavioral therapies such as Applied Behavior Analysis (ABA) are recognized as some of the most effective treatments for children with autism. However, there are some children who have only limited or no response to behavior therapies. I suspect that in many cases this could be due to their underlying medical conditions.

Once a child's medical issues are addressed, behavioral therapies can be very helpful in teaching particular skills, such as language. It generally requires a consistent and intensive approach, but it can be difficult for families to obtain the level of services needed for their child. Speech therapy can also be helpful, but most times kids need more than what is allotted. As a result, parents must do what Marcia did and use that time to learn from the therapist how to implement similar therapy throughout the child's day. Physical and occupational therapy can also be important for children with fine/gross motor problems or with sensory sensitivities.

Educational support is essential for children with autism, but we still have a lot to learn about the best ways to teach and support affected children. Some common problems are low teacher expectations, limited teacher training, and limited classroom support. Also, many higher-functioning children have suffered severe bullying in school, so it is important for the school to have intensive programs to address that issue. Every school must promote tolerance and acceptance of all students. Marcia's book gives some good examples of how to address the issues with our educational system.

I think one of the most critical, and most overlooked therapies for autism is social therapy and support. The core symptom of autism is a lack of social understanding and impaired development of social relationships. In adulthood this often leads to a lack of friends, resulting in loneliness and depression, and is one of the most important issues affecting their quality of life. Too much time spent with therapists can limit the time available for developing relationships with family and friends. It is very important for families to spend time interacting with their child, and to support their interactions with friends via "play dates" and other approaches. Again, Ryan's story shows good examples of how his family encouraged social development and taught him these very important skills.

Overall, I think that this book will give families hope that, once we identify the medical problems in children with autism, a combination of medical/nutritional care and therapies along with a lot of family love and support can help many children improve, and in some cases, like Ryan, recover from autism.

—James B. Adams, PhD
Autism/Asperger's Research Program at Arizona State University
(http://autism.asu.edu)
Adams Autism Research
(www.adamsautismresearch.com)
President, Autism Nutrition Research Center
(www.AutismNRC.org)

INTRODUCTION
DON'T BELIEVE EVERYTHING
YOU'RE TOLD

The one thing children wear out faster than shoes are PARENTS.

—Johren J. Plomp

AS PARENTS, WE find ourselves in a unique, exclusive group, the *Autism Club*. No one asks to become a member, but, because of our kids, we are forced to be in the *A-Club* together. Autism isn't just a medical crisis; it is a crisis that affects every member of the family. The personal anxiety, stress, and social isolation that results from living on *"Autism Island"* is overwhelming. Only another parent with a child on the spectrum understands what it is like to live with autism day in and day out. It's beyond exhausting. Our friends and family don't understand how hard this is or how much we love these kids in spite of how difficult they make our lives. Our kids don't seem to fit anywhere, and as a result they are usually not included or invited to anything. And as much as we'd like to, we can't give up on our children because sometimes we catch a glimpse of the kid we *know* is in there.

We knew something wasn't right with Ryan even before the psychiatrist predicted he would probably end up in an institution. My son was diagnosed with autism at age four. That day changed everything. The doctor gave him and us a life sentence. At first all I could do was cry. I continued to cry about my son's future for years. The diagnosis ripped away every dream my husband and I had for our child and our family. Ryan was stranded on Autism Island, and our family was trapped right there with him.

We were told there was no recovery from autism.

There was no cure. There was no hope.

The grief parents experience after receiving this diagnosis can be paralyzing. Each of us is devastated by the loss of our dreams. But you can't feel sorry for yourself or your child for too long. You don't have time. You have too much work to do. Only a parent has the determination, stamina, and commitment to complete the seemingly insurmountable task of recovery. We are the only ones who will keep working to help our children in spite of how tired or discouraged we feel.

Don't allow this frightening diagnosis to overwhelm you. And don't ever think anyone will volunteer to do this job for you. Your children will not come out of this by themselves. You have to go in there and get them. So, roll up your sleeves, trust your instincts, and do what needs to be done.

And please remember that recovery takes time and a never-give-up attitude. Some people call this perseverance, I call it being more stubborn than our kids. It is not like I woke up one day and BAM my kid was better. Getting better takes time. That was hard for a parent like me who wanted my son fixed before lunch.

I Know You're in There: Winning Our War Against Autism details our family's rollercoaster ride from pregnancy through Ryan's diagnosis and to his life today. This book questions everything we were ever told about autism. Ryan's story isn't about coping with autism. It's not about managing autism. It's definitely not about accepting autism. This book does not read anything like *Chicken Soup for the Autistic Soul.*[1]

I Know You're in There shows you how to fight back and not accept the myths associated with an autism diagnosis. We began Ryan's journey burdened by the medical community's false belief that his autism was incurable and untreatable. We ended our journey enlightened by the knowledge that our son's autism was a complex medical condition caused (for the most part) by an immune system

---

1   The actual title of this great book is *Chicken Soup for the Soul: Children with Special Needs* by Karen Simmons and others. Karen is the director of Autism Today.

that is not working properly. It is long past time to retire the antiquated belief that autism is a psychiatric and developmental disorder because autism is, in fact, TREATABLE.

Ryan now does everything the autism "experts" said would never happen. With medical intervention, focused rehabilitation, and being in the right place at the right time, the only institution Ryan ended up in was the university that awarded him an academic scholarship. There, he joined a fraternity and became president of the Jewish Student Association.

Although Ryan's stellar grades and scholarships surpassed all our expectations, it was not his academic accomplishments that gave us our happiest moments. It was the everyday things that were not extraordinary in the least, except to parents of a child on the spectrum. Ryan was your typical college student. He drank an occasional beer, went on dates, stayed out too late with friends, and sometimes slept through his 8:00 a.m. classes. His parents couldn't have been prouder!

Ryan graduated *magna cum laude* and went on to earn a master's degree with distinction in engineering. NASA awarded him a scholarship for his post-graduate studies as well as a paid summer internship. Ryan is presently a project manager and systems engineer at a major aerospace company. He owns his own condo just a mile from the Pacific Ocean, where he goes out with friends and surfs anytime he can. He loves to travel and has made several trips to Asia and Europe, sometimes with friends and sometimes on his own where he makes friends along the way. Somedays I pinch myself because what I wanted most for him actually happened. He is happy, has friends, and is leading a typical life.

When Ryan was little, we never dared to dream the things he has accomplished might actually be possible. To hope for any future with this disconnected and distraught child was just too painful. Ryan spent every day, all day, plugging his portable radio into every outlet in the house and screamed when anything in his environment changed. Just putting on a new pair of shoes could initiate a behavioral meltdown.

One of the hardest things to deal with when you have a child with autism is that you don't know the rest of the story. You have no clue how things will turn out. Not only do you have an awful day-to-day existence dealing with the behaviors of your child and the shortcomings of our medical and educational systems, but you are frightened beyond words about your child's future.

There were too many mornings I didn't want to get out of bed to face another day filled with autism. The worst times were when my husband Frank and I had no direction or plan. And there were many no-plan and no-hope days when we were hanging on by our fingernails. I searched everywhere for anyone to help us. But at the end of the day, it was up to us. We were Ryan's parents.

My husband and I had to choose. We could let Ryan drift forever into his own world or drag him kicking and screaming into ours. Choosing was the easy part. The hard part was discovering how to help our son and that is what this book is about.

Each child's treatment plan looks somewhat different. There will be variations, but the theme is the same—your child has an immune system that is not working properly. And when it is possible to correct their medical issues, that's when children improve and, for some, full recovery becomes possible. That being said, this is not an easy fix. This is the hardest thing I have ever done. There are no guarantees your child will recover no matter how hard you work at this. I made many mistakes along the way but the one thing I did right was to keep going no matter how bad things got.

In hindsight, it may look like we had a master plan. But most days I was just trying to hang on. I couldn't look too far ahead, or I might have given up. Recovery was one day and one behavior at a time.

There is no magic pill to cure our children. Trust me, I looked everywhere for it. But I did find many snake-oil salesmen with the latest autism "cures" who took our money and then asked for more. Ryan's recovery was not a simple, straightforward path to normal.

No one can MISS a child with autism. They have epic meltdowns in the grocery store and throw award-winning tantrums in restaurants. They do and say strange things. And some children never say anything at all, including "I love you."

And yet there is hope. The solution to the autism crisis seems complicated, but in reality, it is simple if you know the truth about autism. When doctors treat autism medically and reduce the *total load* on a child's immune system, that's when children can learn what they couldn't before. These doctors understand that once you heal the body, the brain follows. But finding the right doctor to treat the subset of autism your child has still remains one of our biggest challenges.

When our son entered kindergarten at almost six years of age, he was in trouble developmentally, and we were in trouble as a family trying to cope with Ryan's intense and confusing behavior. He was in the third percentile for speech and language, and that was just one of his many developmental problems. After years of medical treatment, supported by behavioral and educational interventions, Ryan tested in the eighty-fifth percentile for speech and language by the fourth grade.

Although my kid no longer looked severely autistic and was ahead academically, he still wasn't *typical*. Ryan loved to repeat obscure facts about sharks, electricity, and airplanes over and over again. He had no idea how to decipher social situations, and he was the perfect victim for any bully. The loneliness our son experienced was the hardest part. After he was "with it" enough to realize he was not accepted by his peers, he still wasn't normal enough to know what to do socially. He didn't have any real friends and was rarely invited anywhere.

Recovery is more of a marathon than a sprint. At first, even I didn't think Ryan could have a typical life. During those awkward middle school years, my dream was that someday Ryan could maybe hold a job at McDonald's and live independently. But back then, I wasn't sure that was possible. Who knew that one day he would accomplish all that he has? If I had known then that one day he would be okay, I could have continued without all the tears and anguish.

My fear for Ryan's future continued past the awkward school years and into the beginning of college. I questioned if our family's sacrifices and efforts were accomplishing anything. I worried about the impact of Ryan's issues on my daughter. At times, I wasn't sure if I had the strength to be more stubborn than my son. We worked constantly to lure him away from Autism Island.

Treatment is time-critical because the earlier you start, the less you need to teach your child to catch up. Each child's medical issues must be individually addressed. If an individual's health can be restored by treating hidden viruses and other infections, that's when recovery becomes possible.

And it is never too late to start. Ann Millan wrote the book *Autism: Believe in the Future*.[2] Ann didn't start treating her daughter's autism medically until Robin was twenty-eight years old. And at first, the only reason she did was to stop her daughter's screaming and self-injurious behavior. Now, Robin has a full-time job, drives, and lives independently down the street from her mom. Their success story is a remarkable example of how we must never give up until we find the medical answers to help our children.

This book is written for those currently trapped in the trenches, who are still fighting the autism war and searching for the child they *know* is *in there*. At the end of most chapters is a section called "If I Knew Then What I Know Now." I included this to save you time and to prevent you from making some of the same mistakes we did. My hope is you will see yourself in our family's struggles and know you are not alone in this hell we call autism. Our journey will show just how possible recovery can be for our seemingly impossible children. No parent should accept that their child cannot be helped! No matter how hard the "experts" and your children try to make you, don't *ever* give up!

---

2   You can read Ann Millan's book and Robin's recovery story free on her website at http://www.autism-believe-future.com/.

Part 1

Our Arrival on Autism Island

CHAPTER 1

WE HAD NO IDEA RYAN WOULD CHANGE US FOREVER

The central struggle of parenthood is to let our hopes for our children outweigh our fears.

—Ellen Goodman

A LIGHT DUSTING of snow fell on the older family homes typical of the Midwest. The town of Edina looked like a picture postcard. The rooftops and manicured lawns were covered with the promise of winter. I traveled down the tree-lined street in my standard issue minivan littered with sticky McDonald's wrappers and crumpled grocery receipts. A sharp *click* yanked me back from my mindless thoughts. I frantically looked in the rearview mirror. My three-year old was missing from his booster seat behind me. For a moment, I stopped breathing.

As I turned around, I saw Ryan standing in front of the open sliding door. Cars passed inches from his face. With one hand still on the wheel, I grabbed enough of Ryan's jacket to prevent him from jumping out. After I stopped the car, I did what any mother would do. I shoved him back into his car seat and screamed, "If you ever do that again, I'll kill you myself!" That happened before I knew Ryan had autism. That happened before I knew life would be like that every day, and every day would feel like forever.

Back then, Ryan craved *sameness*. I didn't understand this need. Frank, our daughter Megan, and I enjoyed being spontaneous. We loved to seize the moment, go with the flow, and take chances. This kind of unencumbered life-style terrifies children with autism. But we didn't know Ryan had autism then. We just thought he was difficult and rigid. We thought with enough time he would become spontaneous like us.

We were wrong.

Ryan's never-ending need for sameness was strong enough to compel him to jump from a moving vehicle. This near disaster began with a simple play date. At first, Ryan didn't want to go to Danny's house, and when it was time to go, he didn't want to leave. Ryan had difficulty with *transitions*. He was determined to go back to Danny's so, in his world, things would remain the same. Children on the spectrum have trouble moving from *the now* to whatever happens *next*. Before Ryan, I never had to think about social events in terms of transitions or any of the autism jargon that was to soon take over my life. Megan and I simply had playdates and fun. Those days were gone.

Impulsivity and this rigid response weren't unusual for Ryan. When change inevitably happened, it was hard to anticipate just what he would do or what kind of outburst it would trigger. I didn't know any other mother whose child tried things like that. It didn't matter that the car was moving at a speed that would probably kill him. That was not the first time I lost it, nor was it the only time I had to save Ryan from himself. When these types of incidents occurred, I worried something might be seriously wrong with my son. He confused and frightened me when he did these crazy things.

At other times, Ryan wowed me with his intelligence. I knew he was smart. At only two, he spent hours playing computer games and could operate any piece of electronic equipment in our house. He knew all his letters and numbers. Even though he couldn't say them, he had no trouble pointing to them in books. When it came to anything that captured his interest, his levels of concentration and comprehension were phenomenal. But his interests were limited and a bit odd. Besides letters and numbers, he loved cars and mechanical things. Anything having to do with the electricity and our audio/visual equipment fascinated him. If I had let him, Ryan would have spent the entire day turning every light switch in each room of our house on and off or grabbing my keys and inserting them into every door that had a lock. Ryan loved elevators and objects.

But did he love us?

When it came to interacting with people, Ryan didn't seem to care. He paid attention to us only when we had something he wanted or when he wanted to talk about one of his current interests over and over again. He never said "Hi" to anyone when he entered a room, and he always looked away if anyone talked to him. If I had been honest with myself then, I could have admitted that Ryan and I did not connect in the same way I easily had with my first child.

The exception to Ryan's social disinterest was the dog. Ryan loved to crawl under the table to share dog biscuits with Snooper or use a magic marker to color her blue—the only color he liked. He also spent an inordinate amount of time conversing with the shiny coat hooks in his bedroom closet.

To alleviate my concerns, I convinced myself that Ryan might be the next Albert Einstein or Thomas Edison. I focused on anything that calmed my fears—Albert Einstein developed the theory of relativity, but he was a late talker. Some of his early teachers even thought he might be mentally ill. Thomas Edison didn't utter his first word until the age of four. Both Einstein and Edison had trouble in school, and although we didn't know it yet, Ryan was going to have *big* trouble in school.

Einstein and Edison triumphed and overcame their early oddities. I repeatedly told myself that because Ryan exhibited some of the same strange behaviors as Einstein and Edison, he would grow up to be a genius too. What I didn't know was how many other parents were also having similar thoughts about their unusual children, and that we were already card-carrying members of the A-Club.

Child development experts tell you not to compare your children, but we all do. Ryan was definitely different from his older sister, Megan. From birth to four months, my son screamed most of the time. If Ryan had only cried, I might have been okay. But he didn't know how to cry. Ryan only knew how to shriek. His face contorted as he produced high-pitched, dry-eyed, screams. To console him, we usually tried the big four—we fed him, changed him, held him, or burped him.

Nothing worked.

There was little my husband or I could do to calm him. Most of our days were spent trying to figure out what Ryan wanted or needed. We were like contestants on a game show where only Ryan knew the rules.

In contrast, his older sister smiled at me when I fed her. Megan loved to be held and she cuddled stuffed animals. She gazed at me with eyes that absorbed everything I said or did. Ryan would smile at me occasionally, but most of the time I wasn't sure Ryan knew I was there at all. When I held him and rocked him, his eyes rarely met mine. I never got a reaction or a smile, and most times I gave up trying to interact.

When Megan was little, I talked to her constantly. Our chats were about what we would do when she was older: how much she would love going to school, the dress I would buy her for prom, what college she would attend. It didn't matter that Megan didn't talk yet. She loved listening to my voice and was interested in everything we "discussed." I felt like I was part of a conversation. Ryan didn't seem to care about my plans for his future and most times didn't even look in my direction. There was no conversation.

Since Ryan was my second child, I rationalized that there simply wasn't enough of me to go around. As a mother of two small children, there wasn't any time to relax or escape from the endless to-do list of parenting and housework. Sometimes when I fed Ryan his bottle, I used the time as a way to get a few minutes to myself with the latest *People* magazine. What I hadn't figured out yet was that I was disconnected from Ryan because Ryan rarely connected with me. I rationalized that the problem was all about housework and having too many things to do.

In my quieter moments, I wondered if it was my fault Ryan was so different. Was the reason Ryan didn't look at me or connect with me because I was more interested in the latest Hollywood gossip than in giving him a bottle? Or was it the other way around? The effort it took to meet both my children's needs left me too tired to think things through.

As time went on, it became increasingly difficult to ignore that Ryan was nothing like my daughter. He was different in a way that didn't feel okay. Even as a baby, Megan smiled at anyone and everyone. She'd catch their eye with an impish grin and didn't give up until they smiled at her. Ryan seemed to prefer objects to people. He'd focus on a light switch or a Tupperware container. He spent too many hours babbling to them, connecting in his idiosyncratic way. Some of his best friends were the living room clock and Mr. Shiny Shower Nozzle. We laughed because it seemed silly, and he was cute. We laughed because we didn't know what else to do.

If I Knew Then What I Know Now

It takes time for parents to realize something is wrong. Realization is seldom an "Aha, it's autism!" moment. Knowing is a slow process consisting of wondering, comparing, consulting, discussing, and suspecting. We are confused and consumed by doubts, worries, and rationalizations. A first-time mom or dad who has little experience with babies probably won't recognize their child has the signs that something is not right. Even experienced doctors often can't identify a young child with autism. Not knowing is not a failure of parenting; it is simply part of the autism experience.

Most doctors never took the time to examine Ryan or even talk to him after they learned of his autism diagnosis. They usually said I needed to accept my child, disability and all, and move on with my life—as if his life were already over. They wanted me to make Ryan the *best little autistic boy* he could be and just love him.

I couldn't listen to the things the "experts" told me Ryan would never do. I *knew* Ryan was in there. There were times I saw him clearly. Other times, I only caught a glimpse of the kid he would someday become. During some of the more discouraging times, I just *hoped* he was in there. Frank and I refused to listen to the "specialists" who condemned our son to a life of hopelessness. We set out on a mission to prove them wrong, even though we didn't yet know if Ryan could be helped.

Autism can seem so hopeless.

When the doctors strip you of any hope, it is difficult to keep going. After all, aren't they the ones who are supposed to know about autism? I told myself over and over again that Ryan was okay. I said this to drown out the inner voice that told me he really wasn't. Ryan screamed uncontrollably, refused to adapt to new situations, existed in his own world surrounded by inanimate objects as proxy family members, and exhibited little expressive language. But I continued to tell myself he was fine. In fact, he was more than fine—he was the next Einstein! As a result of my denial, I wasted valuable time not getting him the help he needed. If you think there is something wrong, then there probably is. Don't do what I did and waste time pretending your child is *normal*.

Many of us in the A-Club have similar stories about our initial steps toward the diagnosis. You know in your gut there is something wrong, but you don't want to accept the feeling or fear that accompanies it. You don't want to believe your child is not like other kids, and you want it to be anything other than autism.

You, your family, and your child can survive this diagnosis. Everything you read and hear about autism is not necessarily true. If an expert says your child can't be helped, or to wait and see, run out of their office and find someone else. Many well-meaning doctors told us our child had a lifelong disorder and could never get better. They were so wrong.

Living on Autism Island—Could This Be Your Child?

Autism is a hard diagnosis for anyone to understand and a difficult diagnosis for doctors to make. No one wants this diagnosis. When a child falls and breaks a leg, it is obvious. You can see the broken bone on an X-ray. But autism is not just one thing. It's more like multiple things (or *domains*) that come together in the three-ring circus we currently call autism.

Autism is usually diagnosed by observing a child's behaviors, rather than any concrete scientific tests. Many physicians still believe it is psychiatric in nature. As a result, there is no pee, no poop, no spit, or blood test for autism that is widely accepted by mainstream doctors. Every child with autism exhibits varied symptoms in the three domains of *language/communication difficulties, restrictive/repetitive behaviors, and social skills impairment*.[3] These deficits can result in functional limitations in communication, social relationships and participation, academic achievement, and/or occupational performance. The symptoms are varied in degree and are not all always present in each individual affected. This

---

3   American Psychiatric Association. *Diagnostic and Statistical Manual of Mental Disorders*, 5th ed. (DSM-V). Arlington: American Psychiatric Publishing, 2013.

is why one child with autism often looks very different from another. Dr. Stephen Shore, who actually lives with autism himself said, "If you have seen one person with autism, then you have seen one person with autism."

The autism spectrum ranges from severe/profound to high functioning. A doctor locates your child somewhere on this spectrum. Some experts believe movement in either direction is possible over the child's life span, while others do not. There is no clearly accepted exit point from the spectrum. To be blunt, all the variations are bad. And like your shadow, autism is yours for life.[4] Even though some people with Asperger's Syndrome or high-functioning autism have not been held back from doing some extraordinary things.

To complicate things further, a child may have more than one diagnosis. Children with autism can have multiple medical conditions. Attention Deficit Hyperactivity Disorder (ADHD), anxiety, depression, developmental challenges, and genetic variations are not uncommon diagnostic gate-openers. Combinations of intellectual disability, intellectual ability, learning disabilities, and savant skills also exist, sometimes within the same child. The traditional treatment, never agreed upon by conventional doctors, depends on the complex interactions of the three symptom domains.

But according to leading autism researcher Dr. Joseph Piven,[5] "The issue with autism is that it is not one thing. We call it autism, but some people in the field are starting to call it *the autisms*. Say somebody shows up at your doorstep and they're short of breath. You don't know if they've just run a race, or they just smoked a carton of cigarettes, or they have pneumonia, or they are having a heart attack. That's the situation with autism. We're now discovering that they don't all have the same thing."

Autism should more correctly be called "autoimmune encephalitis," and in simple Dr. Mom terms that means brain inflammation. It is not one thing, but

---

4   Helt, Kelley, et al., "Can Children With Autism Recover? If So, How?" *Neuropsychology*. Rev. 2008 Volume 18: 339-366.

5   Nathe, Margarite, "Signal To Noise." *Endeavors* Volume 28: Winter 2012 pp. 14-19. Piven is also known as Sarah Graham Kenan Professor of Psychiatry, Pediatrics, and Psychology and director of the Carolina Institute for Developmental Disabilities.

rather the cumulative effect of multiple triggers and assaults on the immune system that cause all the issues. Autism is very complicated. But when it is possible to reduce the *total load* on a child's immune system, then they can learn what they couldn't before. Successful treatment of autism is similar for most people. First you must address the individual's medical issues. Once Ryan regained his health, then we had to catch him up on all he missed when he was too ill to learn.

It sounds so simple . . . until you have to do it.

The road we traveled was long and grueling. No freeway directly took us to the coveted final destination of recovery. But some kids can and do get better. Like us, you will hit many roadblocks and detours along this difficult highway. There aren't many rest stops along the way or any places where you can ask for directions. It is hard to find any place that offers sustenance and encouragement to keep going. Exhaustion and discouragement are an integral part of the journey. There aren't one-stop centers that provide what every child needs for recovery. My dream is that one day we will have them. But for now, you must develop your own programs that combine medical, behavioral, and educational interventions.

The important thing is to stay on the road no matter how long it takes or how tired you get. These are our children, so we must never give up. We can't give up when we are exhausted—we can only stop when we are done. Unfortunately, no one is going to do this for us, and no one wants our job. Sometimes, my anger over the situation my family was trapped in was the only thing to keep me fighting for Ryan.

Parents often ask me when I knew Ryan would be okay. Although his autism was much improved by fifth grade, I didn't know he would lead a typical life until much later. I didn't dare to believe he was actually okay even after he was hired by a leading aerospace company. It was a year after he started working there when I finally allowed myself to believe my son made it. By that time, I knew his bosses were extremely happy with his performance and relied heavily on him. Ryan was liked and felt appreciated at work.

Ryan was born in 1988. Back then, autism was considered a rare event nowhere near the epidemic numbers now quoted by the Centers for Disease

Control (CDC). In 1988, routine screening for autism was unheard of. There was no position paper from the American Academy of Pediatrics to guide physicians. In 1988 there were no medications specifically for the treatment of autism. More than two decades later, there is only one medication, Risperidone, and it is used mostly as a last resort to control aggression and not to actually cure anything.

Today, more than ever, we need a new way to help these children. Their behaviors are not simply autistic, but rather symptoms of illness. Children who get effective medical treatment can get better. When effective behavioral and educational interventions are used in conjunction with medical treatment, problem behaviors diminish.

This is why Ryan's story matters. Ryan's journey shows us a new road to travel—the road to recovery.

CHAPTER 2

IT'S A BOY!

We must be willing to get rid of the life we've planned, so as to have the life that is waiting for us.

—Joseph Campbell

WHEN THE NURSE gave us the results of the pregnancy test, I hugged Frank, and we both got a little teary-eyed. We knew our lives together had just changed forever. At first, my husband was deliriously happy. Then reality set in. Frank held his stomach, turned the palest shade of white, and announced he didn't feel well. Frank was pregnant!

Even before we entered the elevator on our way out, Frank started to worry about his ability to provide financially for his new up-sized family. It didn't matter that he had a great job as an airline pilot and good health insurance. The fact that he had supported his family all along was somehow now insignificant. We were having another baby. And my beloved husband was having a cow.

Don't ask me what changed in those first minutes after we got the big news, but for my husband, everything did. Within minutes, the rapid-fire questions started. "What if the flight attendants decide to go on strike? What are we going to do if I get laid off?"

That was my Frank, a man who took his family responsibilities very seriously and worried to excess about finances. I rubbed my stomach protectively.

There couldn't have been a bigger smile on my face when I told Megan the news. Megan, who was almost three, said she had a baby in her tummy, too. She informed us she had a girl baby in her tummy and I had a boy. That way, we would have one of each!

Good news and good food go together in our family. Once Frank got over his initial pregnancy pain, he suggested we all go out to lunch to celebrate. He took my arm as we entered our local coffee shop to make sure I didn't slip on the icy walkway. For Frank, pregnancy equaled being protective. He treated me like I was breakable. I tried to look exasperated, but secretly I enjoyed every minute.

Well, maybe not every minute.

Frank's involvement encompassed all aspects of our pregnancy, including everything I ate. While he contentedly munched on a burger and side of fries dripping with ketchup, he monitored every morsel of food I put in my mouth. He thought it was his job to make sure our child received proper nourishment. "Are you sure you should order that greasy patty melt?" he asked as a disapproving look crossed his face. I ignored him and ordered onion rings to go with it.

A new baby meant a new room. Soon Frank and I were busily decorating and color coordinating Ryan's future nursery. You would think royalty was moving in with all the effort we put into that room. It took almost two hours for Frank to install the closet hooks that were soon to become so much more to us than some place to hang a jacket. The room's theme was *Sesame Street*, and everything down to the crib sheets had to be sewed and coordinated in the bright primary colors that were so fashionable at the time. This was just the first of the many theme rooms in the years to come for our kids. I loved theme rooms. I had trouble understanding when Megan requested not to have one anymore.

When I was pregnant, I never said out loud if I preferred a boy or girl. That was asking for too much. A healthy baby with a complete set of fingers and toes was all that mattered. Like most moms, my fears and hormones sometimes got the best of me. I worried if I had enough love to meet the needs of two kids. How could I love anyone as much as Megan? Nonetheless, I thought it important and comforting that our daughter had a sibling to share a lifetime of memories after Frank and I were gone. Megan had other plans. A new sister was acceptable. A new brother was to be thrown out in the snow.

Before Megan was born, I could sleep through anything and often did. When I asked our family doctor why I couldn't sleep anymore, his answer was simple, "You are a mother now, Marcia." During my middle of the night wanderings, while the rest of the family slept, I thought about my new baby and planned our family's future together. Sometimes, I walked into the nursery and sat in the rocking chair covered with its cheerful *Sesame Street* cushions and looked at Ryan's empty crib. I had the same thoughts most expectant moms have as I slowly rocked back and forth. What will my baby look like? Will he take after Frank or look more like me?

The night before Ryan joined us, Frank was in full-term pregnancy anxiety mode. Instead of being excited about the C-section scheduled for the next day and the joy of Ryan's birth, we were both a little on edge. It seemed like a good moment to cry. So I did, although I had no idea what I was crying about. Frank didn't understand hormones and why I was crying for no reason. My husband became increasingly upset because he couldn't fix the problem for me. Earlier that evening, we had argued over which suitcase I should take to the hospital. Before Ryan, we seldom argued. Was that argument a forewarning of how life with Ryan would change us?

The next morning, Grandma Betty and Megan headed for preschool while Frank and I drove to the hospital. Frank was my rock. Just his presence was calming and comforting. He held my hand during the C-section and kept reassuring us both that everything would be okay.

Although my husband said all the right things while the surgeon made the incision, I still worried. Frank's eyes were fixed on the obstetrician's hands as he delivered our baby. Just as Ryan made his entrance, our family practice doctor made his. Dr. Jim Rhode was more than our family doctor; we were friends. Dr. Jim had switched around his morning schedule, so he could be there in time for Ryan's birth. Ryan's newborn cry was a glorious full-lung scream. Our baby was finally here. I started crying. Frank had a huge grin on his face.

"It's a boy," Dr. Slosser announced.

Ryan rewarded Dr. Slosser's hard work by peeing all over him. I asked Frank if everything was there, and he reassuringly kissed my forehead and said, "Yes."

Frank knew the drill. He had his orders that after Ryan was born he needed to stick with him like glue until the hospital attached that identifying wristband. Frank, ever calm when I was not, placated my silly fear about bringing home the wrong baby. I could see my husband in the adjoining room taking pictures of Ryan while the doctor weighed and checked him. When they returned to the delivery room, Dr. Jim pronounced Ryan to be a perfect healthy boy.

The curtains surrounding each bed in the recovery room yielded little privacy and seemed more like decorative shadows than proper room dividers. I replayed Ryan's joyous birth in my mind as I lay there. I couldn't wait to get to my hospital room and hold our son. I wanted to touch our baby's face and count his ten perfect fingers and toes.

The metallic curtain rings slid noisily as a doctor drew them apart and entered the recovery area next to mine. He quickly closed the curtains as if the fabric somehow provided the privacy that was so obviously missing. His voice immediately captured my attention. His somber tone quietly confirmed that something was seriously wrong. I was only a thin sheet of fabric away when the parents on the other side of the curtain were told their baby had Down Syndrome.

That moment, if there must ever be a moment like that, should have been private. Yet the dreaded onslaught of words kept coming through the thin material that separated our lives. I wanted the doctor to *STOP*. I wanted him to suddenly discover he had made a mistake and say anything except what he was saying. But he just continued with his monotone of doom. Their sobs reverberated throughout the recovery area after the doctor ripped most of the dreams from those parents, The consultation ended with, "I'm really sorry I had to be the one to tell you this."

And he probably was.

My plain, pastel hospital room was a safe haven from the misery and sobs in the recovery room. My sadness for that family abated as soon as I held Ryan for the first time. He was perfect! Perfect! I was grateful we would never—could never— experience the pain I had heard from behind that thin divide.

If I Knew Then What I Know Now

Life doesn't always turn out like we plan. I thought my baby was healthy and okay. What I didn't know yet was that there was no curtain and no barrier separating me and my family from the couple whose child had Down Syndrome. All too soon, my "perfect" child would be diagnosed with autism. Just like those parents, all our hopes and dreams for our child would be instantly stolen. Many children affected with autism look and act like normal babies. Ryan had great APGAR scores. APGAR scores are a total score of one to ten. The higher the score, the better the baby is doing after birth. A score of seven, eight, or nine is normal and is a sign that the newborn is in good health.

There is no APGAR scale for autism.

Some children with autism develop normally, but they later lose some of the abilities and skills they mastered. A regression in any or all of the three domains, *language/communication, behavior,* and *social skills,* seems to just happen. The child that was once *in there* slips away to a lonely life on Autism Island.

CHAPTER 3

LIFE SEEMED PERFECT AND THEN THE DOUBTS STARTED

I wish I could be half as sure of anything as some people are of everything.

—Gerald Barzen

NEVER, *EVER* WAKE a sleeping baby. *No matter what!* That was the new house rule when Megan wanted to play with her new "live doll." Like most newborns, Ryan slept a lot those first few weeks, and like most newborns, it didn't last long. Life with my baby boy was immediately different than it was with my daughter. Ryan soon earned the nickname "Mr. Whiz" because he peed on everyone and everything. We changed Megan's diapers on our bed and never bought a changing table. That didn't work so well with Ryan. All we ended up successfully changing were the sheets.

Megan started to question the existence of her new rival the first night we brought Ryan home. "Mommy, I thought the baby was just going to stay in your tummy. I didn't really want him to come out." Then Megan added something about wanting a sister instead of a brother.

A good way for Megan to delay going to sleep was to ask a ton of questions after her bedtime story, but that night her questions were different. She urgently needed answers about how her family had changed and why she was supposed to love and adore this noisy, hungry *thing* that took so much attention away from her. I didn't tell Megan she should love her new brother. I didn't explain that our world also had revolved around her after she was born.

That was probably what I would have said if I hadn't read *Siblings Without Rivalry*.[6] In that book, the authors instantly clarify how your child feels when you bring home a new baby. What they wrote went something like this: Imagine your husband tells you that he loves you so much, he wants to have another wife just like you. And lucky you, you get to share all your clothes and everything you love most with her.

After reading that analogy, I understood how displaced Megan felt. I didn't try to convince her that I loved both her and Ryan. I didn't deny Megan's feelings. Instead, I went on and on about how important she was to me. In great detail, I told her about all her special qualities that made me love her so much.

Megan asked why Ryan got so many presents, while she didn't get anything. I explained that Ryan didn't have any clothes or toys, so he needed these things. And in our family, we give to the one who *needs* it. She must have understood because when we were at the mall a few days later, I heard Megan repeat my words to Frank's mom. Grandma told Megan to pick out something she wanted. Megan said, "Grandma, in our family we only buy things for someone who needs them. And I don't *need* anything." Megan understood how our family life would be even before we did. It was Megan who taught our family a lesson that rescued us many times in the dark years ahead.

Ryan *needed* so much more.

Our family belonged to the A-Club way before our membership cards arrived. In a strange sort of way, not knowing was the first step on our journey. You have to be one-part experienced mother, one-part developmental expert, one-part behavioral expert, and one-part an unflinchingly, frighteningly honest parent to raise a child with autism. I lacked the skills to be any of these.

When we took Ryan for his eight-week checkup, he passed with flying colors. Of course he did. We all knew he was perfect. Even Megan thought he was perfect—when she wasn't carefully measuring who got more attention. My son

---

6   Faber, Adele & Mazlish, Elaine. *Siblings Without Rivalry: How To Help Your Children Live Together So You Can Live Too*. New York: W.W. Norton & Co., 1987.

charmed Nurse Heidi with his toothless grin and cooing sweet talk. She smiled and talked to my son as she gave him the diphtheria and tetanus injections followed by the oral polio chaser. How could I have let Heidi give him so many shots all at the same time? It happened because our doctor followed the accepted vaccine schedule for babies. I hadn't yet learned to question doing things that could possibly change how Ryan's immune system functioned.

During the middle of the night, Ryan developed a high fever and vomited repeatedly. Frank and I immediately went into what we call *the survival mode*. That's what we do when we have a sick kid. Frank brought what I needed like ibuprofen, a bottle, and a change of clothes before I could ask for anything. I then did the mom stuff, like holding and soothing. After I cleaned Ryan up, I gently rocked and softly sang to him. Ryan looked so sick. I sensed he was in pain. By the next morning he seemed okay, but he slept more than usual. Babies who sleep more are a good break for any tired mom.

Ryan recovered and continued to develop in a manner we thought was typical. His nicknames changed almost as often as the sheets. Newborn "Mr. Sleepy" turned into infant "Mr. Whiz" and then to "Squeak Man" for the adorable noises he made as he woke up. Of course, if we didn't respond fast enough, these adorable squeaks tuned into full-fledged screams. His screams demanded attention. My son demanded that whatever he thought was wrong needed to be fixed *immediately*.

So, we fixed it for Ryan.

Ryan was never content to go with the flow, unless it was his flow. For the holidays, Ryan got a walker. I don't remember if it was Christmas or Hanukkah; we celebrated everything. Frank is Catholic and I'm Jewish, so we call ourselves *Cashews*.

At only four months old, this magical machine called a walker opened a whole new world of stuff for our son. Ryan became quite proficient at maneuvering and getting to new objects. His tiny feet scooted across the floor as he explored his new universe.

When some friends came for a visit with their baby who was close to Ryan's age, I couldn't help but compare. Their kid couldn't even sit up, and mine was actively exploring everything in the house. Their baby seemed content to stay in one place. My kid, who was never satisfied with the status quo, raced around and was more than inquisitive. I was convinced that my son's superior intelligence had to be the reason.

At six months, Ryan used his walker to travel into the kitchen. Next, he planted himself in front of the refrigerator. He screamed until we opened the door, so he could examine what was inside.

Ryan screamed. We opened.

We rationalized this intense behavior as Ryan being our always moving, always screaming, passionate genius. After all, his superior intelligence demanded stimulation. We were sure Einstein must have done the same thing. Even at this young age, Ryan's behavior was frequently extreme and disruptive. *Intense* is the word many A-Club parents use to describe their child's confusing behaviors.

We even invented a family story to explain Ryan's extreme behavior. We surmised Ryan must be a secret member of the Heartstrong family. This was a *Sesame Street* family featured in a clever spin on soap operas. Each episode began with, "The Heartstrongs. A family much like yours, except they feel their feelings very strongly. Let's enter the Heartstrongs' living room for today's emotion-packed episode."

In one episode, Mr. Heartstrong lost his beloved shoelace that he used as a bookmark. Soon, the entire Heartstrong family is sobbing tragically over his loss. Their sorrow instantly changes to jubilation because their son arrives home unexpectedly. They are deliriously happy until they remember the missing shoelace. That thought quickly brings them back to tears. And so ends another stirring saga of joy and tears in the home of the Heartstrongs. And just another day in the home of the Hinds family.

The Heartstrong stories parodied a typical day spent trying to please and placate Ryan. His emotions changed as rapidly as the Heartstrongs'. When he was happy, he was almost giddy with joy, and when he was sad, he was inconsolable. If he didn't like something I did, he immediately let me know. Sometimes when I held him close on my shoulder, he would fling his entire body backwards. I had to be alert and ready so I wouldn't drop him.

If I Knew Then What I Know Now

We didn't acknowledge Ryan's emerging behavior issues. The family completely avoided anything that might cause an emotional outburst because the intensity of his outbursts unsettled everyone. When he was a little older than two, we went to our first *Mommy and Me* class. Like other moms, I looked forward to this as a chance for both of us to make new friends. *Mommy and Me* was not a success. My son didn't interact with the other children and stood out as behaviorally challenged.

Since I couldn't make Ryan do what he was supposed to, we quit the class. We almost always adapted to Ryan's idiosyncrasies and never required Ryan to adapt to us unless it was a safety issue. Sometimes even that was not a strict requirement. We pretended everything was okay. That was how the family dealt with his issues in the beginning. If I admitted that Ryan had difficulties, that meant I had to admit I wasn't doing my job correctly. Could it be my fault Ryan's behavior was so unusual and difficult?

The first *job* of a newborn is to connect emotionally with his mother. I worried when Ryan wasn't as attached as Megan had been. I made excuses for him and blamed myself. But it wasn't anyone's fault. The reality was that the mother/child attachment process was already awry because the neuroimmune issues causing Ryan's autism prevented it from working normally.

Like so many other A-Club moms, I came to believe it was something I did or didn't do, something I ate or didn't eat, and something I breathed or didn't breathe that caused Ryan's autism. On other days, I blamed Frank's family. But autism is not anyone's fault and looking for someone to blame isn't helpful to anyone. My guilt about what I had done or not done to Ryan was simply my expression of an inner dialogue I didn't want to have—a dialogue that said something was already wrong. I didn't want to admit Ryan already preferred things over people. Things never required social skills.

CHAPTER 4

THE SIGNS WERE THERE BUT WE DIDN'T SEE THEM

When you confront a problem, you begin to solve it.

—Rudy Giuliani

RYAN WAS THE toddler from hell! Normal activities of daily life were now confrontations. Doing simple things such as putting on shoes or a coat were more than difficult for Ryan and completely frustrating for me.

Ryan confused me. There were many incidents and behaviors to indicate that my son was struggling developmentally, but I spent most of my time trying to justify his behavior. I pretended his extreme intelligence caused these immense challenges to our family's daily life. Any connection between Ryan having a meltdown over brushing his teeth and Ryan having superior intelligence was questionable. But that's how I coped. Making that connection comforted me and reduced my concerns about him.

Dressing Ryan was always a struggle of wills. He always wanted to play and eat before ever considering getting dressed. I compromised back then and let him eat immediately after he opened his eyes. However, on the days when the needs of other family members meant he needed to get dressed before playing and eating, a battle ensued. "Mr. Touchy Feely" only agreed to clothing that felt soft and hated anything with buttons. Wearing jeans was out of the question, and every tag needed to be cut out of every shirt.

Ryan needed to do things in the same order—always *his* order—and the way that *he* decided they should be done. When I put on Ryan's coat, he wouldn't go outside unless it was zipped all the way to the top. He had to wear a hood and never wore a hat. To protect his hands from frostbite, I had to fight him each and every time to make sure he wore mittens during our cold Minnesota winters. There were so many weird things about our daily life with Ryan. But doing things differently was already *the norm* for us. We didn't notice the absurdity of all the things we did almost subconsciously to prevent Ryan from having another over-the-top tantrum.

In contrast to his intense and quirky behaviors, Ryan could operate any piece of mechanical equipment in the house. He could open any lock—even the broken one on the backdoor that I couldn't get to open. His newest nickname was "Inspector Gadget." Ryan loved to take things apart to study how they worked. The automatic closer on the screen door was just one of his many disassembly hobbies and Frank's reassembly chores. If left to his own devices, hours would pass as he traveled from room to room turning on and off all the lights. My miniature Thomas Edison also spent considerable time turning on and off the bathroom faucets. It didn't take long for him to discover he could only use the cold faucet after a painful experience with the hot one.

Inspector Gadget's new favorite friend, the vacuum cleaner, went with him all over the house. He would push our old, red Eureka and plug it into every outlet. When this new interest started, Frank immediately ran to the store to buy more child protective covers for the outlets that didn't have any. But that barely slowed Ryan down. We tried so hard to protect him. However, he deliberately removed each outlet cover as he ignored our conscientious efforts and dangerously played with electricity. After he was done with an outlet, Ryan meticulously and carefully replaced the protective covers. It was as if to say, "Don't worry, nothing will happen to me because I put the cover back exactly where you wanted." The puzzle that was my son was never easy to understand.

Ryan's moments of obvious superior ability in certain areas contrasted uncomfortably with his outbursts, lack of awareness of dangerous situations, and unwillingness to comply except on his terms. When the *genius* explanation seemed too weak even for us, we justified his behavior by attributing it to the terrible-twos.

A terrible-twos child would be defiant about staying inside against our wishes, right? When we told Ryan he couldn't go outside, it didn't matter if the temperature was ninety degrees or thirty below, he just wanted out...period. We put chain locks on every door to try to make it more difficult for him to escape in order to protect him from the cold, harsh Minnesota winters.

A terrible-twos child would be content to ride a rocking horse or a car that scooted, right? Not Ryan. When he was two and a half, he dragged a chair over to the rack where we hung the car keys. Ryan went into the garage, climbed into the car, and inserted the key in the ignition. Inserting keys in locks was one of his favorite pastimes back then, but we didn't know the trouble it could cause . . . until we heard the car start.

I flew out of the house to try and save Ryan from himself. He was okay, but I can't say the same for all the storm windows that were lined up at the back of the garage. Buying new storm windows for the entire house was actually an inexpensive lesson for us, if you consider what could have happened. At least Ryan wasn't hurt, and we didn't have to replace the garage at the same time as the windows.

These stories of near catastrophes and close calls make it sound like I was an inattentive mother who didn't watch her kid. That couldn't have been further from the truth. I wasn't just watchful—I was vigilant. I was in a constant state of apprehension and nervousness and worried about what could happen in the future.

At the same time, I still pretended everything was okay with my son. Ryan's emotional intensity coupled with his intellectual ability and perseverance made it impossible to predict the kind of danger he would get into next.

If I Knew Then What I Know Now

A garage is a no-negotiation, off-limit space to most children. Cars are also a no-negotiation, off-limit object to all kids, but not for my son. Ryan loved cars, and the pretend kind only kept his interest for so long. That's why we let him play with our real one.

He didn't want to get in the car when it was time to go anywhere, and it was almost impossible to get him out of our car when we came home. So, we left him in the car to play. It was inevitable that one day he would insert the keys in the ignition and drive through the storm windows. In Normalville, Ryan should never, ever have been given the opportunity to play with a real car. But we lived on Autism Island. So, we gave him access to the car and the garage because it kept him happy and out of our hair for a few minutes.

Ryan struggled with each of the domains that were characteristic of autism.[7] He was frustrated and already stranded on Autism Island, hidden from his family. We didn't notice Ryan's verbal and nonverbal communication issues at first because Ryan was able to learn words that named objects (nouns). The way he could assemble words into very simple sentences seemed perfectly normal for a young child. He spoke his first word, "Hi," at six months, which is a little early and more of a reason for celebration than concern. He sometimes spoke in simple two-word and three-word sentences to get what he wanted. If that didn't work, he dragged us over to show us what he needed. That seemed like normal development to us. Like many parents, the more words Ryan used as nouns, the less we worried that there was a language issue.

In fact, we didn't worry about his speech at all.

But communication is more than just learning words and assembling sentences. Communication is a back and forth event where the speaker and the listener engage in the exchange of ideas, information, and emotions. What wasn't normal was the way Ryan used language to communicate. And who and what he communicated with was also odd. Ryan had conversations with objects. When he became obsessed with a new object buddy, he sometimes tuned us out. We had no idea this behavior was actually a sign of autism.

Developing speech is an important assignment for every toddler. Parents expect to have conversations with their child, and when these conversations are absent or unusual, parents worry. Nonverbal communication is also essential to their social interaction. We didn't notice that Ryan was missing many of the

---

7   American Psychiatric Association. *Diagnostic and Statistical Manual of Mental Disorders* 5th ed. (DSMV-5) Arlington: American Psychiatric Publishing, 2013.

essential parts of communication and didn't have any *small talk*. He didn't use what speech therapists call *minimal encouragers*, such as saying "Uh huh" or displaying non-verbal communication like a head nod. He seldom used language to show interest in anyone else. We should have worried. Ryan knew the names of everything, but he did not know how to connect with anyone. He had words, but he was already alone on Autism Island surrounded by his friends Mr. Electrical Outlet and Mr. Shiny Shower Nozzle.

Impairment in the area of social skills was another domain associated with autism. Ryan didn't have many of them. In addition, he lacked ability in other areas of occupational functioning and seemed to be almost indifferent to pain at times. But it was his repetitive behavior that showed the depth of Ryan's autism most clearly—had we been looking. Ryan was super sensitive to sounds and textures in the sensory area of his environment. He excessively smelled and touched objects repetitively, and he seemed fascinated with visual things like lights or movements.

My son was intense, had restricted interests, did the same thing over and over, and had frequent emotional outbursts. We never looked for these signs of autism because of our presumption of perfection. We had already begun to assume that Ryan's behavior was due to his superior intellect. We made excuses and held onto this belief. It was our life raft that kept us from seeing the shores of Autism Island.

CHAPTER 5

HANGING ON BY MY FINGERNAILS

When you reach the end of your rope, tie a knot and hang on.

—Thomas Jefferson

I WILL NEVER know if Ryan was born with autism or if autism was something that the world *did* to my son. I don't know if vaccines and the chronic use of antibiotics for Ryan's never-ending ear infections caused Ryan's strange behavior, but they did impact his immune system—and not in a good way. But in the end, whatever caused his autism didn't really change what we needed to do to help him. He was definitely affected, and I couldn't alter what had already happened to him. His autism was already a pervasive part of our lives.

Ryan had one continuous ear infection from birth. It never completely cleared up with any of the many antibiotics we tried. Ryan was only four months old when he had his first appointment with the ear, nose, and throat (ENT) specialist. When I wasn't blaming my mothering skills or attributing his behavior to repressed genius, I believed my son's ear trouble had to be the reason he was so difficult.

Megan also experienced ear problems, but she was much older when her first set of tubes went in. It took us some time to realize Megan's ear canals were too small and didn't drain properly. Ryan had the same problem, which became evident much sooner. Ryan's first set of ear tubes went in when he was only six months old. Frank and I were terrified at the thought of putting Ryan under general anesthesia at such a young age. We had to help our son, so we did the surgery anyway. I insisted on having the procedure done at a children's hospital where the equipment had safeguards specifically designed to protect younger bodies from accidentally getting too much anesthesia.

During the surgery, I paced the waiting room anxiously. I was frightened and asked Frank over and over again if we were doing the right thing. By that time my question was pointless since the operation was almost over. It seemed to take forever until they called us to the recovery room. I was relieved when I heard Ryan's familiar wailing cry. He was screaming and inconsolable.

That meant he was fine!

Ryan's second set of tubes went in just after his first birthday. This time, his reaction in the recovery room was completely different. I expected that reassuring scream—instead he was smiling and mesmerized by the workings of a copy machine. While I had been scared to death, he was having the time of his life interacting with yet another non-human friend. The contrast was striking.

Life seemed somewhat easier after the tubes. We hoped those simple ear devices would help Ryan become more agreeable. However, two sets of tubes were never enough for my son. Ear infections continued to be a problem. Ryan frequently had to take antibiotics when he was young. Too many antibiotics also mess with a kid's immune system. It wasn't until our son was around ten that his ear canals grew large enough to prevent the persistent ear trouble.

Ryan's post-tube improved disposition didn't last long and became worse after he started crawling. He seemed constantly frustrated and out of sorts. It's hard to be tough on a sick kid. We assumed part of the problem stemmed from him knowing what he wanted to accomplish but his body not yet cooperating. Don't all children experience these same frustrations when they are attempting to master new skills?

Ryan was on time for all his motor milestones and did everything the developmental books said he should be doing. He did things at the right times, but he did them in his own peculiar way. There was language, but it was odd. There was social communication, but it was minimal. There were all kinds of semi-normal behaviors, but they were so intense. We did not connect the developmental dots. We didn't want to.

Ryan was so proud of all his new skills. We were, too. But the more mobile Ryan became, the more proficient he became at getting into trouble. All early walkers are in danger of accidents; however, the intensity of the danger with Ryan was far beyond that of other kids. It became a full-time job to keep him alive to face another day. Electrical cords were one of his favorite things to chew on, and he never passed up any cupboard that had dangerous chemicals inside. He could smell danger! I put childproof locks on everything. I never left Ryan alone in an area of the house for much more than a few minutes, but that was sometimes long enough for him to find trouble.

When things got too quiet, I ran to see where Ryan was. My mom radar was always on high alert with lights brightly flashing—"Check the kid; he's into something!" At nine months old, I found him in the kitchen. He'd managed to get through the childproof lock and into the chemicals under the sink. He had a rim of dark ooze around his mouth. Next to him there was a bottle of Old English furniture polish. I wiped it off, as I frantically dialed the poison control center.

The man who answered my call told me that we were lucky the childproof cap was still on the bottle. As a result, Ryan couldn't have ingested much. He also said that if Ryan had managed to open the bottle, the contents could have killed him. I was so grateful for the childproof cap that I wrote a letter to the company thanking them for putting such an effective device on their product. I put two extra childproof locks on that particular cupboard and on the bathroom cupboards too. I also stopped polishing my furniture.

The stress of trying to keep Ryan alive was getting to me. I felt like a mobile EMS service more than a mother. It was exhausting to be so watchful of my little *NAFOD*. That was yet another one of Frank's nicknames for Ryan. It was an acronym from his Navy days for pilots who had No Apparent Fear Of Death.

On one morning, I told Frank I needed a few minutes to myself. I decided to take the dog for a walk around the block. I came home to complete chaos. Frank was as white as a sheet, Ryan was screaming, and Megan was sobbing. What could have happened in those fifteen minutes to cause such mayhem? Frank had gone to the back of the house to get something for Megan. The next thing he heard was a dull thump, thump, thump followed by Ryan's high-pitched screaming. He ran and found Ryan sprawled out at the bottom of the steep basement steps on the hard tile floor. Out of his fear for Ryan's safety, Frank lost it and yelled at Megan. He told her she should have watched her brother more carefully.

Of course, Megan was only four at the time and couldn't really be in charge of anything more than a teddy bear. Since Megan was not used to being yelled at, she started crying, too. Fortunately, Ryan wasn't seriously hurt and soon calmed down. But Frank was another story. It took him quite a bit longer to regain his composure. Frank feared Ryan's fall could leave him permanently harmed. What made it even worse was that it had happened on *his* watch.

After that, Frank was hypervigilant and made sure the safety gate at the top of the stairs was latched. I was frightened to leave Ryan alone with anyone. In my anxious mind, even his loving father couldn't protect Ryan from himself. I felt trapped, alone, and overwhelmed by all the responsibility. When I did escape from my son, bad things always seemed to happen. And most times, things weren't even so great when I was there and in charge.

Ryan started to walk at about eleven months. I'm not talking about a step or two. He went directly from crawling to six steps in a row. He had no fear of falling and never seemed concerned about hurting himself. Frank was on a trip to Boston when all the excitement started. I told my husband that he better fly the plane faster because his son was walking and he was missing it. We all cheered with delight every time he took a step. But walking meant Ryan now had to be watched *even* more carefully.

Ryan did not limit his difficult behaviors to only the daylight hours. Getting Ryan to sleep started to become more difficult with each passing day. We attributed this new development to separation anxiety and his excitement over all his new motor accomplishments. Whenever we put him to bed, the next thing we heard was a *blood-curdling* scream. He didn't want to go to sleep, and he made certain we knew he wasn't going to sleep. Sleeping issues were just another symptom we failed to recognize. And by that time, we were all too tired to analyze anything.

However, even with all these problems, we had our moments of complete happiness and bliss. Mornings were wonderful. Ryan would sit in his crib and sweetly say, "Mama." Next, he'd make animal noises until I came to get him. His favorite book at that time was *Baby Animals*. We would read it together at least four or five times a day. When I asked, "What does a duck say?" Ryan quacked. He also made snake sounds, kitty sounds, and my personal favorite, monkey sounds.

My mornings alone with Ryan while the rest of the family slept were a time we both enjoyed. Sometimes, Ryan and I tiptoed into the living room, so the rest of the house could sleep while he made animal sounds. I loved listening to him. But now I understand it wasn't really about him and me interacting at all. Making sounds was what he wanted to do. He did this for himself and when it was useful to him. I was just an observer. Whenever I searched for Ryan around the house, I never called his name. He wouldn't have answered to "Ryan." However, if I yelled, "What does a monkey say?" I could track him down by the location of the monkey sounds.

Ryan usually tried to make his way to Megan's room to wake her up and play. Most times, I kept him distracted so she could sleep. However, when he succeeded, he liked to climb in bed with her. But it was not Megan who Ryan really wanted. It wasn't about him being with Megan at all. Once again, she was just another observer in his little world. One of his favorite games was to try and knock off all the pictures hanging on her wall. He loved to watch them swing back and forth. Megan's bed was the road to his friends, the pictures. It wasn't about Ryan cuddling with his sister. I just wanted it to be.

When these quiet moments were over, for the remainder of the day, every day, I could never let my guard down. There was never any relax time. I was on high alert to try to counteract the things my little *NAFOD* got into. I had to do this right! The consequence of not being watchful was that my child could be permanently harmed or dead.

Even so, he was *normal*, perfectly normal.

Ryan didn't see things the way we did. When he was three, he succeeded in one of his infamous escape attempts out of the house. To him this wasn't an escape at all. He just followed his logical path of interest. One minute he was in the kitchen, and the next he vanished into silence. I sent troops out to look for him. Frank, Megan, and Megan's friend, Shannon, all ran in different directions.

They called for him and searched for our missing *NAFOD*. I felt the ache in my stomach grow as fear gripped me. This time, we couldn't find him anywhere.

Frank frantically ran to all of Ryan's favorite hangouts. Finally, he heard a muffled voice say, "Daddy, Daddy." It came from the trunk of our car. Ryan was locked inside, his little hand tightly holding onto the stolen car keys. He was not upset. Ryan expected someone to know where he was and let him out when he was ready to get out. It was impossible for him to be upset about anything when he had a set of keys in his hands and was in the garage with the cars he loved. His expression seemed to say, "Silly you! Where else would I be?"

After a particularly trying day of Ryan trying to escape and me trying to corral him, it crossed my mind that I should do what Doris Day did in the old movie *Please Don't Eat the Daisies*. When she had a kid who got into everything, she put him in a cage that had multiple locks to keep him safe. I considered it ridiculously funny when I first saw the movie, but now it was neither funny nor ridiculous.

Parents are supposed to keep their kids safe, and Child Protective Services or any sane person would never understand why this idea of locking them up was actually necessary. However, if Ryan were safe in a cage, I could take a break. I thought about that a lot. Although we still didn't realize he had it, Ryan's behavior was typical of severe autism. Nor did we know that our survival instinct to avoid anything that made things even more stressful was also typical for families with a kid like ours. Our reaction to Ryan's never-ending, bizarre behavior was to avoid anything that set him off. We gave him anything he wanted to improve the probability of more tranquility in our home.

Ryan was our little autistic mess. His sensory issues expressed themselves in so many ways, and in so many ways we were totally unaware of what and why things happened as they did. An example is our misunderstanding about clothing. Ryan didn't really have clothing preferences; he had clothing needs. He needed clothes to feel a certain way and fit a certain way. If these needs were not met, he could not cope. When he didn't cope, we didn't cope. It was that simple.

No one explained *sensory integration disorder* to us. We had never heard the term. We didn't realize A-Club kids have increased or decreased sensitivity to sensory input from each of the five main senses, and a couple more senses that science was just starting to study. We didn't understand that some kids crave more sensory stimulation, and others are sensory aversive. We were so clueless. So, we continued to battle with him over buttons and zippers day after day.

Likewise, no one explained what *restricted interests* (another symptom of autism) *means in real-life behavior.* A *fascination* with locks, keys, and anything mechanical to the exclusion of anything and anyone else was yet another warning sign that we missed. Love affairs with *objects*, rather than *people*, were just one more sign of his social disconnect. *Transitions* were difficult for my son. One of our biggest problems with Ryan's behavior was he was rigid and insistent on sameness and routine. Again, this is a classic sign of autism.

Looking back, it seems obvious that Ryan had autism, but at the time he was just perplexing to us. We were correct that Ryan showed superior intellectual ability in some areas, but what we didn't understand was that these behaviors did not mean he was gifted. He wasn't a genius or even an autistic genius; he was simply autistic. Our family's orientation to the world changed over time after dealing all day, every day, with Ryan's strangeness. Our *new normal* would have been anyone else's nightmare. It was easier to call it genius and just too scary to recognize what it was—autism.

If I Knew Then What I Know Now

By now, the family unconsciously reoriented our lives around Ryan's intensity and Ryan's safety. We were no longer just his mother, father, and sister. Instead, we were Ryan's twenty-four-hour bodyguards. We were tired, and we were fearful. Tired people do not always have the mental energy to take a step back to see anything clearly. We never recognized how bad the situation had become. There was never time to dwell on any event's greater meaning or significance because the next life-threatening incident was just about to happen. We were simply too busy trying to survive to do anything else. We already became desensitized to Ryan's peculiar behaviors and hypersensitized to his needs.

I used to wonder why Ryan often seemed to prefer getting a negative reaction from me and from others such as teachers and peers rather than being praised for doing the right thing. Over time, this peculiar behavior started to make sense. When he didn't know what to do next, he would do something wrong. My yelling was a reaction he could count on. Keeping things the same was the most important thing for my son. Ryan craved predictability and needed sameness. Most of us want to avoid anyone being angry with us. But kids with autism try to keep everything predictable. That is far more important than someone being upset. Who in their right mind would want to be yelled at? Why couldn't he just listen to me and do as he was told?

Lost, exhausted, and confused, we made the same mistake that most families do. We gave in to Ryan's demands without realizing what we were doing. Instead of making Ryan join our world, we changed our world to accommodate him as a way to prevent more explosive behavior and more family stress. Rather than force Ryan to adhere to family routines, we adhered to his. We helped prolong his stay on Autism Island.

CHAPTER 6

ROAD RAGE IN A BUFFET LINE

Courage doesn't always roar. Sometimes courage is the quiet voice at the end of the day saying, I will try again tomorrow.

— Mary Anne Radmacher

BY AGE THREE, Ryan was merely difficult at home. But when we took him away from his familiar surroundings, he acted much worse. When we went any place that had too many things going on, Ryan would have one of two reactions. He either screamed at the top of his lungs or got that blank stare on his face that frightened me to my very soul. Ryan appeared to be absent from his own body. When that happened, Ryan never acknowledged our presence or anything else in his surroundings. The lights were on, but nobody was home! I couldn't understand why he did this. No one else's child acted this way.

At the grocery store, no one ever said Ryan was cute or said anything positive about my son like they had with Megan. Nobody talked to him because Ryan never looked at, smiled, or responded to anyone. He simply didn't connect. Most times, all I saw was that absent stare until something in his environment changed, at which point his response became rapid, loud, and panicked.

One of his legendary meltdowns resulted from something as simple as Fruity Pebbles being moved to the other side of the cereal aisle. When this happened, people gave me that disapproving look to express their displeasure with a child they knew was spoiled and out of control.

Ryan's outbursts were not only limited to the grocery store. We'd pick our restaurants by how loud we could be. One of our favorites was a local buffet, not because we especially loved the food, but because we rated it a *Five-Screamer*. When Ryan had an explosion there, it wasn't so bad. The restaurant was so noisy, his screaming and weird noises weren't as noticeable.

The stress of raising Ryan created a lot of tension in our home. Frank and I argued all the time. Typical child-rearing solutions weren't working, and the hopelessness of our lives upset us more. We both felt helpless and couldn't understand why Ryan was so difficult. Neither of us could talk to the other about the terrible situation we were trapped in. Why bother to talk when almost every conversation ended with me crying and Frank frustrated because he couldn't fix the situation. Ryan couldn't be fixed because *nothing* worked. There was no consensus and, increasingly, no hope. Frank thought I was too soft, and I knew he was too tough. Poor Megan just got what was left after we were done dealing with Ryan and each other.

We had been arguing about Ryan yet again. It had been another rough one. I was in no mood to cook and certainly in no mood to be diplomatic. When it was time for dinner, we went to the buffet to give us the sustenance to continue the argument for the remainder of the evening. Frank was standing quietly with Megan in the buffet line a few feet ahead of us. My husband didn't want to be anywhere near Ryan or me. So once again, I was abandoned to handle Ryan on my own.

As we waited in line for our turn to pay, the man next to me thought it was his job to tell me how to raise my *spoiled* child. This man didn't seem to care whatsoever that my marriage depended on a good meal. Someone once said, "The only people who are truly sure about the proper way to raise children are those who never had any." That was certainly true of this jerk.

It didn't take much to rev me up that day (or any day) after dealing with Ryan. When the guy said, "Why don't you control your kid?" I instantly snapped back, "If you wanted fine dining, you definitely chose the wrong place. This is a family restaurant." I wanted to yell at him that this restaurant was rated a *Five-Screamer*, but I didn't think he would understand what I was talking about.

Mr. Fine Dining went on to tell me how my child was *out of control*. That's when my husband got involved. Even though Frank was furious with Ryan and me, he wasn't about to let anyone talk to his family that way. We may have hated each other at that moment, but it was still *us against the world* for Ryan. Suddenly, our marriage was okay.

It got kind of ugly. I don't remember all of it, but I do remember the veins sticking out of my husband's neck when he stepped up to protect us. It was like road rage in a buffet line. Eventually, the man left the restaurant, but not before he muttered under his breath that my husband was a wimp. Frank didn't hear him, but I made the mistake of telling him.

My husband bolted out of the restaurant to look for the guy while I remained in line panicked about what was happening in the parking lot. I imagined the headlines, "Northwest Airlines Pilot Arrested for Brawling in Greasy Spoon." I'm grateful Frank never found him. And in a way, I was grateful to that awful man for reminding me how wonderful my husband really was—even when we weren't talking.

Although I would never presume to tell a hungry stranger how to raise their children, I should be fair to the guy in the restaurant line. My kid did look out of control. Parents with autistic children become desensitized to just how bizarre our children's behavior appears to others. After all, for us this is just part of every waking hour. It seems outrageous to let a preschool kid play with electricity or with a real car. But for a family with a child with autism, what would seem strange sometimes becomes normal.

Everyone had ideas on how to raise Ryan—everyone but us. When my cousin and his wife came for a visit from New York, they brought a suitcase full of opinions about me and my son. They were clear and direct. There was *nothing* wrong with Ryan and *everything* wrong with me.

Although I secretly knew Ryan had issues by then, I publicly fronted an attitude that these differences were not deficits. I could agree my child was not normal; he was *advanced*. Ryan would be an Einstein just as soon as he stopped talking to the kitchen faucet. Being advanced seemed like a good tactic to explain away my inner concerns and doubts.

Cousin Bernie wasn't buying it. Bernie was a social worker in a prominent New York school district, and his wife was an experienced fourth grade school teacher. Even so, neither of them recognized Ryan had autism. With all their combined credentials, they never considered the possibility that something was seriously wrong with my child. Instead, their combined training and expertise led them to the conclusion that I was Ryan's problem.

They assumed Ryan's idiosyncratic behaviors resulted from my horrible parenting skills, as they so delicately described them. They proceeded to lecture me on how to raise my son, with an emphasis on clear limits and strict consequences and a second emphasis on the negative impact of being an ineffective, spoiling, overindulgent, clueless mother.

I should have screamed, "Who the hell do you think you are, you condescending assholes!" Instead, I retreated to the safety of my bedroom and sobbed. I hated Frank for rearranging his work schedule to be out of town for their visit (he never liked them). And I hated Bernie and Miriam for what they said. But at the same time, the little voice in my head whispered, "They might be right."

If I Knew Then What I Know Now

In reality, no one was right in our situation. Ryan had autism, and no one knew it. Not me, not Frank, not Bernie, not Miriam . . . no one.

I wasn't a bad mother. Everyone just thought I was.

Children with autism do strange things. And their parents do stranger things in order to cope. We often don't notice that the things we do to survive appear bizarre to other people. It is not about being a bad parent or having a bad child. My son was marooned on his own island. I was trying to figure him out while simultaneously struggling to remain in denial.

I was consumed with self-doubt. Things got worse when my awful relatives jumped into the chaos and announced my kid was spoiled, out of control. Part of me believed Bernie and Miriam when they said I wasn't doing it right and blamed all of Ryan's behaviors on me. What they failed to realize, and what I failed to realize, too, was that parenting by the normal rules just didn't apply to Ryan or to any child with autism. I don't need to provide any examples of what our relatives do and say. For those of us in the A-Club, a million painful moments come to mind.

What most of our relatives don't realize is that their advice isn't helping. We have enough guilt and anguish all on our own. Our personal hell becomes even more intense when well-meaning relatives, doctors, and other experts can't wait to tell us that the reason our children are out of control is because of the things we do, or don't do, or maybe ate, or maybe touched, or maybe... The list of mother-blaming reasons is endless.

If your family believes you are spoiling your child and their strange behavior is your fault, *don't buy it*. Just walk away. And keep saying to yourself...

"Autism is not my fault!"

Rinse, repeat, and say it again.

And keep saying that over and over until you actually believe it. Don't try to explain how things really are. Just continue to do what your gut says your child needs. Yes, you will make mistakes, but you will learn how to get it right, and your self-esteem won't be further eroded by their caustic remarks. It doesn't make a difference if everyone thinks you are the worst parent in the world. It only makes a difference if you let what they say get to you.

CHAPTER 7

NOTHING WAS NORMAL ANYMORE

Just when you think it can't get any worse, it can. And just when you
think it can't get any better, it can.

—Nicholas Sparks

RYAN'S AUTISM WAS changing us as a family, as a couple, and as individuals—and *not* for the better. The frustration about what to do about our problem grew worse as Ryan grew older. Before Ryan, my husband's playful antics and sense of humor lifted the spirits of everyone around him. When we went to refill our propane tank at the hardware store, Frank made the woman behind the counter laugh when he asked her if she would help him with his gas problem.

Just going to the grocery store with Frank was a romantic experience. He loved to embarrass me as he waltzed me down the aisles to the elevator music playing in the store. That was before Ryan, when we both still saw the humor in life and when I could still be embarrassed.

We had no one to give us respite from Ryan. Family was in California, and we lived in Minnesota. There was no way Ryan could be left with a babysitter. No one could handle him. Every once in a while, we would try, but Ryan screamed inconsolably the entire time we were gone. His babysitters never returned for a second attempt.

Ryan became more than a full-time job. Ryan wanted only me, and he usually got what he wanted. Most times, even Frank wouldn't do. The only break I got from dealing with Ryan was when my husband asked, "Hey, Ryan, do you want to go to the Embassy Suites?" That was one of the few things that got our son out of the house without me or a major meltdown. The two of them would happily go to the hotel to ride the elevators up and down. Ryan loved to push the elevator buttons during those infrequent times he wasn't pushing ours.

Elevators were one of Ryan's *restricted interests*. Hotels were the next most-preferred item on his list, probably because they had elevators in them. He used to close the doors of the closet in his bedroom to pretend he was riding an elevator. He made a dinging sound at each pretend floor. Eventually, Megan colored buttons on a piece of paper and taped them to the closet doors. We all helped Ryan with his consuming interests. Back then, elevators and imaginary trips to Elevator Land equaled a few minutes of relief for all of us.

The only other place Ryan wanted to go without me was Jerry's Hardware Store. It was a little higher priced than the big box stores but worth every penny because it kept Ryan's attention and my sanity. Most times it didn't really matter how expensive it was because the boys weren't there to buy anything. We used the store as a distraction to get Ryan out of the house without me. It was retail therapy in the most bizarre way.

Jerry's Hardware, filled with staff more than eager to help with home projects, offered the kind of customer service you don't find anymore. The aisles had everything from pet supplies to any kind of nail or screw you ever needed or wanted. The cleaning supplies lined up in the front of the store gave it a fresh smell. Ryan's preferred section of the store was the electrical department that was completely equipped with all his favorite things: plugs, outlets, and extension cords. Frank watched patiently while Ryan spent many happy, focused minutes attaching all the extension cords together in a long snake. Victorious, the two of them would sneak out of the store before anyone noticed.

Ryan had us trained at home and in public. Avoidance of public places that were stressful for Ryan became second nature. Ryan was hard to control in public. His behavior humiliated us, but Ryan was completely oblivious to the embarrassment his actions caused. When there was an unexpected loud noise, like a siren or school bell, Ryan screamed at the top of his lungs. He sometimes made high-pitched and odd noises that caused everyone to stare at him. We learned to anticipate and avoid circumstances and situations that could potentially cause an outburst. Outbursts, with their screams, hitting, sobbing, and biting were exhausting. Who wouldn't want to avoid them?

We excelled at making creative excuses to our friends to explain Ryan's bizarre behavior: "He didn't sleep well last night. He's coming down with something. He has a new tooth coming in. He's just a bear when he's hungry." We felt like bad parents. We thought we knew how to parent until Ryan came along. No one in our family had any comprehension of how awful life with Ryan had become. The friends we still had didn't get it either.

There was no one to talk to. Whenever I got up the courage to speak to a friend about Ryan and my worries, their eyes seemed to glaze over with disinterest. Everyone got that far away look, similar to the one Ryan had when we took him anywhere new. Nobody wanted to hear about our out-of-control kid for the umpteenth time. Everybody knew he was spoiled, and I was ineffectual. I learned to keep my fears to myself. The isolation this diagnosis brings to parents is just another aspect of our terrible existence. We had officially joined Ryan and were marooned on Autism Island.

This was a mutually lonely and depressing time for me and for Frank. I couldn't even vent to my husband, my closest friend, about what was happening. I tried to talk to Frank about how frustrated and scared I felt. Those discussions were unproductive. Neither of us had any real ideas about how to help our son.

Our talks often disintegrated into an argument, and we, an enamored couple who had once waltzed in grocery aisles, became bitter adversaries. We started out fine and reasonable, but it was impossible to be rational about something that didn't make any sense. There was no logical reason why Ryan acted the way he did.

As time went on, our arguments became as scripted as an autistic rant, with Frank criticizing my parenting and me fighting back by saying he needed to stop spanking Ryan. We both wanted to blame someone or something for the way Ryan acted and it usually ended up being each other. Neither of us ever raised a hand or even our voice with Megan unless it involved a dangerous situation. But Ryan was another story. The unending patience Frank had for his first child flew out the window when it came to his son.

If I gave Ryan a swat on the butt, I knew I still loved him in spite of how hard he was to live with. In moments of despair, I sometimes questioned if Frank even loved Ryan at all since he often was so annoyed with his behavior. I was just as annoyed and sometimes less patient than Frank, but I needed someone to blame. I protected Ryan from the world. At times, this even included protecting him from his own father.

I never fully acknowledged all the accommodations our family made to avoid upsetting Ryan. My son was simply easier when we all did what he wanted. Back then, I thought we actually controlled his outbursts somewhat, but we really didn't. Ryan had us trained, rather than the other way around. Ryan had certain rules in his head about how the world operated. If we did what he wanted, then there were fewer outbursts. We were all under his control.

Ryan's stubbornness, inflexibility, and emotionally intense behavior became part of our family's daily routine. Many of his rigid patterns of behavior centered on and were initiated by his need for me. It wasn't about Ryan loving me and wanting to be with me as much as it was about that Ryan needing my body there in order to initiate the routines and rituals that enabled him to feel secure. I had become Ryan's personal security guard and transitional object in a world he perceived as unpredictable, disorganized, and scary. This is why I was indispensable. As a person, I wasn't really important. It was my presence that mattered, and no one else was acceptable.

Ryan demanded my presence exactly as he wanted it, exactly as it had to be, in a hundred different ways each day. When we drove anywhere, my son had to sit directly behind me. If that didn't happen there were unpleasant consequences for the entire family. Ryan sat on the left side when I was driving. When I was in the passenger seat, he buckled up on the right. This was Ryan's rule. We all learned his rules without a word being spoken. If Megan sat in the wrong place and sat behind me, Ryan predictably screamed, bit her, and pulled her hair. She broke his rule.

Megan quickly learned to do what her brother wanted. I was too busy trying to survive this nightmare to even notice my daughter usually gave in to all of Ryan's demands. Megan spent most of her childhood trying to be the good child to compensate for how difficult Ryan made our lives.

Ryan's demand for sameness affected everything we did. I spent most of Ryan's early childhood making sure his world was predictable. According to one of Ryan's rules, he had to eat lunch between 12:00 and 1:00 p.m. He planned his (and our) day by the time on the clock. If we were off-schedule and it was after the noon hour when we returned home, Ryan refused to eat. When he was hungry, thirsty, or sleep deprived, his behavior became even more difficult. My waves of anxiety increased if we were late. We had to be on time!

Finally, I figured out how to beat my toddler at his own game. If we were late for lunch, I would turn the kitchen clock back to 12:30 when Ryan wasn't looking to avoid an afternoon of crying and screaming. I wanted to treat Ryan like a normal kid, with normal kid discipline, normal kid rules, and positive reinforcement, but he didn't act normal. Ryan called the shots.

Clothes and shoes were another area where Ryan was rigid and rule-bound. His rules and rituals had to be followed, no matter how inconvenient. When we had to go anywhere, we began getting Ryan dressed at least an hour before we needed to actually leave the house. That way we could get him ready on time, in his way, and without a major meltdown.

It wasn't only the sensory aspect of his clothing that derailed him. It was also severe motor planning problems. At five years old, he still couldn't dress himself. Ryan's solution to the nightmare of remembering and negotiating the *how-to-get-dressed* sequence was to resort to a ritualized and rigid routine in order to guarantee sameness. The routine we adhered to was ridiculous. We would put on one piece of clothing, wait a while as he did something he wanted to do, and then try for another. Whenever we bought new shoes for Ryan, they had to sit in his closet for weeks so he could look at them and get used to them. In time, we introduced them into the sameness of his dressing routine. We gave him way too much power and control. And we were way too ignorant of why these behaviors are so common in autistic children.

If I Knew Then What I Know Now

In hindsight, I made many mistakes. I tried to change our world for Ryan, rather than making Ryan change his behavior. We tried hard to make Ryan conform to our world, but it was so difficult and so unsuccessful. He usually won the battle, and most often we gave in. We constantly walked on eggshells and did anything to avoid upsetting him. I even convinced myself that my child seemed somewhat well-behaved given his high-strung personality. Why behave if not behaving means you get everything you want when you want it?

Despite our best efforts to give Ryan the life he demanded, there were times we still couldn't figure out what he required, and that's when the full-scale, epic outbursts erupted. Ryan was smart enough to know what he needed, but he still didn't have the words to tell us. His limited language was a huge part of his behavior issues then, but I didn't understand that yet.

We never used visual schedules or PECS[8] (a picture communication system that nonverbal and preverbal children use to help communicate their needs). This was before PECS existed. There were no pictures to point to, no iPad, nor any special smartphone apps. We guessed at what Ryan wanted in order to avoid a confrontation. We insisted on communicating verbally with a child who desperately needed to communicate visually. I didn't understand why he acted so badly, but now I finally get it. He was extremely frustrated. Ryan didn't have the language to communicate his wants. In the absence of communication, rituals, rigidity, and sameness are the best way for a child to ensure at least some of his needs would be consistently met.

The best way I can best explain the frustration children with autism feel is with a chocolate analogy. Imagine your favorite candy bar is right in front of you and you missed lunch. You are starving. Your blood sugar plummets along with your mood. You try to communicate to anyone who will listen to hand over that chocolate candy bar loaded with caramel and nuts now, but no one understands what you are trying to say. Then someone gives you a pencil. Next, they demand you say "Thank you" for an object you do not want. And when you don't, they give you a swat on the butt. Given this scenario, I might hit or scream too.

Some parents that have children with autism insist their kids do not exhibit behavior problems and are relatively easy to deal with. That's when I question

8   Frost, Lori and Bondy, Andy. *The Picture Exchange Communication System Training Manual, 2nd Edition* Pyramid Educational Consultants, 2002.

how often they unknowingly change the world for their kids in order to avoid their impossible behavior. Most of us make the same mistake. We thought we were making our lives less chaotic by following Ryan's lead. As a result, we were the biggest obstacle to our child's recovery. We bargained with Ryan rather than enforcing consequences for inappropriate behavior. "Ryan, if you get in the car quickly, then we will get an ice cream at Baskin-Robbins." That was us. In time, I learned this was not what was best for Ryan or our family. *Never negotiate with terrorists*, especially when their name is Ryan.

CHAPTER 8

MEGAN HAD THE ANSWER BEFORE WE DID

There is nothing more deceptive than an obvious fact.

—Arthur Conan Doyle

ALTHOUGH I DIDN'T want to admit it, deep down I knew there was something seriously wrong. Ryan's path of development, wherever it was heading, was destroying our family, our marriage, and me. We had ignored, rationalized, justified, minimized, and explained away too much for too long. This child who stared blankly, screamed loudly, and had strange, sometimes dangerous interests, was now hidden behind our family's wall of denial. We were insulated from the world and stranded on Autism Island.

I asked our pediatrician at every appointment if Ryan's behaviors were typical of boys his age. When I questioned why Ryan didn't have as many words as Megan did at his age, all I got was reassurance that everything was fine. Dr. Hobbs said most times boys tend to be more physical and active, while girls are more verbal. I should just stop worrying and enjoy being his mom. I took comfort in this stereotype and that it was just a phase. We explained away all his strange behaviors to feel better about the many, many things he did that we couldn't control or understand. We had a million rationalizations. Our pediatrician helped our denial with his assurances.

Ryan was now at the age where language acquisition and social communication were critical developmental tasks. His language development, like everything else, was uneven and atypical. Ryan's vocabulary was exceptional for words related to his restricted interests, but lacking and sometimes nonexistent in other areas, especially social communication. His communication style was odd, to say the least. He struggled to form more than a simple sentence. He also had multiple issues with articulation, tone, and volume. Yes, he had language, but it was not functional or conversational the way it should have been. His speech was seldom interactive. Instead, he used language mostly to get something he wanted from us or to be able to talk about his restricted interests.

By age three and a half, his favorite toy was a brochure with a map of Eden Prairie Mall. We took this worn and tattered piece of paper with us everywhere we went. He loved it when we read it to him. Our several-times-a-day *conversation* went something like this:

Ryan would hold the brochure tightly in his toddler hands and in Ryan Speak ask, "What does this say?"

I would answer, "Mommy and Daddy love Ryan. And Megan loves Ryan, too."

Then Ryan would proudly puff up his chest and loudly proclaim, "And it says EDEN PRAIRIE MALL!"

To me, this conversation was about social bonding with my son. To Ryan, the conversation was about the joy of a scripted and predictable response. It really wasn't about me or Frank or Megan or Eden Prairie Mall at all. It was all about sameness.

I thought it was a little peculiar that Ryan didn't play with regular toys like other kids. His unusual emotional attachment to his map of Eden Prairie Mall was just another autism symptom I hadn't yet recognized. It was somewhat similar to his attachment to electrical outlets, shower nozzles, and other inanimate objects that were just not as portable as his brochure.

Linus had his blanket. Ryan had his map. We just thought it was funny.

We kept an extra stash of brochures on hand to make sure there were no outbursts if we couldn't find the original one he so carefully took with him everywhere. When Ryan was no longer content with the map of Eden Prairie

Mall, he studied maps of the United States. He knew the names and locations of all the states. When I would ask him to identify the state next to Washington, he would get a big smile on his face and answer, "Dryington." This was just another reason for us to laugh and assume he was a genius—albeit a funny genius with articulation issues.

Kids with autism say the darndest things. When we said to Ryan, "Point to your forehead," he'd point, laugh, and instead say "fivehead." We weren't quite sure if he understood the pun or not. This unique way of looking at the world usually resulted in the rest of us laughing, too. I was convinced Ryan must have inherited his father's odd sense of humor, but I wasn't sure it would serve him well in the future.

Later, Ryan started to echo many of the things we said word for word. He also repeated entire TV commercials verbatim. I didn't know then that this was called *scripting*, which is another sign of autism. Whenever the Glade air freshener commercial came on, he'd run and stand in front of the television mesmerized. Ryan repeated the jingle over and over again, singing, "Plug it in; plug it in," for hours on end. His fascination with this jingle even made sense. Or rather, we made it make sense. Someone was plugging the air freshener into one of his favorite things, electrical outlets.

Pronoun reversal was another sign we didn't recognize. When Ryan wanted me to pick him up, he'd say, "Hold *you*" instead of "Hold *me*." To us, this *Ryan Speak* was adorable! When he wanted to say, "I'm going to do it by *myself*," it came out as "Do it by *yourself*." When I asked, "Do you want to sit and read *Baby Animals* with me?" Ryan beamed and exclaimed, "*Sit me!*" What he should have said was, "I want to *sit with you*."

His lack of communication back then was endearing! We all understood *Ryan Speak*. We knew what he was trying to say. We learned his language because he couldn't learn ours.

Ryan wanted to talk, yet he didn't have the ability. Confusing *"you"* with *"me"* is a temporary error for typical kids, but a complex and puzzling task for children on the spectrum. For them, using the correct pronoun is not simple. Using *"you"* versus *"me"* requires them to understand the social context of an interaction. Ryan couldn't differentiate that he was speaking to a separate person, rather than just another object. Nevertheless, Ryan had learned that using language would increase the pleasure he obtained from his restricted interests.

Around this same time, Ryan developed an intense interest in the hooks in the closet of his room that Frank had struggled so hard to install. The entire family, including the dog, had to go in there several times a day to see Ryan's hooks. If we didn't move fast enough, he would yell, *"Mon, mon!"* That meant, *"Come on—come with me right now!"*

Next, he would push and steer us into his room until we were correctly positioned to view his beloved hooks. We would all act as if we were extremely interested in these shiny pieces of metal. When our adoration was complete and satisfactory, we were dismissed. We went every time we were summoned. If we didn't, he became very agitated and sometimes explosive in his behavior. And none of us wanted to upset Ryan. An out-of-sorts Ryan made our lives painfully difficult.

Ryan's lack of age-appropriate communication was a major source of aggravation for him, too. He knew what he wanted, yet he couldn't say what he needed. He couldn't understand why we *didn't* always respond in exactly the same way to his repeated commands. We kept giving him pencils when he wanted chocolate.

Even Snooper, our dog, bore the brunt of his frustration. Ryan and Snooper often shared dog biscuits under the dining room table together. There was no way Snooper could eat them as fast as Ryan served them up. Ryan would scream gibberish at her until she did what he wanted. Snooper ate her biscuits, not because she was hungry, but because he was yelling at her. He even had the dog under his control.

Ryan's struggles with language and social communication further intensified the impact that his unusual and intense behaviors had on our family life. Of course, Ryan tested the limits. In that way, he was typical. He would climb onto the dining room table to reach the china cabinet filled with precious glassware passed down for generations in my family. That's when I announced we had a new rule. I told Ryan he could stand on the chairs, but the table was off limits. Defiantly he climbed on the chair, put one foot on the table, and yelled in *Ryan*

Speak that he wanted to get on the table. Then, he looked at me as if to say, "Aren't you going to try to stop me?"

I responded with, "Ryan, you can't climb on the table." He yelled back at me in words that only he understood. Then, he would do it again and again. He was stuck, and I was stuck right there with him. After I told him for the umpteenth time not to climb on the table, Ryan did something different. Ryan spoke his first complete sentence, "But I want to." I looked at Frank and asked, "Did he say what I think he did?" My husband just nodded, dumbstruck as I was. Ryan could speak. But, of course, his speech was all about Ryan.

And so was his behavior. In Ryan's mind, he had a right to my presence at all times, and by logical extension, a right to my possessions. What's mine was his. Ryan was always somehow involved when something went missing.

When my purse disappeared, I had a feeling Ryan was responsible. But with his very limited language, Ryan could not be expected to answer the question, "Where did you put my purse, Ryan?" with a sentence like, "It's in one of my favorite hiding spots, Mommy." I asked anyway. His lack of response and blank stare didn't stop me from going back to six different stores to confirm what I already knew; I hadn't left my handbag at a store at all. Ryan stashed it somewhere in the house. Frank later found my purse in one of the cupboards only my son frequented. Ryan's new nickname became "Stash."

Megan usually had more patience with Ryan than I did. On a particularly difficult day, I was yelling at Ryan again. Megan immediately came to his defense and very calmly gave me a lecture. Her sermon went something like this, "Mom, he's not going to learn anything if you *yell* at him. You have to show him the right way to do things."

She was right. We did have to show Ryan the right way to do things, and we hadn't been doing that. We either yelled at him or placated him. And sometimes, when our frustration became too much, I'm embarrassed to say we spanked him. Little by little, Ryan taught us to accept his autism with its peculiar rituals and interests. He endured a smack on the butt rather than let go of an inappropriate behavior. And, with each lesson, we let him go deeper into his own world on Autism Island and further away from ours.

Ryan and his strange behaviors made me feel and act crazy. Still, I wasn't ready to acknowledge that my kid was not okay. Frank wasn't either. Megan was the only one who seemed to have a bead on the situation, although I don't think we ever asked for her opinion. It was easier to convince ourselves that smart people such as engineers, rocket scientists, and maybe our son, often seem a little different. His doctor said he was normal. So it must be me or my parenting skills that were the problem.

In spite of everything, I fiercely loved him. It was more than just motherly love. I protected him like a mama bear from everything and everyone. He needed me differently than Megan did. As you already figured out, in our family, the one who needs more help gets it—except most of our help did not really help my son at all.

We all adapted to Ryan's idiosyncrasies instead of demanding Ryan conform to the rules every family needs to set. Our accommodations ranged from those that seemed almost normal to those that were truly bizarre. I knew Ryan would not come to me if I called him. When I wanted him to come to the kitchen, I simply opened the refrigerator door. That's when Ryan came running. I knew Ryan loved to look inside the refrigerator, and he seemed to have supersonic hearing if it involved one of his restricted interests. If the refrigerator trick didn't work, I loudly asked, "What does a monkey say?" I could find him as a result of the noises he made. Someone watching might have thought my actions were a little strange. But they worked, and whatever worked had taken the place of good parenting.

Uneven development is a hallmark of autism. Ryan struggled in the areas of language and communication, his social skills were rudimentary, and his behavior was less than exemplary. Ryan's limited verbal ability worried me. We did everything to develop language. I read to him constantly. We watched educational TV shows like *Sesame Street* and *Mr. Rogers' Neighborhood* together. He loved anything to do with computers, and we used that to our advantage. We used computer programs to help overcome speech issues. I spent hours working with Ryan every day to provide him with the same enriched learning environment that every child needs.

But when it came to one of his restricted interests like letters and numbers, he was not just normal, but advanced. At age three, he could count and identify every number up to one hundred. He also knew all his letters. This was our proof that he must be a genius. After I bought him a new number book, for some unknown reason, he latched onto the number fourteen. He ran around the house with the book, pointing to the number, and yelling "fourteen." However, this new pastime did little to reduce his fascination with the hooks in the closet. When he went to bed every night, he now had to say goodnight to the hooks in his closet and the number fourteen in his book.

If I Knew Then What I Know Now

Sometimes, it feels as if we are caretakers of an absent soul. But you must remember your child really is *in there*. When I talked to Ryan, he never looked at me, and he seldom acknowledged anything I said. I used to wonder if he actually heard me since he usually acted like I wasn't even there. It was hard to recognize his intelligence when it was overshadowed by his odd, intense, and unpredictable behavior. And I never got the bulletin that my son was still learning, just in stealth mode. It was only later after he recovered that I realized he had been *in there* all along. He just lacked the communication skills to respond or nod his head with understanding that would have made it clear to me that he was learning.

We all need positive reinforcement. Since Ryan didn't respond, it was hard to continue talking to him. I wanted some inkling that I was getting through to him or that he was listening to me and what I said. He gave me *nothing*. Not a look nor a smile. Since I was the only one talking, we never really had a conversation at all. Most times all I got was that blank stare. At the time, it was all about hope and mostly desperation. So, I kept talking to him about the same unimportant things I did with Megan. The difference was that she responded. I hadn't yet realized the profound and positive effect this one-sided interaction had on my son's future development.

When I suggest to other parents they must expose their children to new situations, the typical response is, "It's too hard to take them anywhere." Or "Why bother when my kid can't really understand what is going on, anyway?" I also wanted to hide my kid at home so I didn't have to deal with the behavior issues or people's indignation with how my kid acted.

But that wasn't what *was best* for Ryan.

It's important to take your children to the museum and anywhere that stimulates learning. I continued to expose him to situations that encouraged him to interact with the world even when his behavior caused issues for others in restaurant lines and embarrassed me. I learned to ignore the stares from those parents who had already decided in a few short minutes that I was the worst parent ever.

These children may not talk or show you they understand what you are saying, but you have to assume they do. I cringe when I hear parents talk about how awful their children are *right in front of them*. I worry that they think their child not only has autism but are deaf and stupid as well. Every child wants to know their family loves them and thinks they are good kids. Talk to them like they get it even if you are not sure they do. Nobody (not even me) thought my kid was capable of learning or taking in information, but he was. I often questioned if there was any form of intelligent life in there. You have to believe he or she is *in there* in spite of all evidence to the contrary.

I Used to Know How to Raise Children—Until I Had One by Donna B. (Another Mom in the A-Club)

Full disclosure: Back when I was single, *child-free*, and clueless, I thought I knew best, rolled my eyes and spouted my opinions with the best of them. I had opinions about how I would and could do it better and smarter with my own child. I could raise the perfectly behaved, perfectly coiffed, perfectly smart little lady or gentleman with one hand tied behind my back.

I knew when I became a parent my lifestyle wouldn't change just because I had a kid. Children should be required to adapt and fit into the lives of the adults raising them. That's how my single friends and I saw things. After all, that's what life is, right? Adapting? Although I never directly criticized anyone, it was almost like I had. The look on my face probably said it all.

All that happened before reality came along in the form of a picky-eating, tantrum-throwing, hand-flapping, non-talking, oddly-behaving runaway train that permanently knocked me and my precious opinions off of our comfortable pedestal. *Karma* wasn't just a bitch. In my case, *Karma* had a name, a face, and the sweetest smile, and promptly kicked my smug, opinionated behind from here to Sunday.

If I had a dollar for every time some stranger shook their head and gave me the stink-eye as they said, "Can't you control your child?" or "Somebody slap that kid!" well, I wouldn't exactly be a rich woman, but I could easily host a weekend at Disneyland for a family of five with meals, souvenir hats, and sweatshirts included.

When Aiden behaved oddly, inappropriately, or had a meltdown, some of these helpful people scolded my son because he wouldn't look them in the eye or answer when spoken to. Some even unabashedly informed me that my method for dealing with a particular issue was definitely wrong.

Here are just a few examples: Once in a restaurant ladies' room, an elderly lady looked down her nose as I helped four-year-old Aiden wash his hands and said, "If you wash his hands for him, he'll never learn how to do it himself." *Oh really?* Another time, when I stopped in at Target to pick up some diapers and an antibiotic for one of Aiden's many painful ear infections, the checker (that's right, the checker at Target) narrowed her eyes at my crying child and said, "If he was *MINE*, he'd be in time-out right now." *Um . . . okay. I'd love to have seen her try it.* Another woman thought it perfectly appropriate to inform me, loudly, that my child was too old for Pull-Ups.

But the Grand Prize for the Stupidest, Most Ignorant and Most Ridiculous Comment of All Time (I'm calling it the S.M.I.R.C.A.T. Award—the acronym is mine, but feel free to submit nominations) goes to the woman who, after being politely informed that the reason for my child's behavior was autism, announced, "Well, then, if he's autistic, you shouldn't be taking him out in public." *Seriously? Seriously??? I almost took the witch out with my bare hands.*

I suppose my *Karma* would be useless if I didn't put it to good use. So, I've come up with a list of things for my inner armchair judge to remember next time I have the urge to criticize someone's parenting, child, or children.

Five Important Things to Remember the Next Time Someone Else's Child Makes Me Want to Reach Over and Slap Them:

1. That parent and child are *not* having a good time right now. Don't add to their stress, just because you are annoyed.

2. That child could have a disability or be ill or in pain. The point is, you don't know why that child is upset, not listening, or misbehaving. Don't assume anything.

3. Use this mantra: *You don't know them. You don't know them. YOU DON'T KNOW THEM.* Next, lather, rinse, and repeat the mantra until thoroughly cleansed of all other internal commentary.

4. Instead of criticism, offer help and/or sympathy if it seems appropriate. Leave them alone if not.

5. Save your opinion for the next time you do jury duty, where it might actually do some good.

CHAPTER 9

I CAN'T PRETEND THIS ISN'T HAPPENING ANYMORE

Running away from any problem only increases the distance from the solution. The easiest way to escape from the problem is to solve it.

—Rishika Jain

My pretending days ended after our preschool conference. Miss Lisa gently held my hand as she told us she thought something was wrong with Ryan. She said, "Ryan is not interested in, nor interacts with other kids." Ryan's preschool teacher explained that while most three-year-olds don't really play *together*, they do play *next* to one another. Although she never said it, even I knew typical children play with toys instead of hooks and shower nozzles. I felt my stomach tighten and my eyes mist as Miss Lisa talked about my son. She didn't use words like *gifted* or *talented* or *advanced*. She said *"wrong."*

And *wrong* didn't sound like a synonym for *genius*.

I now realize how difficult it was for Miss Lisa to tell us about Ryan. We had known Lisa for a long time. She had been Megan's preschool teacher and was almost like family. We knew she had Ryan's best interests at heart. I knew she was right, but I still hoped she might be mistaken. Although she told us what we didn't want to hear, I couldn't continue to ignore Ryan's behaviors.

He wasn't just eccentric and intense. My baby was not okay!

Ryan began preschool with Miss Lisa at age three. Almost every public-school district in Minnesota had a Family Center where excellent preschool programs and parenting classes were offered. We were about to use every resource they had. Ryan attended preschool with me one day each week and by himself for a second day. On the Mommy-and-Me day, I played with Ryan in Miss Lisa's classroom along with the rest of the mommies and children for a half-hour. Then, all the moms (and sometimes Frank) went to another classroom to learn about parenting. The challenges every parent needed to master, like effective discipline, were some of the many topics discussed.

My husband loved going to class and being *one of the girls.* He enjoyed himself when other moms looked to him as the *expert* on the dad's point of view. Frank was a part of our daily activities in a way most dads couldn't be. When he wasn't flying, Frank was with us all day long. Many dads only get to see their kids after a long workday when everyone is hungry, tired, and cranky.

More important than the parenting tips we learned, these classes provided a connection to other parents. It felt almost like a support group. The Family Center also had a lending library. The classic *How to Talk So Kids Will Listen and Listen So Kids Will Talk*[9] was just one of the books that improved our parenting skills with Megan. It didn't work as well with Ryan. When I attended these classes with Megan, I felt like we were doing okay as a family. As a result, I felt more secure in the methods I used to parent Megan. The classes helped me parent better. I left each class feeling confident and reassured that I was a good mom. But with Ryan, these classes had the opposite effect.

Our life with Ryan and the confusion his behaviors created was never covered in any parenting discussion. When we talked about children and the things they do, Ryan did not fit the pattern of a child developing in a typical manner. No one else's child was so fascinated by the number fourteen. My son would run around the house yelling "fourteen" over and over again. He even had to say good night to the number fourteen every night before bedtime.

---

9   Faber, Adele & Mazlish, Elaine. *How To Talk So Kids Will Listen & Listen So Kids Will Talk.* New York: Avon, 1982.

Soon we dropped out of Mommy and Me because of Ryan's behavior, even though I desperately needed preschool to be a success. It wasn't. The other children in Ryan's toddler class liked school. They liked being with each other and playing with all the exciting toys. Ryan just wanted to go home. Most times he got that blank stare and tuned out when we were at school. He didn't interact much with anyone; not even me.

I couldn't help but notice the difference between Ryan and the other kids. He played with objects instead of toys. When he did play with toys, he did it in his own unusual way. He would take the cars or trains and line them up in a perfect row. He didn't participate in art projects, mold Play-Doh, or fill and dump water into cups at the science station. There wasn't much social interaction in anything my son did. Ryan wanted no part of school even though I was there with him. After going to class with him for a month, I never wanted to go back. I didn't want to see how different he was from the other children. It became increasingly difficult to pretend he was okay after seeing the way he acted. Sometimes after class, I came home and sobbed.

Even with all the evidence, none of this stopped the *Queen of Denial*. I now clung to the fact that Ryan was one of the best-looking boys in his class. Somehow, the monumentally unimportant detail that he was handsome made me feel better. I needed to hold on to anything that made Ryan okay.

I further deluded myself with the observation that Ryan loved the musical part of school. Every time Miss Lisa and the other kids sang, when the singing ended he announced too loudly, "ALL DONE!" The other parents laughed when he did that, and their nervous laughter encouraged him to repeat this behavior after every song. I think it must have been obvious to everyone, except me, that Ryan had problems—*ENORMOUS* problems.

If I Knew Then What I Know Now

The conference with Miss Lisa was our wake-up call. Although we had hinted to our pediatrician there was a problem, we finally demanded a referral to some kind of an expert. Without much discussion, Dr. Hobbs sent us to a psychiatrist. I later found out she was the leading authority on autism in the Twin Cities area. I still wonder if our pediatrician knew all along that Ryan was a member of the A-Club. Maybe Dr. Hobbs didn't tell us Ryan had autism because he thought it kinder to leave us in the dark for as long as possible.

In 1992, most doctors at that time believed nothing could be done to alleviate the symptoms of autism. This lack of understanding continues today. The majority of doctors still don't believe our children can get better, nor do they know much about any of the medical interventions that significantly help our children. There must have been a lot more autism in the Twin Cities than Frank or I realized because it took several months to get an appointment with the specialist, Dr. Goodman.

Part 2

A Diagnosis and a Prescription to Nowhere

CHAPTER 10

PLEASE LET THIS BE ANYTHING ELSE

Always listen to the experts. They'll tell you what can't be done and why.
Then do it.

—Robert Heinlein

We entered Dr. Goodman's office, not knowing what we would hear and afraid of what she would tell us. But we needed to know anything that would explain the enigma of Ryan.

Dr. Goodman was tall and thin. She had shoulder-length hair surrounding her stoic, expressionless face. She'd occasionally smile politely, but her demeanor lacked warmth or any reassurance toward Ryan or his worried parents. The atmosphere felt dismal and grave. It was kind of like a funeral without the casket.

Ryan immediately went to Dr. Goodman's desk and picked up her telephone to study how it worked. He followed the cord to the wall and socket. Next, he became interested in the radiator and started to pace back and forth repeatedly in front of it. Dr. Goodman introduced herself and tried to connect with Ryan several times, but Ryan never responded. I wanted to speak up and make excuses for his strange actions, but I remained silent. I wondered if anyone else could hear my stomach churning. My head began to ache. I didn't want to be there. Who in their right mind takes their four-year-old to a psychiatrist?

What Ryan did next seemed almost appropriate, and this gave me a glimmer of hope. He went to a toy kitchen area and started cooking at the stove. He served his pretend food to everyone in the room, including Dr. Goodman. Still, he never answered any of her questions or looked at her. Ryan started to talk to himself about some of his favorite topics of conversation. He sounded like a broken record when he repeated and repeated his standard lines about the hooks in his closet. Today, just when I needed him to act as ordinary as possible, Ryan distinguished himself by making silly comments about his rubber iguana collection and hotels, particularly Embassy Suites.

Dr. Goodman's written report described his speech and behavior this way: "Ryan is a four-year-old male accompanied to the clinic today by his biological parents because of concerns of developmental delay. It should be noted that Ryan has some delayed echolalia as well as verbal perseveration." That's Doctor Speak for Ryan says the same things over and over again. She also noted in her report, "He has intermittent staring spells. He makes no attempt to socialize with the interviewer, but follows simple commands given to him. He is more socially appropriate with his parents and will frequently crawl into his dad's lap for a hug. His eye contact with the interviewer is mixed and he seems to have purposeful gaze aversion at times. His eye contact with his parents is quite a bit better." Again doctor jargon for saying my son had poor eye contact. Her report went on to say, "For the majority of the time he wandered somewhat aimlessly around the examination room not particularly interested in any toys. He makes no attempt to play in an organized way with any objects except the toy dishes. He frequently expresses that he is bored and wants to go home. Then he proclaims he is, *All Done.*"

As part of this initial visit, Ryan was given a Peabody Picture Vocabulary Test to measure receptive language skills. According to Dr. Goodman's evaluation, "His overall score was 27 giving him a standard score equivalent of 71 which put him approximately at the third percentile for speech [in his age group]." Her report also stated, "Ryan is preoccupied with unusual objects such as the telephone and the heat vents. He has intermittent self-stimulatory behavior with a mirror available in the office." That was more *Doctor Speak* to explain Ryan engaged in repetitive behaviors that had no apparent purpose. He touched the mirror over and over again and spun it.

It didn't take much time for the psychiatrist to drop the bomb that Ryan might have pervasive developmental disorder—not otherwise specified (PDD-NOS).

We had no clue as to the enormity of what she was saying. We didn't even know what PDD-NOS was, but it didn't sound good. PDD-NOS didn't sound like a synonym for genius, either.

It took me three weeks of middle-of-the-night reading to figure out that PDD was the term doctors used so parents don't freak out about the A-word. It's almost as if PDD is your consolation prize; "Congratulations, contestant, we have some great news for you! Your child has something that kinda looks like autism.[10] Consider yourself lucky, your child is only *a little autistic*!" I also learned autism is a very, very serious diagnosis.

There was no cure.

Dr. Goodman wanted to refine her diagnosis with further psychological testing and sent us home with a carful of ominous looking forms to complete. These tests consisted mostly of subjective questionnaires to be filled out by us and by his teachers. They seemed repetitive and stupid to me. How were these tests ever going to help my kid?

After giving us the PDD-NOS diagnosis, it was two long months before Dr. Goodman could fit us in for a second appointment to discuss Ryan's test results. Two months seemed like an eternity when you were waiting for anything that might help your child. During that time, I was in a state of deep depression. I walked around in a daze, going through the motions of being Mommy, but not really present at all.

10　PPD/NOS is a diagnosis found in the previous edition of the *Diagnostic and Statistical Manual of Mental Disorders, 4th Edition (DSM-IV)*. It is an atypical form of autism used for "severe and pervasive impairment in the development of reciprocal social interaction or verbal and nonverbal communication skills, or when stereotyped behavior, interests, and activities are present, but the criteria are not met for a specific PDD" or for several other disorders. Children with PPD/NOS may or may not receive a label of autism depending on the results of further assessment. American Psychiatric Association & American Psychiatric Association. *Diagnostic and Statistical Manual Of Mental Disorders:(DSM-IV-TR)*. Washington, DC: American Psychiatric Publishing, 2000.

I felt like I lived two separate lives. I was the mom who made dinner, washed the floors, and gave Megan a ride to school. I was the mom who pretended to friends and family that everything was okay, but in reality, I was scared out of my mind. What if I can't help Ryan? What if the doctor isn't wrong and Ryan really does have autism? When those thoughts snuck into my head, I couldn't sleep, and fear was the only emotion I felt. Ryan's life was at stake. I wasn't sure if my little boy would ever play baseball or learn to ride a bike. Would he ever get married or have someone to love and share his life?

Somewhere, in the midst of this inner turmoil and despair, I recalled my discussion with Megan the night Ryan came home from the hospital, "In our family, we give to those who *need* it." Since Ryan *needed* me, I became a mom on a mission. I had to help Ryan, but I had no idea how to do that.

We turned to our pediatrician, Dr. Hobbs, for help. He had always been there in the past for even the smallest problem with our children. His great bedside manner made us laugh whenever we went for a checkup. But after he received Dr. Goodman's report, he suddenly didn't have any smiles or any jokes for us. He was awkwardly silent and, worse than that, he became absent. Shortly after Ryan's diagnosis, he transferred us to a different doctor in the practice. He said Dr. Zada was better equipped to handle Ryan's autism.

I felt lost and confused by Dr. Hobbs's actions. Why did he abandon us? Was it that he had trouble dealing with our suffering? Looking back, he probably felt as helpless as we did. Nobody knows the right words to say in these kinds of situations. Maybe he saw Ryan slipping away and believed there was nothing he could do. I know my desolate crying jags in his office must have made him uncomfortable. When did I become such a sniffling idiot? I had always been a strong, assertive woman, but somehow my helplessness over how to help Ryan washed away my strength and left me crying way too often.

To be fair, I now realize Dr. Hobbs didn't believe there was anything he could do to help Ryan get rid of his autism. Even so, being discarded by the doctor we trusted the most left us completely alone.

After Ryan started on his road to recovery, part of my healing was to write Dr. Hobbs to explain how his abandonment made me feel.

Letter to our Pediatrician
June 11, 1995

Dear Dr. Hobbs:

When I first learned of my son's autism, I looked to you for help and guidance. You always took care of my children when they were ill. After Ryan was diagnosed with autism, everything changed. My son no longer had an ear infection that could be easily fixed with a quick dose of antibiotics. You decided we should become Dr. Zada's patients. Although Dr. Zada is a very nice person, you were the doctor who had cared for my children since they were small. You were the one I trusted with their lives.

Fortunately, I found answers to help Ryan elsewhere. However, I still find it sad that in our time of need, you were unavailable. Maybe you left us because you didn't know what to do or maybe the tears I cried in your office made you feel uncomfortable. Or maybe, you thought our situation was hopeless.

I think you're a dedicated doctor, but didn't know what to do, so you did nothing. I want you to understand how this made us feel. Maybe then, you won't abandon other families in their time of need. I know you truly care about your patients, but sometimes we all need a wake-up call.

Many parents with children on the spectrum lose valuable time because they are continually reassured by their pediatrician that everything is okay. You told us there was probably nothing wrong and we should wait awhile. This is what I wanted to hear, but not what was best for my child. It was only after I insisted that you send us to a specialist, that you did. Not all parents are assertive, and nobody ever wants to admit their child has a problem.

I would guess that there are many children in your practice that are still undiagnosed. If these children do not receive early intensive intervention, they will pass certain developmental stages that may never be regained.

Sincerely,
Marcia Hinds

Dr. Hobbs never answered my letter. I wasn't even sure that he received it until after one of our subsequent visits to the office. On this visit Dr. Zada was unavailable, so Dr. Hobbs took care of Ryan. He looked me straight in the eye and said, "Good letter." By that brief comment, I knew he was aware that he should have been there for us. I hope my letter helped him become a better doctor for other families struggling with such a serious medical condition.

The two months of waiting were finally over, and we were back in Dr. Goodman's office with its dark wooden desk and silly toy kitchen. Dr. Goodman bluntly stated the assessment test results confirmed a diagnosis of autism. She informed us in cold, unfeeling medical terms that most children with autism end up in institutions or group homes. The psychiatrist smiled when she revealed the *good news*, "With a little luck, Ryan could end up in the basement of some company running a computer and not having to deal directly with people."

I sat in stunned silence. In that instant, I became the mother in the recovery room on the other side of the curtain being told there was something wrong with her child.

Something unfixable.

I thought we had dodged a bullet when Ryan was born healthy and pronounced *perfect*, but that just wasn't true. It had never been true, and the bullet hit us right between the eyes. With just one sentence, we were no longer the *perfect* family, and were exiled to Autism Island without a lifeboat or rescue plane in sight. Ryan had autism, and the psychiatrist said there was *nothing* we could do. Her advice was to "wait and see how he turned out" since autism was a developmental disorder no one truly understood.

I was crushed by her diagnosis and unable to ask any questions. I hit overload and shut down, staring blankly into space almost the same way Ryan did when there was too much going on. Fortunately, my husband had the presence of mind to ask Dr. Goodman about programs to help our son. He looked to the psychiatrist for information on where we should start. Frank's first questions were about schools and special education. She said special education was not for Ryan because most kids with autism don't fit in either special education or regular education. Special education preschools would not address what Ryan needed nor would regular classes. It was starting to sound like he didn't fit anywhere except alone on Autism Island, with no hope for any future.

Dr. Goodman had virtually no suggestions on how to help our son. She did, however, have a very clear mandate for us as his parents. We were to accept the reality that Ryan had autism and move on. Our expert in the autism field seemed oblivious to our pain. She never offered hope, interventions, or any possible solutions.

When we left the psychiatrist's office, I was dazed, confused, and defeated. Frank steered me toward the car, opened my door, and buckled my seatbelt. Tears of frustration began to flow.

Ryan *couldn't* have autism! She *couldn't* be right!

I had never felt that kind of pain before. Our world was crashing down around us, and all this doctor seemed to care about were her superior diagnostic skills. She acted as if PPD-NOS was a good diagnostic outcome, considering that my child was incurably *damaged, broken... UNFIXABLE!*

I began screaming and swearing at the top of my lungs. Frank, ever calm in a crisis, made an emergency landing on the side of the road and tried to calm me down. Without any discussion, both of us knew we would never go back to that doctor again.

A few long hours later, I recovered from the worst of what was to be a multi-year series of my own mini-meltdowns over Ryan's autism and the impact it would have on him and our family. Again, without discussion, my husband and I decided we would not accept what this expert said. We were grief-stricken and felt a tremendous sense of loss. Our dreams about Ryan's future were shattered along with what was supposed to be our *perfect* family.

Nevertheless, we weren't about to wait and see how Ryan turned out. Not *our* kid!

I *used* my anger toward Dr. Goodman many times in the years to come when I had nothing left to give Ryan and he still needed more. Anger and outrage kept me going many times when Ryan's autism left me unable to breathe. Anger worked when I was too exhausted to get up another day and fight. All I had to do during the desperate times was revisit that day in Dr. Goodman's office. I would get angry all over again and would continue my mission to prove her wrong. I was determined to show her that my son would be okay. Her inaction taught us an important lesson. Even though there were professionals to help us, we would be the ones *ultimately responsible* for the decisions affecting Ryan.

I was sure the psychiatrist was wrong. I prayed she was wrong. And I had never prayed in my life. I didn't want to accept Ryan had the A-word. I couldn't understand how an autism diagnosis resulted from filling out billions of forms and a twenty-minute observation of Ryan, but somehow it did. None of the assessment tools the psychiatrist administered proved my son had autism. Wasn't there some sort of a blood test? Couldn't you see Ryan's autism on an EEG or an X-ray? If it was so invisible, how come it took only twenty minutes to diagnose?

I wondered why this happened to our family? In my less lucid moments, I thought it might be better if Ryan had been diagnosed with cancer. That way my son might have a fighting chance and we would have a shred of hope that he could be helped. I bargained with God and fate. I promised him if he helped my son, I would help everyone with autism.

This new reality that Ryan could end up alone and institutionalized was what I worried about the most. "*Institution*" became a word that haunted me for years. "*Group home*" sent me into a physical and mental panic. What if I got sick or died? What would happen to Ryan if something happened to me? If I got in a car accident, who would do all the crazy things I did for him? No one but Ryan's mother would put up with him and all his antics.

The images these thoughts conjured left me sick to my stomach, weak, unable to breathe, and in a panic. During many of these moments, I would frantically distract myself by cleaning the floor or scrubbing a toilet. Anything that was a normal activity done by normal people comforted me. Cleaning the floor was something I could control and accomplish. My house was cleaner than it had ever been before.

But my mind was a total wreck.

To reassure myself that Ryan would be okay even if I died, I came up with a list of women Frank was *allowed* to marry if something happened to me. I wanted him to marry someone who loved Ryan and accepted him, warts and all. They didn't even need to love Frank. My husband knew I wasn't kidding when I talked about his *future bride*. Frank never questioned my sanity when I said these kinds of things. How crazy is it to pick out someone for your husband to marry if something happens to you?

If I Knew Then What I Know Now

Ryan's diagnosis was made when most psychiatrists and doctors believed autism was a rare and incurable *mental* disorder defined as a *forever* condition with no hope for recovery. And yet, twenty years after Ryan was first diagnosed, autism is still not treated medically by most doctors. A child's autism diagnosis is still largely based on clinical interpretation of behavioral observation and parent surveys. That needs to change.

This diagnosis needs to be based on objective empirical evidence as opposed to subjective surveys. Tests like brain neuroSPECT or functional MRIs, targeted blood work, and genetic and epigenetic lab screening should be used to determine conclusively what is and isn't functioning correctly in a child's brain and immune system. There are blood, urine and excrement tests that will help provide answers to guide the treatment your child needs. Autism will be treated scientifically and medically if you have a doctor or immunologist who has not stayed behind in the old paradigms.

The word "autism" simply identifies a collection of symptoms that look different in every kid. We need to change what the general public and most doctors still believe about autism. Maybe if we just stop calling it "autism" and start calling it what it is: a messed up or dysregulated immune system, the kids would get the medical treatment they need and deserve.

Some kids appear to be ill all the time, while others never seem to catch anything at all. The common thread is they all have immune systems that are not working properly. Sometimes their immune systems are underactive and don't respond. And other times, their systems work overtime to fight off infections that are no longer a threat.

Nevertheless, the common belief among most conventional doctors continues to be that autism is a dead-end developmental disorder. This couldn't be further from the truth. It is not simply a developmental disorder; it is a medical disease caused by an immune system that is sometimes over- and/or underactive. It should never be a life sentence to a special education classroom or a group home. Autism is medical and treatable!

CHAPTER 11

OUR INITIAL SEARCH FOR ANSWERS

Progress always involves risks. You can't steal second base and keep your foot on first.

—Frederick B. Wilcox

ALTHOUGH I COULDN'T accept Ryan had this dead-end diagnosis of autism, I could now accept that something was wrong with my son. It was almost a relief to find out I wasn't a bad mother, and I wasn't crazy—at least not completely. Still, I secretly hoped the autism diagnosis was wrong and that the "not otherwise specified" part of Ryan's PDD-NOS diagnosis was a secret doctor code that meant Ryan would turn out to have something else. Something with a nice, tidy cure. This all had to be a mistake.

By this time, and because of Miss Lisa, the school district became involved. Of course, they felt it necessary to administer yet another round of educational and psychological assessment tests. I didn't understand how these assessment tools would help Ryan. Still, I just blindly followed their instructions because I didn't know what else to do. These people were the experts, and we were just Ryan's parents who filled out lots of forms. The bottom line was that Ryan was now a *special education* student.

Meanwhile, Frank and I did what most parents do after they get an autism diagnosis. We started down the conventional treatment road searching for any expert who could help us or, better still, change Ryan's diagnosis. The first stop on this thoroughfare to disappointment was an appointment with Dr. Paine at the Minneapolis Clinic of Neurology. It took more than three months to get an appointment with the acclaimed pediatric neurologist we *needed* to see.

As we entered his office, Frank's hopes were high and mine were stratospheric. Ryan had his bag of object friends to keep him occupied and was looking perfectly normal in what I hoped was a way that suggested our old friend named *genius* rather than our new enemy named *autism*. We just knew this renowned doctor would help Ryan. But within minutes, he became just another disappointment with the medical profession. This man did not even give us ten minutes of his time or bother to do a cursory physical examination of our son. As soon as he read Ryan's history and diagnosis, he couldn't push us out the door fast enough. Was Ryan's autism really that obvious to everyone but us?

His very first words were simply, "There is *nothing* I can do to help you." Stunned, I asked if we should do an EEG, another test, or anything else. What about urine, excrement, saliva, and blood tests?

Please God, anything else.

This doctor couldn't even look me in the eye as he replied that autism is not a medical condition but a developmental disorder and doesn't show up on physiological tests. He never even considered that Ryan could have something else that mimicked autism. That was what I was really hoping for. A nice little benign brain tumor would have been great! All that was left was the enormity of silence surrounding the word *autism*.

Ryan had the A-word. End of story!

Maybe we didn't know how to cure Ryan's autism, but I hoped we could fix some of his bizarre behaviors while we searched for the miracle cure. Perhaps a psychologist could help? Jackie Rains was warm and welcoming. Again, Ryan needed to be evaluated even though we had already filled out ten million forms for Dr. Goodman and our school district.[11]

---

11   The speech specialist from our school district had her own barrage of tests. They included: *The Clinical Evaluation of Language Fundamentals-Preschool (CELF-P), Expressive One-Word Picture Vocabulary Test-Revised (EOWPVT-R)*, and *Test for Auditory Comprehension of Language*. The Occupational Therapist gave him the *Bruininks-Oseretsky Test of Motor Proficiency (B-O)* and *The Test of Visual Motor Skills (TVMS)*.

I was starting to become *form phobic* and questioned why professionals wasted so much time on these paper evaluations when all we really wanted was medical treatment and anything that would help our son. Why fill out forms when anyone with any expertise in autism could tell Ryan was a member of the A-Club as soon as they laid eyes on him?

Nonetheless, Ms. Rains insisted, and we complied. I soon discovered she actually understood that a standardized assessment form doesn't tell you much when you are dealing with a child with autism. Their strengths and weaknesses are so scattered. She videotaped Ryan and observed how he responded to tasks she asked him to complete.

Jackie could get Ryan to pay attention in a way no one else had—including us. She knew how to engage my kid who usually didn't respond. It didn't take her long to figure out how smart Ryan was. That surprised me since his intelligence was hidden deep behind his odd behaviors. I thought his family members were the only ones who knew. Ms. Rains treated him with respect and not like a damaged autistic child who didn't understand anything. Even though Ryan lacked communication skills, Jackie Rains saw through all the noises, biting, and strange behavior. Jackie saw what I saw. She knew he was *in there*. Maybe Ms. Rains could throw Ryan a life preserver to help my son and my family escape from Autism Island.

Jackie devised a comprehensive treatment plan. It included trained staff members who came to our home to work with Ryan on age-appropriate basic life skills, such as feeding, dressing, and toothbrushing. Ryan was not even close to mastering these simple activities of daily life. Speech was also supposed to be part of the remediation plan. Unfortunately, while the staff she sent to our house looked strong on paper, they were weak on technique. Ryan wanted no part of learning what they wanted to teach. They couldn't control him or get him to do much of anything.

After I suspected Jackie's therapists weren't helping Ryan, I started to make a habit of entering the room unannounced. I usually found them socializing with each other instead of working with my son. One time, Ryan wasn't even in the room with them, and they were clueless as to where he was. I was paying big bucks for these undertrained *professionals*, and they weren't doing anything of value—not even giving me a break. It wasn't long before I stopped using these *therapists*, but I did stay with Jackie Rains to help me. I still needed her.

Jackie went with us to school Individualized Education Program (IEP) meetings, held parent support groups, and hosted all kinds of informational seminars. Although she offered no real concrete ideas or staff that was of any real assistance to my son, she did help me cope with the stress associated with Ryan's autism. Just her presence made me feel like I was doing something. At least I wasn't still alone on this highway to nowhere.

Megan and Jackie were both telling us as loudly as they could that Ryan's autism could be helped significantly if we focused on teaching him how to behave. Even so, I was not yet ready to hear their message. Ryan's non-response to Jackie Rains's behavioral "experts" suggested to me that Ryan's autism was too profound to respond to simple behavioral interventions. I went back to searching for the cure.

Ryan's autism introduced us to a new circle of acquaintances—other A-Club parents. Some seemed to be travelers on a very different treatment road than we were, and each road seemed to be as unique as the child. One such road was the *biomedical approach*. It had the word *medical* in it, so it sounded good to me. Anything was better than these endless assessment tools and subjective rating scales that led to no action or real solutions. We had filled out a million of them and Ryan still could not dress himself. When Frank and I asked Ryan's psychologist about biomedical interventions such as diet, megavitamins, anti-yeast therapy, and allergy/intolerance tests, Jackie advised us that most of the time these interventions didn't work. She added that they could even cause harm. We shouldn't go down that path. We shouldn't waste our time or money. So, we didn't. She was costing enough.

Of course, all of this occurred in 1993, back in the beginning of what is now called the *Autism Epidemic*. That was back in the Stone Age of medical treatment for autism. I'm not sure if Jackie had any real knowledge of the emerging and innovative interventions available for children with autism. We asked her about employing the Lovaas method (applied behavior analysis or ABA). Jackie was so opposed to it, she told us she would not continue to work with us if we employed any of those *abusive, dog-training techniques.*

The experts we took our son to were definitely credentialed, but not really effective in changing anything for Ryan. Biomedical had been banned by our psychologist. Where did that leave us? We decided to try *conventional*. We needed a conventional therapy that was not as mainstream as psychiatry, was more helpful than psychology, but was definitely not as controversial as biomedical. Just like in *Goldilocks and the Three Bears*, we wanted a therapy that was just right. So Maria Chavez, an occupational therapist (OT) from Minneapolis Children's Hospital, became the newest member of Ryan's growing treatment team. Ryan was four at the time, and her evaluation scored him in the second percentile on the age-normed *Miller Assessment for Preschoolers*. This test measures basic motor skills and a child's awareness of sensations. It also measures coordination as well as verbal and nonverbal skills and how they influence the completion of complex tasks.

There was much variation and scatter in his scores. His verbal skills scored a bit higher than his nonverbal skills or his coordination and motor skills. But they were *all bad*. That is typical for kids with autism. Maria's observations during testing reported, "Poor motor planning skills due to impaired tactile discrimination and poor joint muscle body position sense." She also noted in her written report, "...delayed visual-motor skills with probable visual perceptual difficulties."

That meant that Ryan was in *serious* developmental trouble.

Maria said Ryan could not sequence the steps needed to complete a multistep task; he had sensory integration difficulties and significant perceptual issues. But he wasn't a total disaster because he scored in the *second* percentile. Statistically, there were only two percentage points of kids who scored lower than he did. And that meant he was only ninety-eight percentage points away from being a genius.

Our next-door neighbor happened to be Sandi Reese, PhD, OTR/L. Sandi was a department head at the University of Minnesota and responsible for training and credentialing many of the occupational therapists in the Twin Cities area. Even though I thought we were friends, and even though she knew Ryan well, she never once suggested I take Ryan to a specialist or hinted that something might be wrong with my son.

Sandi dealt with children in the A-Club on a daily basis. Given the speed at which other professionals diagnosed Ryan, there was no way she wouldn't have recognized Ryan was a member of the club. It was hard to understand why she hadn't offered to help. Ryan needed so much, and I was desperate—desperate enough to put aside my anger toward her to ask for help. Perhaps she would reassess Ryan and discover that elusive brain tumor.

Sandi's evaluation noted, "The visual world appeared to be a confusing place for him. At times, he did not seem to recognize familiar people in new environments." Both Maria and Sandi said in their reports that Ryan was hypersensitive to certain sounds, particularly loud noises. They further described him as showing symptoms of *sensory defensiveness*. He had extreme deficits in motor planning, which contributed to his inability to dress or feed himself. He also did not participate in hygiene activities like brushing his teeth or washing his hands. Frank and I did all of these for him. Now, at least we knew why we had to do these things.

But there was no "B" for brain tumor. It was still an "A" for autism.

Occupational therapy now seemed like our best option. Maria truly cared about Ryan, and I liked the way she worked with him. She made therapy fun and motivated him to want to do more. She used his love of counting and his restricted interests in hotels, elevators, and escalators to help him focus on his therapy goals.

I carefully studied what Maria did when she worked with Ryan. Our health insurance only covered ten sessions of OT and, when our measly allotment expired, Frank and I continued with what she started. We set up obstacle courses in our basement that had Ryan's favorite computer game at the finish line. We bought a swing like Maria used and hung it in our basement. During bath time, he played with squirt bottles with different colored water to help develop his fine motor skills and hand strength.

The activities Maria did with Ryan taught me how important it was for him to exercise and to move his body in a coordinated manner. We added swimming to his therapy program. We enrolled Ryan in a group lesson at the local pool. He glued himself to the wall at the side of the pool. Instead of looking at the instructor or other kids, he touched the designs on the tiles in his peculiar, repetitive way. It was so hard to watch the other kids smiling and splashing and eager to learn. A few were scared of the water, but no one acted as *weird* as our son.

Ryan clutched the pool wall as if his life depended on it and made grunting noises that sounded like something out of *The Exorcist*. They were loud enough to wake the dead, and when he made them, all eyes at the pool automatically shifted to Ryan. I halfway expected his head to spin around. In hindsight, I now realize he used this disruptive behavior to escape from things he found unpleasant, like almost drowning in front of a group of total strangers. He knew what he was doing and how to control us and the situation. His noises attracted so much attention that we were forced to take him out of the pool, so the other children could continue their lessons.

Ryan won this round!

With time comes understanding—even understanding of very confusing things like autism. We were asking Ryan to do something he was not yet capable of. There were too many sensory and social events happening at the same time in a group lesson for Ryan to learn how to swim. He made bizarre noises because he hadn't mastered the speech necessary to tell us about his frustration and fear. If you think about it, he was really quite smart to be able to figure out how to escape this situation. But, once again, we were hit straight-on with the pain that comes when you realize your child is not like other children—and may never be.

Swimming lessons needed to become less about swimming and more about *showing* and *teaching* Ryan how to meet our expectations for his behavior instead of us always meeting his. Megan's wise words once again whispered in my ear, and this time, I listened. We needed to teach him the right way to behave, and her words became our guide.

We switched to private swim lessons with a smaller, quieter, setting and individual instruction. Pam, his new swim teacher, was unfazed by grunts and growls. I did not know how to explain why it happened, but Ryan always seemed much more focused and *with us* after this kind of vigorous and coordinated exercise. It was after a swimming session that I really began to get my first glimpse of the kid who was *in there*. Swimming became fun for Ryan. He might be stranded on Autism Island, but the exercise and coordinated movement from swimming seemed like a way back to the real world.

Although swimming was great for Ryan, it is a solitary act. Ryan desperately needed to develop social skills. So, we searched for something that involved exercise and a social component. A huge trampoline for the backyard became part of Ryan's OT-inspired therapy program. In addition to being useful to help develop Ryan's gross motor skills, the trampoline was a powerful *kid-attractor*. All the neighborhood kids came to jump and play.

Doctors cringe when you tell them you have a trampoline, and personal injury attorneys start to salivate. Potential injuries were of great concern to us, but we had found something that might work, and we were going to bounce with it. Bouncing gave Ryan exposure to more social situations and provided the sensory stimulation that typical kids experience all the time because they actually *move* their bodies instead of *staring* at their fingers or closet hooks all day long.

Ryan's occupational therapy sessions showed us that sustained, coordinated, intentional physical movement made Ryan's autism symptoms decrease in frequency and intensity. At the same time, his more normal-looking behaviors increased. Exercise and movement became important to making him more like other kids. This was the closest thing we had to the miracle cure I kept praying for. And I didn't have to take out a second mortgage to get the same results the occupational therapist did. We could do these kinds of activities on our own several times per week. All it cost us was our time, snacks for all the kids, and the major frustration that came from working with Ryan.

Our therapy scorecard went something like this:

Psychiatry . . . fail. Psychology . . . incomplete. Occupational therapy . . . still in progress.

CHAPTER 12

NO INSTANT CURES AND MANY MISSTEPS

The simple things are also the most extraordinary things, and only the wise can see them.

—Paulo Coelho

I WONDERED WHAT else might be out there to help my son. My hunger for more therapies that would positively impact Ryan made us sitting ducks for every instant cure that came along. If bouncing Ryan on a trampoline decreased his autism symptoms, why couldn't straightening his spine do the same thing?

I should have run out of Dr. Snap-Crackle-and-Pop's office when I first laid eyes on him. He was unconventional, downright bizarre, and his eye contact was worse than Ryan's. He ordered hair fiber tests and prescribed tons of supplements we could purchase only from him. It appeared his goal was to become independently wealthy off my son's condition. My fear for Ryan's future made me stay through several visits. It is still hard to admit I was stupid enough to believe this crazy doctor could actually help. I want to forget the experience so much that I can't even remember his real name. Frank, ever logical and sane, tried to stop me, but there was no reasoning with a crazy, frantic mother. Not all chiropractors are like this, and many have great solutions for what ails us, but Dr. Snap-Crackle-and-Pop was not one of them.

The chiropractor scored "D" for deranged.

That experience didn't stop my next effort to get a nice pair of rainbow-colored eyeglasses that were supposed to end all of Ryan's autism issues. This search for *the cure* started with a flight to Duluth to see an eye doctor who prescribed Irlen[12] prism glasses for Ryan. We spent a small fortune on these glasses, but after all our efforts, my son, aka *Mr. Touchy Feely*, wouldn't even consider putting them on. I have no idea if they would have helped, because they sat on the kitchen counter instead of the bridge of his nose. Exhausted, I wasn't about to force the issue. Ryan already wore me down, and no one could make him do what he didn't want to do without a real fight. Since I wasn't up for more tantrums, we gave up on the glasses before we actually gave them a real try.

Prism glasses scored "F" for failure (at least for my kid).

When I thought about these therapies with my head instead of my heart, the idea of glasses curing autism just didn't make sense. But at this stage, I would have tried anything and everything to prove to myself we weren't giving up on Ryan. Sometimes, throwing money at autism gave me a sense that I was doing something...anything. *Hoping* I was helping my son was the next best thing to *actually* helping him.

I believed in the potential of these therapies because there was nothing else for us to believe in. Many of these so-called experts fed on our fears, and some well-meaning ones may have actually thought they were helping. Prism glasses taught us a cheap lesson that saved us a fortune in the long run because, while they helped some kids, they didn't help ours. We learned to be more selective in the future.

I was constantly distracted by my determination to find a cure—not just a therapy. Improvement was not enough. I wanted his autism gone. My disillusionment with multiple therapies and their multiple failures left me almost as stuck as Ryan. Megan's words still resonated in my head, but I didn't know where to look for more and new effective therapies that could show Ryan how to behave differently. Megan wasn't just talking about Ryan's challenges—she

---

12 Irlen, Helen. *Reading by the colors: Overcoming dyslexia and other reading disabilities through the Irlen method.* Garden City Park: Avery Publishing Group, 1991.

was also talking about mine. Her words lead me to the idea that I had to behave differently if I really wanted Ryan to behave differently.

Megan's words led to the invention of the *Marcia Method* for treating autism: "*If You Don't Feel It, Fake It*" therapy. I discovered I could change the way Ryan acted just by changing my behavior toward him. It took a year or so after he was first diagnosed to discover this effective therapy. This method started with a little experiment to see just how much my dark thoughts and moods affected him. When he was crabby or out of control, instead of acting scared or defeated, I cranked up the rock and roll music and started dancing around the house like I didn't have a care in the world. No one can be depressed or defeated when that kind of music is playing. I changed the way Ryan behaved and I changed his mood by acting happy instead of getting angry and frustrated.

Sometimes, instead of upbeat music, my therapy consisted of ignoring bad behavior and changing the scenery just before Ryan was about to meltdown. I'd take Ryan, and anyone else who happened to be at our house, for a walk or bike ride. If I didn't feel like doing either of those things, I threw everyone in the car and we would go somewhere else that might improve our attitudes. Sometimes we went to the park, the lake, or the McDonald's playground. We'd go anywhere that got us *out* of the house and into a more positive environment. Even though Ryan never wanted to go anywhere and change was difficult for him, once we got there things improved.

The problem with the *Marcia Method* was that it was all an act. Although it helped Ryan's disposition, I still felt desperately alone and anxious. I acted like I was happy when I really wasn't. I was still racked with fear and anxiety about my son's future. That fear was always there.

In the process of being Dr. Mom, head therapist and OT provider, sometimes I forgot Ryan needed me to just be *his mommy*. He wasn't only a research subject whom I was attempting to fix. Ryan also needed to be my son, who just wanted to be loved by his mom. When I remembered this important fact, I sometimes cancelled whatever therapy I had scheduled for the day. For a while, I got to be the mom who pushed her kid on the swing at the park or went for a swim in the community pool. I needed that, and Ryan needed it, too.

When days were hard, I'd give myself a talking to. I needed to be the *nice mommy*. I forced myself to have patience with Ryan's extreme and bizarre behaviors. It was necessary to treat him like a kid instead of the lab rat he so often became. Some days, I would force him to hug me, and I would try to hide the tension I felt when I realized how unnatural the hug felt to both of us.

I'd say, "Ryan, you *have* to hug me. I'm your mommy, and it's *your job!*" I got to be an expert at hiding my true feelings. When I said these things, I never wanted a hug. More often, I was totally exasperated by his *weird* behaviors and noises. But hiding my true feelings didn't always work, and sometimes I couldn't even fake it. On those days, I was not the *nice mommy*.

When a hard day turned into a day from hell and I was thoroughly exhausted and didn't want to continue, I would give myself a pep talk. I was my own coach in the Autism Olympics. My mantra became, "Even though Ryan *is* weird, he is *really* smart." This was my downsized version of the *"He's a genius"* story from his infancy. That's when I replayed all those old tales in my head about Einstein, Bill Gates, Jacques Cousteau, and Thomas Edison. I remembered all my old rationalizations about how these guys didn't really fit, but they did okay. That helped to calm me somewhat and helped me keep going when I didn't have anything left to give.

Another therapy I used to remain sane was to do something nice for someone else, especially when I didn't want to. On those days, I'd try to help another parent who was a member of the A-Club. Although I was drowning myself, helping someone else got me out of my pity party. It gave me something other than Ryan to focus on, as well as something good and tangible to do. I learned that helping others was not only about helping—it made me feel better.

And there was always the never-ending search to find *the cure* for Ryan. That was therapy too because *I WASN'T GIVING UP!*

If I Knew Then What I Know Now

We listened to many people who had numerous and varied ideas of how to help us. The ideas sounded good, but the reality of our situation was that most of these things were detrimental to Ryan's care, our family, and to my mental health. These supposed experts drained our pocketbooks and, even worse, wasted valuable time.

After expert chasing for more than a year, I finally settled down and did my homework about the validity of any particular treatment. I learned to use my head instead of my fear. I finally realized if something sounded too easy or too good to be true, it probably was. There were no superhuman experts armed with instant cures. There was no miracle cure for autism. There still isn't, and I'm *still* looking.

Therapy was the best option I had found. Our lives were now a treadmill of speech therapy, occupational therapy, social skills therapy, school and classroom therapy, swimming lessons, trampoline play dates, and a whole host of other things. Actually I didn't want to do any of these things. I really just wanted to be Ryan and Megan's mommy, but that was no longer an option. We had too much therapy to do.

I fantasized about finding a one-stop shopping center that provided the entire medical, behavioral, and educational interventions every child with autism needs. If that had been available, maybe I could have relaxed more because it would have eliminated the constant searching for the next *instant cure* that might help Ryan progress. In the process, our family would have been protected from the people who were just trying to make a buck off our misery. That place still doesn't exist two decades later, but I am still hopeful. And someday, I might even start one.

But for now, parents still have to construct their own programs with only minimal guidance. I believe this is part of the reason more children haven't fully recovered. There are so many medical treatments and rehabilitation plans that need to be integrated into one encyclopedic individualized plan in order to teach each A-Club child all they need. Recovery also involves luck and great timing. We need to be in the right place at the right time and do things in the right order for long enough for the interventions to work.

Helping Ryan was such a huge undertaking that sometimes I didn't take care of the most important people in my life. Frank was often neglected. Worse than that, he was sometimes an easy target for my frustrations about Ryan. I knew he would be there for us, no matter how bitchy I was.

Not only did I ignore his needs, but I was also unreasonable in my expectations. When I read a book that Frank hadn't even heard of because he was flying planes and earning money to pay the therapy bills, I was angry when he didn't understand the new *must-do* technique we needed to implement with Ryan. My expectations for my husband weren't fair. I spent every waking hour working to help Ryan and expected my husband to do the same. It didn't matter that Frank provided the income to make it possible for me to do this full-time. I still got mad that the hunt for a miracle cure was my responsibility and left up to me— *all* to me. Even though Frank had a full-time job and other obligations besides Ryan's multiple therapies, I was a crazed woman on a mission, and nothing rational seemed to matter.

I tried to include Megan in our activities, but at times she was only included as a part of the things I did to help Ryan. And sometimes, I couldn't tell if any of these therapies helped at all. Since so much family time revolved around therapy appointments and the other autism-related activities we did, I was concerned about the long-term effect on Megan. I constantly worried that my family's sacrifices wouldn't actually help Ryan anyway. In the process of trying to help him, was I sacrificing my other child?

Frank had been the love of my life. After Ryan's diagnosis, there was never any time for us anymore. Before Ryan, I thought about Frank and how much I loved him all the time. After Ryan's diagnosis, I thought about Ryan and what Ryan needed all the time. Frank had no time for me, and I had no time for him or anything that strengthened or helped sustain our relationship. We couldn't even get away for a date night because of Ryan's behaviors and needs. Most times there was an ocean of tension between us. Even our once active sex life seemed to disappear along with our hopes and dreams for Ryan. We were both tired and running on empty.

Although Megan and Frank were still a part of everything most important to me, they most often took a backseat to Ryan. Ryan was in the driver's seat and I was sitting right next to him, holding his hand, trying to find directions off Autism Island.

Megan always tried to be *the good child* because Ryan wasn't. She was sometimes too patient and never demanded what she *should* have received. Meeting her needs usually came after I was finished with Ryan, and after I was finished with him, there usually wasn't much left. I didn't want to treat my daughter and husband like they came second, but I did. Ryan definitely *needed* me more than anyone else ever did. I forgot that for Megan and Frank, this felt like *forever*.

I also forgot to thank Megan for her wise words—words that had resulted in the best treatment for Ryan so far. Megan, with her quiet love for her brother, was more of an expert on how to do things than all the specialists we consulted and wasted a small fortune on.

Part 3

Searching for Solutions

CHAPTER 13

THINKING OUTSIDE THE LUNCHBOX

Vegetables are a must on a diet. I suggest carrot cake, zucchini bread, and pumpkin pie.

—Jim Davis

THE STRESS OF losing our dreams for our son was taking its toll on me, on Frank, and on Megan. Ryan seemed oblivious to our distress. I couldn't accept that Ryan might be stuck on Autism Island forever, but I didn't know how to help him escape. I continued reading anything and everything I could about autism every night into the wee hours of the morning. I didn't sleep much and was wound pretty tight. My husband was concerned. Frustrated and worried, Frank told me I couldn't continue to do this twenty-four/seven. I almost snapped his head off when I said, "What am I supposed to do? Do you think I want to be doing this? I'm Ryan's *only* hope!"

I searched for anything that would help my son. I read books and medical articles well above my comprehension level. Almost everything I read said autism was an untreatable developmental disorder and not many of the "experts" agreed about anything. There were many conflicting theories about autism except the one that autism remained difficult to understand and was totally incurable. That was back in 1993. Many still believe that today, but more and more researchers are starting to accept the immune connection with autism. I continued to bargain with God for a nice, tidy, curable anything-we-could-fix. But God wasn't budging on his autism diagnosis.

Frank and I realized the conventional psychiatric approach was a dead-end road to Nowhereland. It was always the same prescription Dr. Goodman gave: " . . . accept autism and move on." Frank and I had made a joint decision to improve Ryan's condition and *never accept it*. We would not leave Ryan stranded on Autism Island. We would not *move on* without our son.

Mostly because we didn't know what else to do, we put aside Jackie Rains's opinion of biomedical intervention and slowly started down that path. This less-traveled road would make all the difference in Ryan's future. Frank and I are people who embrace conventional things. This new world of biomedical treatment seemed mysterious and unusual. I was more than suspicious.

One afternoon, after an unproductive week of searching for Ryan's miracle cure, I came across an article from the Autism Research Institute (ARI) in San Diego, California. I contacted them, and they sent me an information packet that caused me to question everything I already *knew* about autism. When I called the ARI for clarification, the telephone was answered by Dr. Bernard Rimland himself. He was a research psychologist and the founder of ARI. I didn't know who he was, so I wasn't overly impressed by his name.

I *should* have been.

Dr. Rimland was among those who founded the Autism Society of America (ASA). He was also a card-carrying member of the A-Club because his adult son, Mark, had autism. Dr. Rimland left ASA to start ARI, an organization with a biomedical emphasis. He knew his son's autism was NOT caused by a refrigerator mother. Dr. Rimland knew autism was both medical and treatable. He had extensive knowledge of every autism treatment available, proven and unproven.

Dr. Rimland and I had an immediate connection, the kind that comes from fighting the same enemy and the same war. We both understood the loss of hope for our children's future and my need to do something—*anything*.

Dr. Rimland didn't suggest blood tests or MRIs or anything else I associated with traditional medicine even though he was an expert on the subject. Instead he asked if Ryan drank milk and consumed much dairy in other foods. I answered, "Only from the time he wakes up until he goes to sleep." He suggested I take Ryan off milk products for a week and then give him a glass of milk and see what happened.

I had no idea if this man knew what he was talking about, but he was kind, and I was desperate. I was not convinced eliminating dairy from Ryan's diet would change anything. What could a cow possibly have to do with curing autism?

I never did give Ryan that glass of milk the following week. The change in Ryan's behavior was astounding. He was more tuned-in and more responsive. His weird noises, screaming, biting, and pinching lessened in frequency and intensity. The first significant step toward Ryan's medical recovery I owed not to doctors with impeccable credentials and beautifully appointed waiting rooms, but to a quiet under-funded researcher with peculiar theories about cows.

Life without milk was definitely unconventional. Hadn't we all been told milk is essential for proper child development? I had never really been concerned about nutrition before. I was the kind of mom who gave her kids cereal packed with sugar for breakfast. Our favorite foods—and almost everything we ate—were prepackaged and contained dairy. We ordered pizza at least once a week and loved eating out. I was a junk food addict, and Frank was no health nut, either.

Suddenly, everything changed. I was no longer sure what to feed my child. What food could I use as a substitute for dairy? Did this mean we would all have to eat health food? I wasn't even sure what a whole grain was. Even worse than *elective malnutrition*, I feared I might have to cook two different meals for my family. If you knew how I felt about cooking, you'd have some idea how unhappy I was about this turn of events.

My unofficial PhD in nutrition began as I read every label in the grocery store. I worried about every mouthful I put in my son's body. Would Ryan get enough calcium after I removed milk from his diet? If I couldn't find a packaged substitute, would I have to cook? I was convinced I would be chained to the stove, cooking obscure foods from scratch. Apparently, fixing Ryan's autism was hidden somewhere in my cooking pots. And if that meant me turning into Julia Child, I would do it.

I, Marcia, would cook.

I had no idea at that time how important Dr. Rimland's words were for me, our family, and Ryan. I was clueless as to how seriously dairy affected Ryan until I systematically eliminated any food containing dairy (casein) and saw the marked change in his behavior. But dairy was not the only food contributing to Ryan's autism. I started to watch him a little too closely, and over time, I learned I could often tell which food changed his behavior. Ryan seemed to react to so many foods. His ears sometimes turned beet red after eating something to which he was sensitive, and his behavior became unmistakably more *autistic*. I couldn't relax. If I didn't get it right, every meal, every snack, could potentially make his autism worse.

Dr. Rimland became my new best friend. He was the man! Frank was still around, of course, but Bernie was always just a telephone call away, and he could help Ryan. Even though Dr. Rimland was extremely busy trying to help all children affected by autism, he always made time for anyone who needed him. And I really, really needed him.

When Dr. Rimland answered the telephone that first day we talked, I had no idea what a driving force he would become in changing the course of our lives. He steered us toward real medical interventions for autism and away from the dead-end conventional ones. During that first conversation, he patiently explained to this mom what I needed to do to start to heal my son. I'm sure I was only one of a million discussions he had with half-crazed mothers where he explained the connection between diet and autism for the gazillionth time. Even so, during that crucial conversation, he made me feel like I was the first and most important person he had ever talked to about this.

After Bernard Rimland passed away, I missed his calming voice and the talks we had. When I think of the thousands of families he helped, I am overcome with emotion. The example he set with Mark, his own son, remains a great lesson to all of us. Mark is an accomplished artist,[13] a savant in this area. Mark's father showed many of us that it is important to find our child's strengths and

---

13   Landalf, Helen & Rimland, Mark. *The Secret Night World of Cats*. Lyme: Smith and Kraus, 1997.

celebrate their accomplishments. Bernie taught by example and made the autism journey easier for so many of us. When we were drowning, he threw us the life raft we needed to begin our journey off Autism Island.

Meanwhile, back in the dairy-free zone, Ryan's improved behavior and greater engagement with his family had convinced us that the inconvenient and unconventional biomedical approach was the way to move forward. I was ready for the next step when Dr. Rimland recommended we see Dr. Sidney Baker in New Jersey. Dr. Baker was instrumental in starting Defeat Autism Now! (DAN!) with Dr. Rimland and many others. It was Dr. Baker's medical protocol that DAN! doctors first used when ARI developed its treatment recommendations for autism. Today, DAN! doctors have evolved into the Medical Academy of Pediatric Special Needs (MAPS) certified doctors.[14]

We boarded the plane for New Jersey as soon as we made it to the top of Dr. Baker's waiting list. Besides being knowledgeable, he seemed ethical and truly wanted to help. He was also expensive and did not accept insurance. We took a deep financial breath and walked into his office ready to receive *the cure* for autism.

To my delight and astonishment, Dr. Baker actually wanted some of Ryan's blood. He wanted to assess Ryan's immune system for its reactions to various foods. I was so happy to finally meet a doctor who wanted to do scientific testing.

In the meantime, our *cure* was an antifungal medication and an even more restrictive diet for Ryan. Dairy was still off-limits, and now we also needed to reduce his sugar intake. Ryan could no longer eat unlimited fruit or have any fruit juice at all. Both contained too much sugar, and sugar encouraged the growth of intestinal yeast. The theory was intestinal yeast contributed to the autism symptoms.

If Dr. Rimland had odd theories about cows, his friend Dr. Baker had even odder theories about sugar and yeast. I wondered why our regular pediatricians

---

14   The MAPS website is www.medmaps.org. Doctors who have completed training courses and treat autism medically are listed there. *Caution:* Not all doctors are created equal. Some of them, even the certified ones, do treatments that may impact our children's immune condition in a negative way.

didn't recommend these dietary changes for children with autism. When I asked Dr. Hobbs about special diets for children with autism, he confessed that he really didn't know much about nutrition. He said in medical school all he got was about a half hour of training in proper nourishment and diet. I didn't know much about nutrition either, but even I had more training than that. Not knowing much about yeast before, I soon became a very reluctant student of *Candida albicans*—yeast.

In a nutshell, Dr. Rimland's theory is that dairy and other individual food intolerances cause *leaky gut syndrome* (Leaky gut, or intestinal permeability, is a condition in which the lining of the small intestine becomes damaged, causing undigested food particles, toxic waste products, and bacteria to "leak" through the intestines and flood the bloodstream). According to him, this is the engine driving the autism train. Dr. Baker's DAN! theory points out *Candida*, or yeast, grows because of the overuse of antibiotics due to the leaky gut. The antibiotics unintentionally kill the good bacteria in the gut along with the infection it was prescribed to eliminate. Sugar acts as high-octane fuel for this engine. Ryan had been on antibiotics for most of his life to treat chronic ear infections. He also gravitated toward sugar like a moth to a flame.

Maybe, just maybe, Dr. Baker was worth listening to—maybe.[15]

Dr. Baker prescribed an antifungal medicine called Nystatin, which was supposed to reduce the amount of yeast in Ryan's gut, and a broad-spectrum probiotic to restock his gut with the bacteria that are desirable. Dr. Baker went on to explain that all of us have some yeast, and when our immune system is healthy, the yeast is kept in check. When the immune system is not working right, or a child is given a high-sugar diet of foods like fruit and ice cream, an overgrowth of yeast can result. As a result of his frequent ear infections and the repeated, chronic use of antibiotics to treat them, kids like Ryan were way overstocked in the yeast department.

My life became all about yeast control.

---

15   Conniff, Richard. "The Body Eclectic." *Smithsonian*, Volume 44, No. 2, January 2013 pp. 40-47.

But, instead of getting better, Ryan got worse. I couldn't understand why he became such a mess. A little more than a week after he started Nystatin, Ryan acted more autistic than ever before. I immediately called Dr. Baker. He apologized and told me he forgot to tell me this regression might happen. He described what was happening as really *great news*. Ryan was going through "*die-off.*" The Nystatin was killing the excessive yeast in Ryan's body, and as the yeast died-off, it dumped toxins into his system. It was going to take a week or two for die-off to be over, and then he would get much better. After I hung up the telephone, I questioned what kinds of drugs this doctor was on in addition to the drugs he had Ryan on. This all seemed as crazy as Ryan's current behavior.

I had been so encouraged after our first consultation with Dr. Baker, but now Ryan was swimming backwards toward Autism Island at breakneck speed. Dr. Baker's explanation might have been *great news* if I hadn't had to deal with my son's deranged behavior. In addition to making noises, hand-flapping, and grinding his teeth, he seemed almost drunk: acting silly and laughing inappropriately at the wrong times. He was all high energy at one moment and had no energy the next. I began to have serious doubts whether we were doing the right thing.

During the die-off period, we just hung out and didn't try to learn anything at home or at school. There wasn't much point in trying to teach him anything. I took Ryan out of school and out of his therapy sessions. He looked sick, and I assumed he felt sick. I was sick with worry.

Ryan's die-off lasted almost ten days, and I wasn't sure either of us was going to live through it. After the die-off was over, we saw a more focused and alert kid. My son was actually getting closer to the ballpark where the normal kids played, but he still was not ready to join in the game.

Another A-Club Mom's Experience with Die-off

My son always had the worst fungal kill off. It always started immediately and lasted three-four weeks, far longer than our doctor anticipated. There were times when I wanted to pack it in. It was hard to believe that a medication that is not in any way related to an anti-psychotic/psychotic pharmaceutical could actually cause my kid to act so bizarre and out of control. My son would roll around on the floor kicking and screaming. He'd crash into lockers at school, spit, get very silly, stim more[16] and appear almost like he was drunk.

All this *craziness* from a usually very polite, well-mannered, sweet boy was hard to deal with. It was very, very frightening to watch. We felt so helpless and frustrated as he appeared to be regressing after so much progress from the antiviral. It was a total nightmare and certainly the most difficult part of the protocol for us. Our doctor advised us to "stick it out and hold on" because it would be brighter on the other side.

Just when I thought we couldn't take it anymore, he gradually got back to being himself, only better, clearer, brighter, and happier. And all those horrifying behaviors became a distant memory!

I learned to be more compassionate during die-off. I catered to my son who was sick and felt really awful. I kept him out of school until the worst was over and made no demands on him. I had to quickly get over my own fears that the regression might be permanent. I started him on a probiotic during this time and flushed his system with water, water, and more water. Also I tried to get him to do some serious exercise like running, swimming, playing ball, or anything else that accelerated his metabolic process.

I know it's hard right now but be extra patient and loving with them. Have faith that it will be okay and trust these doctors who have been through this before. In the time frame of recovery, die-off doesn't last long. It is actually a good sign to have a severe reaction. That indicates that the bad things in your child's body are being stirred up and cleared out. This awful time definitely helped my child have a happier and healthier future! Hang in there. It will be over soon.

---

16   Self-stimulatory behaviors, also known as "stims," in children with autism are behaviors that can include rocking, pacing, aligning or spinning objects and hand-flapping. They are characterized by rigid repetitive movements or vocal sounds and noises.

The *anti-Candida* diet and DAN! protocol was challenging. In addition to the no-dairy and low-sugar we were already doing, we had to eliminate every food to which Ryan's food intolerance tests showed a reaction. There wasn't much left to eat. Certainly, not much that was any fun.

Dr. Baker's regimen for dietary supplements was equally difficult. It is easy to prescribe supplements, but not easy to get a child too young to swallow pills to take them. There was a mile-long list of supplements supposed to help cure his leaky gut and reestablish the proper intestinal flora. There was also a mile-long list of strategies I used to get Ryan to swallow these crushed-up pills. I remember I put Ryan in the bathtub and broke open the fish oil pills to rub into his skin. Ryan smelled like a sardine with autism.

Although this doctor helped Ryan, we were in Minnesota; he was in New Jersey and often unreachable when there was a problem. Appointments were done by telephone, and even if Dr. Baker had taken insurance, telephone appointments were not a covered expense.

When I wasn't giving Ryan supplements, I was cooking food no one wanted to eat. We could never go out to eat because I had to make everything from scratch, adjusting recipes to eliminate every ingredient Ryan couldn't have.

In time, Ryan didn't want to follow the protocol Dr. Baker prescribed. He lost his appetite and did not gain any weight for over a year. I started giving him French fries with every meal to fatten him up, but even that didn't work. Although Ryan's behavior was better, we couldn't go on living on a diet that was so difficult and tasted like low-sugar cardboard.

Dr. Baker was sympathetic and suggested we should relax the diet to try to restore my son's appetite. I didn't know what to do. If I kept him on the diet, I was hurting him because he wasn't thriving or gaining weight. If I took him off the diet, the foods he ate made him act more autistic. This treatment plan wasn't working anymore, and in time we stopped seeing Dr. Baker in spite of how much he initially helped us find some of the answers.

Doctors Rimland and Baker were pioneers and humanitarians. Pioneers have to take risks, take detours, and even find their own paths. Their maverick approach and professional bravery took us in a direction that was wonderful and rewarding but not sustainable *for us*. If I was going to let these doctors cure my son, my son needed to want to participate in their protocol. Ryan, however, was saying "NO" to the diet and supplement road they built.

I went back to my midnight reading looking for new, more accessible answers to help my son. I was trying to be Ryan's "*supermom*." But I kept running into *kryptonite*.

If I Knew Then What I Know Now

To honor Dr. Rimland's memory, over the years I have tried to pay it forward and do for others what he did for us. That is one of the reasons I wrote this book. Dr. Rimland devoted every waking hour to changing how the world viewed his son, Mark, and all our kids. He was a wonderful inspiration to so many and is sincerely missed.

Dr. Rimland and Dr. Baker promoted the then-radical idea that there is a brain-gut connection in humans, and the functioning status of this connection is essential to explaining and treating autism. They knew that immunology and autism are connected somehow. However, in my opinion, these autism experts didn't extend their paradigm far enough. That was where we needed to go to help Ryan. We would have to visit the very edges of unconventional medicine.

The more I learned about biomedical interventions, the more I began to believe a broken immune system was the culprit responsible for everything my kid suffered from. Bernie Rimland was convinced a *leaky gut* was the cause of autism. He thought bacteria, toxins, incompletely digested food, and waste not properly eliminated may leak from the intestines into the bloodstream. According to Dr. Rimland, the result can be autism and brain dysfunction. I have come to believe that these issues are just the secondary symptoms of neuroimmune dysregulation, rather than the main cause.

CHAPTER 14

EVERYBODY HAD A THEORY BUT NOBODY AGREED ON ANYTHING

Life can be like a roller coaster . . . And just when you think you've had enough and you're ready to get off the ride and take the calm, easy merry-go-round . . . You change your mind, throw your hands in the air and ride the roller coaster all over again.

—Stacey Charte

ALL THE MONEY and therapy thrown at Ryan's autism didn't bring any real answers for him. Improvements were a long way from solutions, and what he gained was not enough to sustain us or offer a guarantee that Ryan would escape a future in some sort of institution. After all our searching, not much was really resolved concerning Ryan's autism. It was *still* there.

After Dr. Baker, Ryan was a little better, but that only made me want more. We just needed the right treatment. We still didn't know what that was, but we now believed that it existed somewhere, someplace, and if we looked hard enough, we would find it. Afraid of what the future held for Ryan, I continued the search for the cure while I lived with perpetual anxiety.

We were all alone on Autism Island, surrounded by experts who each had a piece of the lifeboat we needed for escape. But some pieces were still missing and no one had the complete plan on how to build the boat. What I needed was a new expert with a new cure. Someone who had the complete blueprint to build what we needed to get off the island.

Megan's words returned to my mind: "Mom, he's not going to learn anything if you *yell* at him. You have to *show* him the right way to do things." Ryan's behavior was still out of control although to a lesser degree. Maybe a behavioral plan was the place to start while we searched for that elusive cure.

Ironically, Frank and I had both been behavior therapists as undergraduates at the University of California at Los Angeles (UCLA) before we were married. We worked under Dr. Ivar Lovaas, the father of applied behavior analysis (ABA) for children with autism.

I'm not even sure of my motivation the day I called Dr. Lovaas to talk about Ryan and our horrible situation. He was very kind, but even this renowned *expert* and father of ABA therapy didn't understand the emerging biomedical interventions concerning autism. I told him Ryan was on a casein-free, low-sugar diet. I asked him for his thoughts on what we were doing. Dr. Lovaas told me he didn't believe diet changed anything for kids with autism.

According to Ivar, ABA was the *only* proven and effective treatment for autism. He had tried some dietary interventions such as eliminating sugar from the children's diets, but he no longer did that because it didn't make kids normal. My mind returned to Jackie Rains's rant concerning ABA. She was so opposed to Dr. Lovaas's *proven and effective* treatment for autism that she told us she would no longer work with us if we employed these techniques with Ryan. Dr. Lovaas was similarly negative concerning dietary interventions.

I put the telephone down feeling totally defeated. Every professional had a little piece of the puzzle, but they seemed to only understand their piece. We still didn't have anyone who knew how to build the entire lifeboat we needed to escape. Most of these "experts" felt *their* ideas were the *only* ones that worked. And they certainly weren't listening to anyone else's ideas. No one even considered combining some of the pieces together that worked a little. Although everyone had a theory, nobody played well with others. There was no consensus on how to help my son or even if autism could be successfully treated at all.

Conventional doctors offered nothing but a diagnosis and a destination to nowhere. Psychologists offered endless rating scales, held your hand, and dispensed Kleenex. Occupational therapy was grossly insufficient to address Ryan's multiple needs. And the unconventional doctors had treatment protocols so difficult to follow, they couldn't be maintained.

To a non-scientist like me, who only passed college chemistry by copying Frank's homework, the newly emerging biomedical studies seemed as confusing as autism itself. I had no idea what research path to follow or how to bridge the gap between research, treatment, and applying the treatment within the realities and restrictions of our daily life with Ryan. At the same time, I had to sift through research papers like a detective searching for a clue, any clue, to help Ryan. Isn't that what the doctors are supposed to do? And have I mentioned that this was all pre-Internet?

I considered stopping the late-night searches for answers. I was almost ready to invest in intense therapy for me and buy stock in Kleenex to help me accept that Ryan could be a *nice little autistic boy* in a group home when my copy of *The Advocate* arrived. That was the newsletter from the Autism Society of America. In it was a letter to the editor from another mom. According to Bryce Miler, Dr. Michael Harvey helped her son with autism talk for the first time. I tracked Bryce down, and I kept calling until I finally reached her.

THE ADVOCATE *Newsletter of the Autism Society of America, Sept.—Oct. 1994*

Bryce's Letter to the Editor

My husband and I are the parents of a three-year-old son who was diagnosed as "autistic" six months ago. We were told to see a well-known authority, "the specialist of specialists" in this field. We saw her prepared for the diagnosis of "autism" but not prepared for the information she would give us. She stated that there was absolutely positively no cure for "autism" and that it is useless to try and find one. When asked if it was possible for our son to live a "normal" or even "semi-normal" life she said that he would never be anything but "autistic" and that "autistic" people cannot ever have what you and I would consider a normal life.

When we asked about using the Lovaas treatment for children with autism, she emphatically insisted that these children are now physiological disaster areas and that our son would be much worse if put through that kind of therapy. Her treatment plan for my son was to put him in a "normal" preschool with "normal" children. In her opinion, that was the best therapy for these children and all the other therapies available will not show the results that inclusion in a normal preschool would.

I have worked with many other doctors and therapists in the last six months and none of them has been so blatantly insistent on her views being "the only game in town."

We joined a parents' group and heard from parents who adamantly explained the dramatic results their children have experienced from ABA therapy with absolutely no negative effects. Then and there we decided to go with the therapy based on the Lovaas program. We now thank God every day for this therapy as my son may never be cured but has begun to do so many new things that we are sure he would not be doing without it.

During that same meeting we were also given the name of a pediatrician who was treating "autistic" children for food allergies and other medical problems which has allowed the children to work and think better. We thought my son might have allergies, so we saw Dr. Michael Harvey who determined that my son was highly allergic to milk and would later discover that he had a newly identified retrovirus which could be causing the immune dysfunction that was apparent on other tests.

This virus had been found in other "autistic" children and could be having negative effects on his brain. We were given a medicine to treat the virus and within eight days my son spoke his first words. Dr. Harvey's ideas regarding the immune system and its role here are very encouraging, although he is very careful to clarify that all he is trying to do is help maximize the potential for these kids and that by alleviating some of the medically treatable problems, these kids will be able to work and think better. My son has changed so dramatically in a two-month period with Dr. Harvey and the behavioral therapy that we have felt joy now comparable to nothing else we can describe. We are not saying that he will be cured but such dramatic progress is very encouraging to us.

We encourage parents to keep an open mind and not to listen to professionals who insist that we would be much better off just accepting the "autism" for what it is and not looking for a breakthrough that might allow our children to have much better lives. I think most parents feel as we do that it is not the problem of accepting our children as "autistic," it is the fact that we do not want to lay down and accept this life for our children. We would love and cherish our child if he had no arms, no legs, and was "autistic" on top of it, but we do have to desperately work to try and give our child what we have—a nondisabled life or something close to it. Wouldn't we all want someone fighting for us if we couldn't fight for ourselves?

—Bryce Miler
Simi Valley, CA

Bryce was calm and convincing. She quietly countered my skepticism and distrust with the facts about her son's continuing and astonishing improvement. She talked about her hope that he might someday be cured, the same hope I once had. But her hope was alive and infectious. Mine was tattered and in desperate need of something fast. Since we were going to California to be with our families for Thanksgiving anyway, what harm would it do to make an appointment to see Bryce's miracle worker? After that phone call, we were back on the roller-coaster ride and holding on for dear life.

That call to Dr. Harvey's office changed Ryan's life forever.

If I Knew Then What I Know Now

Being a parent of a child with autism is like an extreme sports balancing act. You're almost like the guy on the *Ed Sullivan Show* trying to keep all of those delicate porcelain plates spinning on sticks at the same time. The challenge is we have to realize some plates are more important than others. I probably spent too much time keeping the Dr. Baker plate going, when it might have been smarter to work on spinning the ABA plate.

Even as you focus your entire existence on spinning these plates, you have to be open to new opportunities. When I read the article in *The Advocate*, I could have easily blown it off. But something in it clicked for me. I decided it made sense to try, and I went for it.

CHAPTER 15

FINALLY A DOCTOR WITH A PLAN

Even if you are on the right track, you'll get run over if you just sit there.

—Will Rogers

OUR ANNUAL THANKSGIVING trip to see family in California was already planned. Otherwise, I'm not sure we would have made the appointment to see Dr. Harvey. By this time, I had *almost* given up on the medical profession. I feared another dead-end consultation. Bryce's miracle might be only for Bryce.

I didn't give the office much lead time when I called. Fortunately, there had been a cancellation Thanksgiving week that worked for us. This was just one of the many coincidences that became life-changing events and made it possible for Ryan to get better.

Luck and timing were very much a part of our son's recovery.

Dr. Harvey started his medical career as just another conventional doctor. He started his practice as your garden-variety pediatrician as opposed to specializing in children with autism, attention-deficit/hyperactivity disorder (ADHD), or attention-deficit disorder (ADD).[17] He was best described as a pediatrician with a specialized practice and not as an autism specialist.

---

17   For an understanding of ADD, see Rabiner, David. "Sensible And Perplexing Changes in ADHD Diagnostic Criteria, www.sharpbrains.com, June 25, 2013. Note that DSM-V now places ADD under the heading of neurodevelopmental disorders.

His pediatric focus on autism and ADHD occurred because of an accidental discovery on his part. Ellie, his wife, was extremely ill with chronic fatigue syndrome (CFS).[18] As he was trying to heal her, he noticed the similarities between his wife's labs, symptoms, and issues and those of his patients. Ellie's condition helped him to connect the dots and form a then-radical hypothesis that a dysregulated immune system was the common culprit for the medical issues associated with children with autism.

That moment of insight and making the *immune connection* changed Ryan's life forever.

Dr. Harvey came to believe that *autism* was simply the label for the collection of behaviors that resulted from a dysfunctional immune system. Accordingly, autism is treatable.

Dr. Harvey believes if a child's immune system is not too compromised and can be repaired, that's when recovery becomes possible. In his attempt to help his wife and patients, Dr. Harvey studied autism, ADHD, ADD, CFS, and Tourette's syndrome. Over time, Dr. Harvey developed what was (and still is according to many conventional doctors) a radical treatment protocol for these diseases. And it continues to evolve. The common factor is that these diagnoses are all variations of an immune system that is not working properly.

His dedication to helping our children is accompanied by an equally passionate determination to change how children with autism are viewed. He insists our kids *are* ill and is adamant they *are not* irreparably damaged goods. Dr. Harvey doesn't even want anyone to use or say the A-word when describing our children.

This banishment of the A-word sometimes creates confusion when he refers to our children and uses his own term, Neuro Immune Dysfunction Syndrome (or NIDS), while the rest of the world still calls it "autism." Dr. Harvey insists that you can call it *anything* you want, but *don't* call it "autism." I use whichever term helps get across the pivotal idea that our kids can recover and lead productive lives.

18   See cdc.gov/cfs/ for a general overview of information.

What's in a name? . . . EVERYTHING!

NIDS is a whole new way of thinking about autism. And with that new thinking comes new possibilities when you combine medical treatment with effective, focused, behavioral and educational rehabilitation. Think NIDS, and there is the possibility of full recovery. Think *autism*, and you're left with nothing. I haven't met anyone who has recovered from autism, but I have met children who have recovered from this neuroimmune condition Dr. H calls NIDS.

We began with Dr. Harvey close to the time he began to focus his practice on children with autism, ADHD, and ADD. When we first went to see him in 1993, he was ahead of his time. To this day, doctors and parents either adore him or hate him. There is no middle ground with Dr. H. He is direct and tells it like he sees it. I like that about him. I don't have much time for experts who cling only to their piece of the lifeboat and don't have enough backbone to question conventional wisdom. Although I will always be indebted to Dr. Harvey for saving my son, his passion for helping our children is both his gift and his curse. As much as Dr. H is dedicated to our children, his strident personality *sometimes* gets in the way of helping. You need to have your own backbone stiffly in place when you visit his office.

Dr. Harvey told us on that first visit what I already knew to be true.[19] Ryan didn't really have autism even though it sure looked like it. Ryan's new doctor felt that classic autism was extremely rare and what most kids suffer from is immune dysfunction. I didn't really understand what NIDS meant back then. I didn't care. What mother wouldn't be thrilled to hear their child didn't really have autism and that we should just stop calling it that? I didn't have that curable whatever-I-had-been-praying-for, but I had something else.

I had HOPE!

My kid is sick, and there *is* hope that he can get better. Finally, I found

---

19   The protocol we used to help Ryan regain his health is medically complex and requires a physician to administer and monitor treatment. While the following chapters describe Ryan's journey and experiences with this protocol, the text should not be interpreted as medical advice.

someone who not only wanted to help Ryan but also had a way to do it. And he didn't think I was crazy—at least not yet.

Although Dr. H was very intense, I liked him, and I admired him for fighting the world to save my child and others like him. Before, it was Frank, Megan, and Marcia against the world for Ryan. Now we were no longer alone.

I could tell by the questions he asked that he had read every word of the volumes of Ryan's medical history I sent before our visit. He didn't brush us off with comments like "I'm sorry, there is *nothing* I can do." Instead, he spent three hours explaining what he thought autism really was and how we should go about helping Ryan's immune system heal.

He went on to say, "You can't tell me that a child who develops normally up to a year or two suddenly regresses without a medical condition prevailing." I didn't interrupt to tell him I thought Ryan had autism from the time he was born. I wasn't going to stop the momentum of this man who might be able to help us, so I just nodded my head in agreement.

Dr. H went on to explain that the number of autism cases had increased dramatically. He said it was scientifically impossible for autism to increase in these epidemic numbers if it had been caused solely by genetics or a brain damaged condition. That is epidemiologically impossible. He was convinced autism is a medical issue, and the increase in affected children can only be explained by *a disease process*.

Over the years, we've had many hours together when we both ranted about the failings of the medical community, but Dr. H outdid me with what he had to say that day. He began one of his many impassioned speeches (I've now heard them a billion times) about how the medical profession is ignoring what is wrong with our children. These mini-lectures all start differently but share the same underlying message that our children *are ill* and desperately need help. After we signed up for his services, we heard similar speeches over and over again at every appointment. It's part of Dr. H's treatment protocol.

It took me several months to decipher and truly understand what he was saying. This man is smart and often spoke in *Doctor Speak* that was way above my level. The term NIDS that he coined to describe Ryan's broken immune system and complex medical condition was not easy to understand. Of course, it was complicated. He's a doctor, so the term he came up with had to be long, complicated, and just as hard to understand. Many times, I stopped him in mid-sentence to ask him to use simple, nonmedical terms I could comprehend.

In *Mom Speak*, my slant and interpretation of what he believed about NIDS is that kids with an autism label are not damaged permanently. He said Ryan had a dysregulated immune system. Sometimes, Ryan's immune system didn't respond *enough* or didn't respond *at all*. Other times, that same dysregulated immune system worked overtime, fighting off infections that were no longer a threat. This is why some children with the autism label get ill easily, yet others never appear sick at all. Dr. Harvey gave me hope. If Dr. H could help Ryan's broken immune system repair itself, my son could recover and lead a normal, productive life.

Immune Dysfunction Explained in Terms We Can All Understand
by Kathy Robertson (RN, MSN) [20]

What is common to individuals with autism forms of Attention Deficit Hyperactivity Disorder (ADHD) and Chronic Fatigue Syndrome (CFS) is a dysfunctional immune system. This can be triggered by a plethora of

---

20   Kathy Robertson (RN, MSN) is the former director of the Northern New York Autism Clinic. She has a daughter with autism and works with the Northern New York Autism Foundation. Kathy is published in the *American Journal of Nursing, Maternal Child Nursing, Ladycom,* and the *7th MEDCOM Medical Bulletin.* She facilitates workshops on the Bio-Medical treatment of Autism to Health Care Professionals and parents in the US and Canada. She was contributing editor for the *Journal of Nursing Jocularity* and wrote a weekly Health Care Advice Column in the *US Army Newspaper.*

things: viruses, retroviruses, yeast, bacteria, allergens, chemicals, trauma (both physical and emotional), etc.

Once some of these pathogens invade the body, they replicate (set up housekeeping in the cells) and continue to trigger the immune system. Sometimes the body gets them under control and things will seem to stabilize for a while. However, when another trigger comes along (seasonal allergies are a common one), the problem starts all over again.

Once the immune system is triggered, it sets off a chain of events that causes an abnormal biochemistry that can result in the symptoms that we have labeled autism, ADHD, and CFS. I am going to quote a great sage from the south, Dr. Bruce Russell. This renowned autism expert said, "Complicated problems have complicated answers."

We certainly see a subset of young children who can be treated for one thing, for example HHV6, and they do brilliantly for the most part. However usually with most children, more than one thing needs to be addressed as the child ages and the symptoms multiply.

Dr. Doris Rapp explained it like this, "The immune system is like a pot of boiling water on the stove. Raise the heat and the pot will boil over." If the multiple triggers that cause autism, ADHD, and Chronic Fatigue in an individual can be addressed, the child can greatly improve and even recover completely.

The only way that you are going to know what is going on with your child is have him evaluated by someone who understands how the immune system works and knows how to treat autism medically.

If I Knew Then What I Know Now

There are a growing number of doctors, scientists, and researchers who now know autism and other related problems are medical rather than psychiatric or developmental. More and more doctors are starting to treat autism medically.

Ryan's recovery proves autism is a changeable medical condition. Although my son is now a very typical young adult, getting there took more than a decade filled with mistakes, guilt, wrong turns, and frustration as we tried to make sense of it all. Ryan only began to make significant progress when we abandoned the idea that autism was a developmental disorder and embraced the idea of medically treating his dysfunctional immune system. It was the NIDS approach combined with intensive rehabilitation that helped my son recover from autism.

Other parents are often the best source of finding a doctor who specializes in treating autism medically. Although most doctors do not call their treatment protocols NIDS, those who treat autism effectively use similar medical protocols. The number of physicians who understand the immune connection has increased. But the doctors who effectively treat the underlying medical issues that cause our children's dysfunctional immune systems are still hard to find.

The PANS/PANDAS Physicians Directory is just one source for finding a doctor. The Medical Academy of Pediatric Special Needs (MAPS) website is another good starting place to find a doctor skilled in treating autism. The physicians certified as MAPS doctors take courses and receive special training.

But these websites are only a starting point. You will know when you have found the right physician by results. If your child doesn't substantially improve after six months, then it may be time to start the search again.

The downside of the MAPS doctors is that many use a lot of supplements which are expensive and difficult to sustain when you have young children who don't yet know how to swallow pills. In addition, sometimes they don't use the more effective prescription medications long enough. They mistakenly believe that a short course of these medications is all that is needed.

Some children are able to stop these prescriptions when their immune systems start working again. But as of yet, my son isn't one of them. Ryan has been on an antifungal prescription since he was about five and an antiviral since he was ten. He still takes them as an adult, but the good news is he has never had an irregular blood test. These medications have never affected his liver or kidney function.

I used to be one of those parents who never wanted to use prescription drugs. But I changed my mind. Now I think we should use whatever works. MDs or DOs who use both supplements and prescriptions are the best kind of doctor.

And sometimes your local immunologists and functional medicine doctors are quite adept at treating autism. The doctor who helped my son most was not an autism specialist or listed on any website.

Some of our children need strong medications rather than supplements. I am thrilled for those who have recovered their kids with only the use of supplements. But that didn't work for us, maybe because I couldn't get my son to take them all. There were just too many.

And it is very important to remember, all doctors who treat autism *are not* created equal. You must always proceed *with caution*. Some protocols may not address the subset of autism your child has. And some physicians, even the autism specialists, may do treatments that impact our children's immune systems negatively.

For Ryan, antiviral and antifungal medication had a huge impact. When I first looked up the side effects, I was terrified. I soon realized that if my son is going to have a chance at a typical life, I needed to do something, anything, and had to take a risk.

When you are frustrated with your pediatrician for not treating autism medically, take a breath and remember that treating autism medically is still in its infancy. Doing anything medically that is still unproven and not conventional opens visionary doctors to all kinds of potential risks. Often these doctors, whom we so desperately need to help our children, fly below the radar and don't advertise what they do. This often makes them difficult to locate.

Recovery began by rebuilding his immune system and helping him regain his health. But just doing the NIDS protocol without any intensive rehabilitation wouldn't have been enough. Years of behavioral and educational interventions were necessary to correct Ryan's deficits in speech and social skills. We had to catch him up on all he missed before he was able to learn like other children.

CHAPTER 16

TESTING, TESTING, 1-2-3 AND MORE TESTING

I hate tests. It's a really lousy way to judge a person's ability.

—Bill Paxton

DR. HARVEY IMMEDIATELY set about assessing the status of Ryan's immune system. If his theory was correct, then Ryan's immune system should not resemble that of a healthy person. It should be a mess, and the name of that mess was still called *autism* by the rest of the world.

The first step was to run extensive blood tests to determine what was and wasn't working in Ryan's system. As many parents know, blood tests equal needles, and needles equal meltdowns. I came equipped with bribes. We had a new toy car for when the procedure was over, and I promised McDonalds if Ryan sat still for the blood draw we had renamed the "skin prick." Dr. Harvey's staff was quite proficient at doing this after dealing with so many difficult children.

They efficiently took eight vials of blood, leaving my son vampire pale. That was only part one of Dr. H's protocol that assessed Ryan's current level of functioning. Step two was much more daunting. While other families ate leftover turkey, we headed to Harbor-UCLA Medical Center for a neuroSPECT scan.[21]

---

21   SPECT scans are similar to positron emission tomography (PET) scans. SPECT scans have some advantages in autism patients who may also have, or are suspected of having, epilepsy. SPECT scans have lower resolution than functional magnetic resonance imaging (fMRI) scans.

We didn't even know what a neuroSPECT scan was, but it sounded like it could help Ryan, so we were on board.

Not only did we have to battle traffic on the crazy Los Angeles freeways, but the test procedure was awful. So was the cost. At that time, SPECT scans were relatively new and not standard medical practice. Insurance never covers the cost of anything new. But I learned insurance companies are kind of like our kids: you have to outlast them if you want to win. And you must fight paper with paper. We were thrilled when any part of Ryan's medical expenses was covered by insurance. The only reason the tests Dr. H did were partially covered was because his office billed them under the immune diagnosis code—not autism. Things billed with the autism code were never covered by insurance at that time.

Even though we had already accepted that fighting Ryan's autism was financially draining, and a seemingly endless, war, it changed our way of looking at things. Who in their right mind would be ecstatic about finding good deals and spending less money on medical intervention? We were.

Worse than our concern over cost was the effort it took to get a noncompliant five-year-old with autism to stay completely still for the first twenty minutes of the test. Carmen, the technician, put Ryan's head in a big, scary tube that made noise and looked like something from *Star Trek*. Once again, when I could no longer cope, Frank took over. If he couldn't get Ryan to stop moving, we would have to sedate him (and me) in order to complete the test.

It took us the better part of the day to finish the neuroSPECT. Frank accomplished the near impossible feat of keeping Ryan totally, completely, utterly still while the test was being administered. He read Ryan his favorite books, told him stories, and did whatever it took. This was one entertaining dad, and Ryan's stressed-out mom couldn't do much more than sit there dazed and shell-shocked. This was not the Thanksgiving vacation I had planned. Frank promised Ryan a piece of pie from Marie Calendar's after the test was over if he remained still. We were all emotionally exhausted by the time we collected that sugar fix.

That test was torture and I wondered how my new hero, Dr. Harvey could put us through this agony. But we were somehow strangely comforted by the possibility that soon we would be looking at objective medical test results to show if my kid really did have autism. There would no longer be any question about Ryan's diagnosis.

Ryan's neuroSPECT scan measured blood flow to different areas of his brain. The test results, as interpreted by radiologist Dr. Ismael Mena of Harbor-UCLA Diagnostic Imaging Center, revealed decreased blood flow to the parietal and temporal areas of Ryan's brain. His report read, "In conclusion, findings suggest: Autism???" Without having met my child or having any knowledge of his medical history, Dr. Mena, who specialized in reading these scans, could see Ryan's autism. If autism was a developmental or psychiatric condition, how could he see it?

I didn't understand fully what the report meant until Dr. Harvey explained it. He said that Ryan suffered from autoimmune encephalitis. That meant the areas of Ryan's brain responsible for cognition, speech, and social skills were not getting enough blood flow. Inflammation in my son's brain compromised the blood flow. If the brain is swollen and inflamed, the blood can't get through. The parietal lobe, an area responsible for sensory processing and some language functions, was affected. The blood flow to the temporal lobes was inadequate as well. That is the part of the brain responsible for organizing sensory information as well as higher speech and language functions. Good blood flow equals good thinking.

Suddenly, the light went on for me.

For the first time, I felt a sense of clarity about my son's behavior. Ryan's difficulty with speech and language had an explanation. The reason Ryan was so behind in speech and the reason he acted just plain weird was because parts of his brain weren't getting the blood they needed. Ryan's sensory issues with clothes now also made sense.

CHAPTER 17

DR. HARVEY, AKA THE COOKIE MONSTER

There are no shortcuts to any place worth going.

—Beverly Sills

DR. HARVEY GAVE us hope again. We still had a war ahead of us, but at least now we had what was starting to look like a battle plan. Our family returned to Minnesota armed with regimens of blood tests and telephone appointments every six weeks. During those appointments, we talked about what worked and what we needed to try next.

The real problem was my son's immune system wasn't working correctly. It was sometimes underactive and sometimes overactive. Our first goal was to cool down Ryan's immune system. We needed to remove anything that created stress and caused his immune system to react. Ryan's allergy test looked like he was allergic to everything, but he really wasn't. The reason he reacted to such a large number of foods was because his broken immune system left him trying to maintain his balance while standing on only one foot. It was easy to push Ryan over when he didn't have two feet firmly planted on the ground.

Dr. Harvey prescribed a diet that consisted mainly of *no* dairy, *no* whole wheat, *no* chocolate, and *no* infractions. We used an allergy/food intolerance blood test to guide us on what Ryan could eat. Anything that was in the highly reactive column of the allergy test needed to be eliminated from his diet.[22] Sometimes I was almost afraid to feed him. It was difficult to know what was okay for him to eat since he reacted to so many foods. We changed Ryan's diet and once again eliminated all dairy. We had relaxed this after he failed to gain weight back when we were still with Dr. Baker.

Clinical evidence is important. Dr. Harvey showed me in black and white why getting rid of dairy was necessary. These appeared in the "significant" category on his allergy tests. Ryan had to stay away from anything to do with cow's milk or cheese, casein, and lactalbumin.

Most moms want real-life evidence. I got that, too, and at the worst times. My son melted down whenever he accidently ate something that contained even the smallest amount of dairy. Any infraction in the diet caused behavior problems and worsened his autism symptoms. Sometimes, his ears turned red, his strange noises increased, and he was much, much harder to deal with. If I unknowingly gave him something that contained dairy, a more thorough reading of the food label confirmed what I already knew from observing the change in Ryan's behavior.

For Ryan, gluten was not an issue. Dr. Harvey told me to buy the cheapest dairy/casein-free white bread I could find. According to Dr. H, the more processed the bread, the easier it would be for Ryan to digest. This seemed confusing because it went against everything I knew about eating right. Suddenly, almost all the rules about nutrition *didn't* apply anymore—at least not to my kid. Whole grains were out. Wasn't that what we all need more of? The foods from the health food stores were no longer okay for Ryan. My son had the highest possible score for garlic on these tests. We removed garlic from his diet and our house. Egg whites were also not his friend according to these allergy blood tests.

Dr. Harvey was not the only doctor who understood the immune connection with allergies and behavior. Dr. Doris Rapp was one of the first pioneers to

---

22   These allergy tests are not as reliable as most doctors would like. Dr. Harvey only used them as a starting point.

explain how things worked in her books years earlier.[23] Dr. Rapp said too much stress on the immune system from food allergies (internal triggers) and environmental concerns (external triggers) changed behavior in children. Children's behavior can improve dramatically when you remove these triggers.

On *The Phil Donahue Show*[24] in the same year Ryan was born, Dr. Rapp demonstrated how a compromised immune system caused behavior issues that looked like psychiatric issues (e.g., autism, hyperactivity, depression, aggression, learning problems, etc.). She had video that showed how children's behaviors disintegrate when you give them something they are allergic to. Phil Donahue got 140,000 letters from desperate parents as a result of the program. That show changed lives. But thirty years later, the medical community still hasn't caught up with the forward thinking of medical pioneers like Dr. Rapp.

I watched that show with Dr. Rapp when it first aired in 1988. By the time I realized my son had autism, I had long forgotten the important things Dr. Rapp said four years earlier. If I had remembered them, I could have helped Ryan sooner. Recently, I watched that same *Phil Donohue Show* on YouTube again. What Dr. Rapp said way back then still holds true today. After I watched it again, I wanted to kick myself. But we can't look back or feel guilty about our mistakes. We need to make the best decisions with the information we have at the time and always move the train forward.

Dr. Martha Herbert and Karen Weintraub explain our dilemma and provide real solutions in their book, *The Autism Revolution*.[25] In it, Harvard clinician

---

23   Dr. Doris Rapp, *Is This Your Child's World?* New York: Bantam, 1996; *Is This Your Child?* New York: William Morrow and Co, 1986; *The Impossible Child in School—at Home* Aylesbury: Allergy Research Foundation, 1989; *Allergies and the Hyperactive Child* New York: Simon and Schuster, 1979.

24   Dr. Rapp's 1988 appearance on the *Phil Donahue Show* can be seen on YouTube. Search *Phil Donohue: Misdiagnosed Allergies*. Dr. Doris Rapp is another visionary. She has dedicated her life to providing the science, research, and information as well as solutions for children affected by both the typical and atypical forms of allergies.

25   Herbert, Martha & Weintraub, Karen. *The Autism Revolution: Whole-Body Strategies For Making Life All It Can Be.* New York: Ballantine Books, 2012.

and researcher Dr. Herbert said, "Autism is not a hardwired impairment pro-grammed into a child's genes and destined to remain fixed forever, as we're often told. Instead, it is the result of a cascade of events, many seemingly minor: perhaps a genetic mutation, some toxic exposures, a stressful birth, a vitamin deficiency, and a series of infections." Accordingly, it is the total load of chal-lenges on a child that causes the behaviors associated with autism and usually not just one thing that causes the problem with the immune system. Sometimes removing a few of these stressors makes a huge difference for a child. That's what happened with Ryan.

As his immune dysfunction lessened over time, so did his autism symptoms. The medical explanation was that Ryan had hit a point where his immune sys-tem was less reactive and fragile. His *allergy pot* was not boiling over as quickly as Dr. Rapp put it. When Ryan was allergy tested again in 1996, the improved results were dramatic. They showed he didn't react to as many foods. He no longer appeared to be allergic to everything.[26] The only food that remained in the high range was cow's milk, and his reaction to that was lower than before. Cheese, casein, and lactalbumin moved into a lower range of reactivity. Ryan had been off-the-charts allergic to garlic on his first test, but now Ryan was no longer reactive to garlic at all. So, we tore up his vampire card and celebrated at an Italian restaurant.

Eating a meal is never just about eating the food and following a diet is never just about what is eaten. It is usually about what is not eaten, and once again, there were too many "*nots*" for my comfort zone. Little did I know, my new hero, Dr. Harvey, was about to make our war easier and more difficult at the same time. The doctor-mom interpersonal indigestion was about to turn into a food fight. Dr. Harvey had his medical view on diet and autism. I had my mom concerns. His theory clearly states that food, immunology, and autism are linked. I can't dispute that.

---

26   The only food that Ryan still reacted to was cow's milk, but the value had contin-ued to decline (756, 371, and 358) until it just barely crept into the "intermediate" range. And the reference values for milk were much lower (371 versus 756).

But according to Dr. H, you have to do it right every time, at *every* meal, and *for life*.

My view also centered on how much time I would have to spend cooking. The things Ryan couldn't eat always had a negative effect on him because he hated when he couldn't eat what most people could. As important as diet is to our children's recovery, we have to live in the real world, and in the real world, if you are fortunate enough to have your kid invited to a birthday party, he should get to have a cupcake even when we have to deal with the behavioral consequences later.

Helping Ryan meant we all had to eat differently. The rest of the family didn't eat forbidden foods in front of Ryan (although sometimes we ate them when he wasn't looking). We all switched to drinking water at every meal. That turned out to be a healthier alternative for everyone. The added bonus was the money we saved on drinks in restaurants.

Dr. Harvey threw his diet rules at me, and I hurled my modified version back at him. Dr. *Cookie Monster* insisted that Ryan's sugar consumption needed to be even more limited. Even though I knew he was right about too much sugar, I still put one *"evil"* cookie in Ryan's school lunch each day. Yes, I was guilty of giving that cookie to my child, but I had my reasons. Any physical gains resulting from less sugar became insignificant if you took into consideration the consequences of Ryan not having that cookie. Ryan shut down whenever he felt different. He stopped eating and growing on Dr. Baker's diet. I didn't want that to happen again. He needed that cookie fix so he would be included socially when the kids at his school lunch table compared what everyone brought for dessert.

I believed the diet was essential for Ryan, especially when it came to completely eliminating dairy. Dr. H and I were in complete agreement on that one. However, Dr. H's advice about sugar went against everything I knew to be true about the way my son worked and what needed to happen at school during lunch.

The recurring argument with Dr. H about that cookie was awful.

Megan arrived home from school and ran up the stairs to see why I was screaming into the phone. Megan never heard me talk to anyone that way, except maybe Ryan when he was younger and still very affected. She asked who I was talking to. I mouthed, "Dr. Harvey." Megan nodded her head with understanding. She knew nothing was wrong. This was just how Dr. H and I communicated. It was the nature of our intense relationship. It finally dawned on me that this long-running argument could be avoided if I didn't tell Dr. H. about that stupid cookie. With age comes wisdom. I just stopped confessing about the cookie in my son's lunch. In time, I also stopped telling the good doctor about other things we couldn't agree on.

Many kids with autism are so food obsessive that they self-restrict their diet to no more than five or six different foods. Ryan didn't do that. But there were a few foods (like sesame seeds on a hamburger bun) that were *never* acceptable. I don't know for sure, but I now suspect the reason he didn't self-restrict his diet was because I fed Ryan until he was almost seven. By first grade, he could eat by himself at lunchtime. But I often still helped him at other meals.

What I didn't realize then was that Ryan's motor planning issues left him unable to decide which foods he should eat or in what order he should eat them. I wondered if other kids with autism also had this problem. Could this be part of the reason so many of our children restrict their diet to only a few foods? Dr. H believed that in some kids, a lack of ferritin or an iron deficiency is also a contributing factor to their self-imposed dietary restrictions.

When he did begin to feed himself, he compensated for his poor motor planning and communication problems by copying what Megan ate. When she took a bite of meat, he took a bite of meat. When she took a bite of potato, he took a bite of potato. If you think about it, that was a smart way to compensate for this deficit, but I didn't see it that way at the time. I just thought he was being difficult and wouldn't feed himself. Sometimes, what we perceive as stubbornness and being rigid isn't really that at all.

One day, when Megan's plate accidentally slipped off the table, Ryan picked up his plate and threw it on the floor, too. I was really upset when he did that. What I didn't understand back then was that my son had to watch Megan in order to know what to eat and when to eat it. He even copied her when her plate accidently fell off the table. I only saw that Ryan broke one of my dishes on purpose. And I was furious since I was already one dish short because of Megan's mishap. But I said nothing. Instead, I served up more food and cleaned up the mess. All the weird things our kids do can make us crazy if we let them. But sometimes they do them for reasons we don't often understand.

What I should have done was directly teach that kind of motor planning to Ryan. My ignorance helped us stay stranded on Autism Island longer. I spent each meal spooning food into my child's mouth. And only Megan had it right. She was busy at each mealtime showing Ryan what to do.

If I Knew Then What I Know Now

Dr. Harvey had strong views on diet then, and his dietary restrictions have become even stronger over the years. He was adamant that extreme diets don't cure autism and is equally adamant his dietary requirements are not extreme. I tend to differ. His dietary restrictions were dairy, whole wheat, milk chocolate, and sugar when Ryan first started the protocol. Now, carbs are extremely limited. Citrus, berries, tropical fruits, and everything red are no longer allowed. Some children can't have peanut butter or nuts. His new additions to the diet protocol make things even harder on families.

If your child does not recover as quickly as Dr. Harvey would like, then he is certain you are doing the diet wrong. His next demand is a food diary. This includes everything your child eats for a week. What he fails to understand is how difficult life with a kid with autism is for parents like us. Mostly because he doesn't have to live with one. For parents, there is never an extra minute in the day, and most times we are just trying to survive. And if there ever had been a spare minute, I thought it would be better used to teach my kid what he hadn't learned yet. I never sent a food log the multiple times he requested it. I understood the diet requirements and writing down what my child ate didn't make me comply with the dietary restrictions more. We never cheated when it came to dairy, but I can't say the same about that *"evil"* cookie in his lunch or the cupcake at special occasions.

In my *Doctor Mom* opinion, diet is not the only thing that causes big issues in our kids. Diet isn't the only thing we need to control to help them heal. Environmental allergies to pollen and other things are sometimes overlooked. We need to always be searching for anything that might help alleviate stress on our kids' immune systems. Are you using a laundry detergent they are allergic to? Is there mold in your basement? The things that can affect their immune system are endless. Ryan constantly had strep throat when he was younger until we had his tonsils and adenoids removed. That operation gave his immune system a huge boost. Getting tubes in his ears so he didn't need to take so many antibiotics was another thing we did right.

Now that Ryan is better, there isn't much in the food department that can throw him off. He eats almost everything other people do, but he hardly ever consumes dairy and is pretty good about limiting his sugar intake. Cows are still off limits, but now things are easier because goat's milk, goat's yogurt, and goat's cheese have been added to the mix. If he has an offending food (for him, ice cream) he does have some slight gastrointestinal distress, but it doesn't affect his mind anymore. I suppose it's possible that Ryan might be even healthier if he followed the diet to the letter and all the restrictions that Dr. H decreed as needed, but Ryan would have trouble complying with the stricter dietary rules.

I used to be concerned that if Dr. Harvey continued to make the diet too restrictive, then parents would stop it completely—kind of like I did with Dr. Baker's DAN! diet. Nevertheless, setting aside all the disagreements, we are both united in our belief about diet and the immune connection. Dr. H's diet prescription was a cake walk when compared with some other diets in the autism community; it just didn't include the cake.

CHAPTER 18

GETTING BETTER TAKES TIME

If everything seems under control, you're not going fast enough.

—Mario Andretti

WITH THE DIETARY restrictions now in place, Dr. H methodically proceeded to his next step and added an antifungal medication to Ryan's treatment. At first, I questioned this new move. Wasn't this what Dr. Baker had done? Were we simply retuning to a previous approach that hadn't worked well enough to justify the time and energy needed to implement it? I was a bit wary before I realized the treatment approach was different. Dr. H didn't use Dr. Baker's never-ending regimen of supplements. In fact, he told me to immediately stop every supplement Ryan was taking, except what he ordered. Me being me, I secretly kept a few things in place until I learned to trust Ryan's strange new doctor.

Dr. Baker had prescribed leucovorin (a prescription grade of folinic acid) for my son. It is quite common for individuals on the spectrum to have a gene mutation commonly referred to as MTHFR (methylene-tetrahydrofolate reductase). This gene provides instructions for making an enzyme called methylenetetrahydrofolate reductase. And if your name is Ryan and you don't have it, it is much harder for your immune systems to get rid of the toxic substances we are all exposed to. Leucovorin seemed to counteract that issue. It helped Ryan's body methylate better and get rid of the toxins. At that time, I didn't understand any of this. All I knew then was that after starting leucovorin, Ryan's speech improved dramatically, so I secretly kept it in place. He and I both take that medication now.

The antifungal medication ketoconazole was much more potent than the nystatin Dr. Baker had used. When I researched the side effects of this medicine, I was terrified. I read it could damage Ryan's liver. Once again, I questioned if we were doing the right thing. But Ryan was extremely ill. I reasoned if my son were ever to have a real chance at life, some risk and strong medicine might be necessary.

I hadn't yet recognized that Dr. H's regular blood tests were done partly to check that the medicines didn't cause any problems. Dr. H would be alerted to possible liver or kidney problems before any permanent damage could occur. If I had understood this at the time and if I had trusted this doctor and if I had better understood his protocol, then maybe I would have been less crazy—but probably not.

After starting ketoconazole, Ryan had terrible, horrible, epic die-off. I had to watch him act certifiably crazy, while simultaneously praying that he was getting better. Ryan appeared to be more affected by autism than ever before, if that were even possible. It was back to super-autistic Ryan with a sideshow of alternating goofy, hyper, and lethargic behavior. Our past experience with die-off left me a little more prepared, but I don't think you are ever ready to see your child go backward and suddenly become more autistic.

This time, we just had to hang on.

This horrendous second round of die-off left me tired and increasingly impatient with Dr. H's conservative one-thing-at-a-time, scientific method of doing things. It was just too slow for this crazy, obsessive mother. I wanted Dr. H to fire all the cannons at my son's broken immune system and fix him today— preferably before lunch!

When my impatience exploded during one telephone consult, Dr. Harvey calmly reminded me that Ryan had been sick for a long time, and it was going to take some time to make him better. He was right, of course, but I was still tired and also tired of waiting. Dr. Harvey didn't have to live with Ryan, *we* did.

I was *Chicken Little*, and the sky was always falling. I worried about what to feed Ryan and what long-term effect an ever-growing list of prescription medications would have on Ryan's body. It seemed unnatural to give such a young kid so many pharmaceuticals even though I had actively searched for that magic pill for years. Would all these meds hurt his development? Would he grow properly? Hundreds of questions rattled around in my head. I looked all over to find a doctor who could help, and now we had one. But I still couldn't completely trust him because he was a doctor. Dr. H was even more stubborn than I was, and I wasn't too good at giving up control. I needed to protect my son from the world even if that included the doctor whom I hoped would help him.

Recovering from autism is a *S-L-O-W* process, and I am not a woman who likes to wait. It is not like after you start this protocol you wake up one day and *BAM!* your kid is better.

It is more like one day your kid is a little less bizarre, and you have one less thing to teach him. Some days, I didn't notice the positive things Ryan accomplished. I was so focused on his negative behaviors that I usually forgot to notice what he was doing right. At the same time, I was overwhelmed by how much I still needed to teach him. Everything Ryan missed or lost while he was ill had to be systematically retaught. What we did could be compared to the comprehensive therapy a stroke victim needs in order to recover. This grueling work angered me as much as anything else associated with this diagnosis. Why did I have to teach Ryan all those things other kids just knew and learned on their own?

Recovery took more than two decades of rehabilitation. When we first started treatment with Dr. Harvey, I never imagined Ryan was capable of accomplishing all that he has. Avoiding a group home was all I hoped for, and independent living seemed like a totally out-of-reach goal.

Most of what I did during these years was not because I truly believed the medical and nonmedical therapies would make a difference for Ryan's future. I wanted to be able to tell myself I did everything possible before I had to find institutional placement for him. After years of trying, years of exhaustion, and a marriage in shambles, I worried constantly that all our sacrifices couldn't save him.

Ryan's treatment with Dr. Harvey lasted many years, and over these years, Dr. Harvey and I continued to have intense arguments. Every time we changed a medication, I worried. I watched everything Ryan was going through a little too closely, and these obsessive thoughts consumed me.

I couldn't decipher what the blood tests meant. I had just enough medical knowledge to make me suspicious and in a constant state of apprehension. I worried that Dr. H might overlook something on Ryan's blood test. He had a lot of kids to help, so I thought he could miss something important. And since he usually didn't take the time to explain Ryan's blood results or the rationale for the treatment he prescribed, I had no idea what any of this meant.

It took some time before I could relax about Ryan's medical treatment and Dr. Harvey's protocol. It took even more time to realize Dr. H was on top of things. Now that I had found someone to help Ryan, I needed to learn how to let him help. Over the years of our relationship, many times our conflicts revolved around his determination to cure Ryan one step at a time and my determination to make him fix Ryan *NOW!*

As you may have gathered, it takes a lot of faith to follow this protocol and even more faith to be a client of Dr. Harvey. You have to believe in his motivation and his medical ability, not to mention the tenacity needed to keep fighting for your sick child. Ryan's passionate and cantankerous doctor saw himself as the commanding general. To him, I was simply as a lowly foot soldier in the war against autism.

Just as Ryan began to improve and just at the very moment I began to feel as if I could let go of some of my fear for my son's future, Dr. Harvey would add a new medication or alter a dosage. At first, Ryan sometimes regressed. With each medication change, there was a period of adjustment before we saw any gains. It was ten steps forward and two steps back as we advanced across the autism battlefield. My problem was that I seemed to focus on those backward steps. And it was often impossible to tell if any deterioration in behavior resulted from a change in medication, a problem at school Ryan couldn't tell me about, or if he was about to come down with some illness.

I panicked whenever Dr. Harvey changed anything in Ryan's treatment plan. That meant changes to our family dynamics as we adjusted to the newest version of Ryan. Ryan's autism already wreaked havoc in our home, and we didn't need any new turmoil or stress. Every time Ryan took a backward step, I worried I was losing my son again. Dr. Harvey did have a strategy, but sometimes he forgot to tell me what it was or explain the next move.

Dr. Harvey decided to proceed with the next step of the NIDS protocol. And I wasn't going to be happy about it. He told me about this new addition when we made our yearly California visit. He wanted to introduce an SSRI (selective serotonin reuptake inhibitor) like Prozac. Many moms resist when he proposes this part of the protocol, and I was no different. Without a moment's hesitation, I informed him (and not too calmly) we would not give Ryan those kinds of drugs. I was fine with odd diets, odd therapies, odd behavior, and an odd lifestyle. I was even okay with taking an SSRI myself to cope with Ryan's autism. But having Ryan take an SSRI . . . somehow *that* was going too far. At that time, I thought these kinds of drugs were used for depression and only for people who couldn't cope with life.

He was ready for me and my objections. He answered my concerns in an unusually calm and caring voice. He asked me if my child had diabetes, would I hesitate to give him insulin? Dr. Harvey explained the reason for his use of an SSRI was as an *immune modulator*. Given at an extremely low dose, it could improve blood flow to the affected areas of Ryan's brain. On the way home from the visit, my husband and I talked about whether we should do this. We finally came to the conclusion we had to trust this man who already had helped our son so much. Now Ryan was more tuned in, the behavior outbursts happened less often and were less in intensity, and my son started to learn the things he never could before.

Back then, I thought my kid wouldn't get better if I didn't get things right on the first try. I hadn't yet realized that U-turns are allowed with autism treatment. I failed to realize that I could stop the SSRI if it wasn't helping since I was the one in charge of administering the meds.

The SSRI was almost an immediate success. Ryan's kindergarten teachers, who were unaware of this new medication, reported tremendously positive changes in his social skills. I never explained to his teachers what we did medically. They may have believed children with autism could improve, but they never thought children with autism could recover. Telling them Ryan was taking an SSRI would further label him as more disabled and me as more insane.

Now, the fragmentary but more normal behaviors observed at home started to occur at school. He always improved at home first, where he felt secure and loved. Within a few weeks, his teachers were sending home very positive reports. But I didn't comprehend just how much he improved until I witnessed it for myself.

When I had been the classroom helper in the past, it was an emotional struggle to be there. This time was different. I followed the conga line of kids chatting as they traveled down the hallway to the music teacher's room. Ryan looked up at the librarian, Mrs. Bales, as he passed her in the hall. His face broke into a huge grin, and he said, "Hi." Ryan had never said "Hi" to anyone.

Any other parent wouldn't even notice this, but to me it represented a world of new possibilities for Ryan. Ryan's behavior had become more typical at school. I started to have hope for his future, which was something I desperately needed. Ryan started singing songs I never heard before. When I asked where he learned them, he announced, "At school." I was both shocked and thrilled. He started learning a few other new skills without any pre-teaching at home.

Three weeks later, I called Dr. Harvey for our scheduled telephone appointment. "Okay, okay, you were right, and I was wrong!"[27] I hated having to admit to Dr. H that he was right about anything. It was not like he took the compliment with any semblance of humility.

Still, Dr. H was not yet finished tinkering with Ryan. He had changed Ryan's diet, prescribed antifungals, convinced us to start Ryan on an SSRI, and now he wanted to add an antiviral medication. Why?

---

27 Using SSRIs continues to be a contentious choice within the autism community. Children whose symptom profile suggests pediatric autoimmune neuropsychiatric disorders associated with streptococcal infections (PANDAS) should be evaluated cautiously. For a fact sheet on PANDAS, see ocfoundation.org. Parents may wish to discuss the following excerpt with their doctor: "However, children presenting with PANDAS may be more sensitive to behavioral side effects (aggression, hyperactivity, sleep problems and even suicidal thinking) but may tolerate at smaller than usual starting doses. Some children with the first episode of obsessive-compulsive disorder (OCD)/PANDAS will have the symptoms improve gradually after infections were treated. SSRI use should be discussed with a doctor in order to weigh the benefits against the risks." See also www.pandasnetwork.org.

Dr. H explained that Ryan's blood work from that initial visit long ago showed Ryan had been infected with human herpesvirus 6 (HHV-6), human herpesvirus 4 (HHV-4), and Epstein-Barr virus (EBV). Although these are common infections, his HHV-6 titers were very high, and his immune system was actively and constantly trying to fight these infections. This viral burden contributed to Ryan's pot boiling over. A lower viral load should turn the heat down on the stove and help Ryan get even better. Ryan began taking the generic for Valtrex. About a year later, we switched to the generic for Famvir (another antiviral medication) after he built up a tolerance to the first one. Once again, there were improvements in all aspects of his life as well as ours. Antiviral medication became a pivotal part of Ryan's recovery.

But back in these early days, we were frequently adjusting Ryan's medications. When Dr. H changed Ryan's meds, he called it *refining*. I called it *fiddling*. I sometimes wondered why we couldn't leave well enough alone. Ryan was improving. My assumption was that if we kept going without these constant changes, Ryan would continue to improve, and our family could focus on something other than complying with the latest cocktail.

I really didn't understand the dynamic and interrelated nature of the immune system and the complexity of what Dr. H was trying to accomplish. Whenever the body builds up a tolerance to a medication, a change is needed to continue the positive results that medication initially provided. Whenever Dr. H changed Ryan's meds, Ryan's body needed time to adjust. Whenever he varied the dose of anything, Ryan's behavior often regressed for a period of time before it progressed.

Regression scared me!

Sometimes, after starting a new med, Ryan had bathroom accidents at night. Every time Ryan took a backward step, I'd get that sick feeling in my stomach. We had made so much progress. He was starting to care about things, he wanted friends, and he was interacting with others at school. Now he could follow simple instructions and was starting to learn some things without my direct teaching. Now we had so much more to lose. What if he just kept going downhill? What if he didn't come back this time?

Eventually, I learned through observation that the longer we were on the treatment plan, the less reactive Ryan was to everything. Whenever Ryan built up a tolerance to the antifungal or antiviral prescriptions, we had to change to another medication that did the same thing. For Ryan, they usually stopped being as effective at the one-year point. Our clue that a medication was no longer working was when some of Ryan's autism symptoms returned. For the antifungal meds, we switched between the generic for Diflucan and the generic for Nizoral. And for the antiviral meds we switched between Valtrex and Famvir.

As Ryan's immune system became more regulated, his autism symptoms continued to diminish. But I never quite got over the fear that Ryan's regression caused me. Even though progress was just around the corner, I still worried my son could be lost and might sail away to Autism Island permanently.

Two years after we started the protocol, we returned to California for our annual family Thanksgiving trip. We had an appointment with Dr. H and he ordered a second neuroSPECT scan scheduled. I sometimes wondered if Dr. H sat up nights thinking of new ways to torture Ryan's mother since the first neuroSPECT scan was so difficult to do.

I was surprised when the second test turned out to be relatively easy for Ryan. He was older now, but what really changed was that his immune system was partially recovered. As a result, his behavior was more typical. At age seven, he barely resembled the five-year-old affected by severe autism that he had been when we did the first scan. Now, Ryan had no trouble following directions or staying still for the test.

The neuroSPECT results removed any doubt I still had about the cause of Ryan's improvement. The inflammation in Ryan's brain had decreased significantly, and blood flow to the impaired areas had improved dramatically. Increased blood flow meant increased function. Dr. H explained that when the blood flow improves, children can learn what they struggled with in the past.

If I Knew Then What I Know Now

Just getting Ryan to take the medications at the beginning of his medical treatment was a major accomplishment. He was still too young to swallow pills, and some of the medications only came in adult sizes. I tried what seemed like a hundred different ways to solve this problem. Mary Poppins finally provided the solution to my dilemma. She was absolutely correct when she said, "A spoonful of sugar makes the medicine go down."[28]

I would break the pills into small pieces or crush them. Next, I surrounded them in a nondairy frozen dessert like sorbet. Finally, I put this concoction on a spoon. After he swallowed it, I followed it with a water chaser. As he got older, I reduced the amount of dessert camouflage. Eventually, Ryan learned how to swallow pills without the sorbet. That was a big day in our house, and we celebrated accordingly.

Even though Ryan was on a low-sugar diet, I simultaneously helped him with medication and hurt him by using sugar to do it. I had yeast guilt. But in reality, the amount of sugar was not enough to worry about. The benefits of the medication more than made up for any adverse effects from the sugar.

Initially, it was hard to tell which interventions were working. How can you tell a medicine is working when your child has limited verbal ability and prefers his own inner world to the one where everyone else lives? Improvements in speech take time, and the results were not immediately apparent. It takes *at least* three years for most typical kids to acquire speech and even longer for those with autism. Behaviors changed gradually despite my insistence that change needed to be immediate and profound.

It is not just one thing that makes a kid better. It is a combination of many things. When a child is improving so slowly, you don't even notice the changes. It is kind of like when your children grow taller. It's impossible to realize your kid grew two inches when you are looking for that growth on a daily basis. It is only after you make that mark on the wall and measure their height that you can clearly see they are taller.

But I never missed it when Ryan did something wrong!

---

28   On my website is a blog post called, "Three Easy Steps To Make The Medicine Go Down." It will help you teach your children how to learn how to eventually swallow pills. In it is a brilliant video by Norma on how she gets the meds down with her daughter who had a brain injury from a motorcycle accident.

Ryan's bizarre behaviors often overshadowed the fact that we truly were making progress. I didn't notice his improvement in speech because I was too busy noticing his tantrums in the mall. What I also didn't realize is after our children start to recover, they usually pick up developmentally right where they stalled out. All children must go through the same developmental stages, no matter what their chronological age. That means if a child was two when typical development stopped, they resume their development at age two. And two-year-old behavior doesn't look so good in a seven-year-old body. For parents of older children, the terrible twos in an eighteen-year-old body can be very frightening.

Sometimes, parents mistakenly perceive the start of development and improvement as new behavior problems. What appears to be a new behavior issue can actually be a good sign. You may think your child is acting worse and that the protocol doesn't work. You think your child is regressing. All those thoughts went through my head, but that wasn't what actually happened. Remember this mantra and say it over and over again whenever your kid starts backsliding: "Regression often comes before progression." A twelve-year-old who is two developmentally is much harder to deal with than a zoned-out kid who doesn't care about anything.

When my medically treated kid started to wake up and develop again, then ABA, compliance training, and consistent parental guidance were needed to teach consequences for inappropriate behavior. Discipline for Ryan at age five was similar to discipline for a typical two-year-old. You have to meet your child at the age they are developmentally.

Part 4

Escape from Autism Island

CHAPTER 19

APPLIED BEHAVIOR ANALYSIS—TO DO OR NOT TO DO, THAT IS THE QUESTION

The first step to getting anywhere is deciding that you are no longer willing to stay where you are.

—Author Unknown

WE WORKED WITH Ryan every day to teach him all the things he didn't know. We started this before we started any medical stuff. After the change in diet, our concentrated efforts actually started to work. It became easier to see the kid in there more clearly, and my son was better equipped to learn. But we still needed to figure out the best way to teach our son. Our rehabilitation went into high gear about the time Dr. Harvey came on board.

Every day my child remained autistic was another day not learning what he needed to know. We had to reach that kid. My son never learned the things most kids do because it just wasn't possible for him to learn much of anything before his immune system started to improve. When he finally started to move in the right direction, he still didn't act like any kid I knew. His strange, autistic behaviors were ingrained. He had done them all day long for years. I was told these behaviors helped him cope with our unpredictable and confusing world. Still, the way he acted didn't make sense to us or anyone else.

Ryan needed more if he was going to fit in our world. But . . . more what?

The real question was how to teach him all that he missed before it was possible for him to learn. The problem was that our world was full of people—not objects—and he barely understood a word we said or the things we did. He still didn't know how to communicate when something was wrong, he couldn't follow more than very simple one step directions, and dressing and feeding himself were still out of the question. The enormous number of things he didn't know how to do were still there, although we worked with him every day. Of all the nonmedical therapies we had tried, ABA seemed the obvious choice even though Jackie Rains, our psychologist, chastised us for even considering it, and Dr. Harvey compared it to dog training. When they both weren't looking, we began to use the ABA techniques we had learned in college.

As I mentioned before, Frank and I both took a course in behavior therapy from Dr. Ivar Lovaas when we were still undergraduates at UCLA. That was years before we married. Taking Lovaas's class was one of those accidental, life-changing events. Neither of us realized the impact this class would have on our lives or on the future of our unborn children.

When we were undergrads, many of the classes at UCLA were overcrowded. All the classes Frank wanted were full. Frustrated when he couldn't find anything to fill a hole in his schedule, I suggested we go see what Ivar Lovaas's class looked like. I heard it was good. Frank wasn't really interested in the class, but we were in the early stages of dating when he would still do anything to please me.

I held his hand as we walked together to Franz Hall to see what Psychology 170A was all about. Dr. Lovaas had the entire class engaged and laughing within minutes. The longer we sat there, the more fascinated we were with what he had to say. Even though my own schedule was complete, I dropped one of my classes so I could also enroll in this one. I wasn't sure how this class was going to help Frank be a better political science major, but I thought it might be fun to take a class together. Frank was interested in the class, and I was interested in Frank.

After completing this introductory class, we took the next more advanced class and became behavior therapists. There we worked with autistic children in the UCLA Young Autism Project. This class changed everything for me. I had been clueless as to what I wanted to do when I finally became a grown-up. I loved working with these kids and knew I made a difference in their lives. I now had a goal, so I needed to get a teaching credential in order to continue doing this important work to help children with autism. I did finally get that teaching credential, but I instead went on to work with typical elementary age kids. However, you must be careful what you wish for.

Frank and I anguished over the burdens of the parents and the children we worked with. There were many discussions about how hard it would be to walk in their shoes. We came to the conclusion that a child with autism was one of the worst things that could happen to a couple.

Being labeled "behavior therapist" is not the same as actually being a behavior therapist. After just one introductory class of behavior theory taught by Dr. Lovaas, we were thrown into the fire doing ABA with children who were severely affected. Our limited training and experience led Frank and me to falsely believe that if a child had any speech at all, he couldn't have autism. The children we worked with were on the very severe end of the spectrum. They lacked most of the everyday skills needed for independent life. Their behavior was extremely bizarre. The majority of these younger kids had no speech at all. This heart-wrenching group of obviously impaired children was what we thought autism was. When we compared Ryan to our memories of what autism looked like in college, we knew Ryan *couldn't* be autistic.

We were so wrong!

As therapists, we were given a lesson plan or drill to work on with a child. We repeated the same lesson over and over until the child could consistently demonstrate mastery. At least twice a week for two hours at a time, we worked with an assigned child under the supervision of a graduate student from the UCLA Young Autism Project. But our supervisor was rarely in the room with us and didn't directly teach us much of anything. We only met very occasionally to discuss the children under our care.

Instead, there was a notebook at the child's home filled with any updates and new drills we needed to work on. We checked the book for instructions from our graduate supervisor and then simply repeated assigned drills over and over again, reinforcing the targeted behavior. We were mostly on our own to figure things out. We received class credit in place of a salary, and parents were billed exorbitant amounts for our "professional" services.

When Frank worked with Billy, it took more than six months for him to say the phrase, "I like it." The drill was simple. Frank sang a popular song at that time, "That's the way, uh huh, uh huh . . . " Billy filled in the blank by singing the ending, "I like it." I never knew Frank could be so musical until he started ABA. Jason, my student, referred to everything, including the holes in the wall, as "A baby lamb." Susan, a seven-year-old, didn't speak at all. She rocked uncontrollably and masturbated until she bled.

We thought Ryan couldn't have autism because sometimes he spoke. But he didn't have functional language. Ryan never answered me when I asked a question. He mostly used his limited vocabulary to get something he wanted. But he didn't resemble the head-banging, self-mutilating children we had worked with so many years before. It had to be something else. At the time, I couldn't even bring myself to say the A-word out loud.

I still cringe at the memory of a remark I made to Frank before we actually knew Ryan was on the spectrum. Ryan was in his crib with its cheerful *Sesame Street*-themed covers. He lay on his back and stared at his fingers. Then he wiggled them again and again in front of his eyes. I laughed as I said jokingly to Frank, "Looks kind of autistic, huh?"

When we became therapists, UCLA was considered to be ABA Central—the best program in existence. ABA earned the reputation as an effective intervention for kids with autism. So, why wouldn't we want to add on a therapy that worked and that we were supposedly trained to administer?

Although Frank and I were desperate for help after Ryan's diagnosis, we made a conscious decision not to go to Dr. Lovaas for several reasons. The first was that, from time to time, I had tried to use ABA with Ryan, and the results were mixed. Ryan didn't respond consistently to these methods. These were the same methods that were specifically designed to elicit a consistent response. Dr. Harvey's autism theory explained this conundrum perfectly: Ryan couldn't consistently respond to ABA because he was too ill at that time. It was the same for Billy, Jason, and Susan, but I didn't realize that then. It took months and months to teach our UCLA kids anything or to get any response at all.

Secondly, we hadn't received enough ABA training to really help Ryan. We were good at implementing drills, but we were not trained to create drills. We didn't know how to pinpoint the most important thing you need for teaching. You need to find what the child finds most reinforcing and motivating. If you can motivate them, they *will* learn. Thirdly, I convinced myself that Ryan couldn't have autism, and, therefore, ABA was not the correct therapy for him. My logic was monumentally wrong, and my denial acted as protection from the inner terror I felt whenever the A-word was mentioned. At that time, I was still in search of a nice, tidy brain tumor.

Also, there were many aspects of ABA we witnessed at UCLA that disturbed us. In the early development stages of ABA therapy, inappropriate behaviors were eliminated by the use of a negative consequence: a slap on the hand, yelling, or other punitive responses. I never used these methods with the children I worked with although I was instructed to do so. I was not about to use them deliberately and intentionally with my own child. Frank and I didn't believe in corporal punishment. Hitting a child was *never* acceptable, especially since there were so many other methods that worked better. We always knew this when it came to Megan. We didn't believe in hitting Ryan either, but I can't honestly say we always kept our emotions, frustrations, and anger in check with him. Our beliefs about no spanking sometimes went out the window when it came to dealing with Ryan.

What Frank and I (along with much of the medical community, such as Dr. Harvey and Jackie Rains) did not realize was that ABA had evolved considerably from those early days. Archaic, punitive methods were no longer used. Today, when done correctly, ABA is totally positive. Good behaviors are rewarded and inappropriate behaviors are mostly ignored. If done properly, it is just good teaching.

It was not until I read Catherine Maurice's book *Let Me Hear Your Voice*[29] that I learned how much ABA had changed from fifteen years earlier when we were "pretending" to be behavior therapists. Catherine Maurice used an

---

29   Maurice, Catherine. *Let Me Hear Your Voice: A Family's Triumph Over Autism.* New York: Knopf, 1993.

intensive behavioral approach to recover her two children with autism. Her story eased our antiquated fears about ABA. It still is a good read and demonstrates how effective ABA can be when done correctly. It gave me a reason to keep going. That book gave me hope for my child's future.

Once Frank and I decided to reconsider the ABA option, there was still the issue of finding a qualified therapist. ABA was not yet offered by any agency in Minnesota. ABA also was not even offered in our neighboring states. *Of course, it wasn't.* That would have been too simple. So, I called Ivar Lovaas at UCLA to explain our ironic family predicament. Ivar suggested we take a trip to see William Dyer in Iowa. William had been Dr. Lovaas's right-hand man at UCLA.

I was beginning to feel our journey toward Ryan's recovery was like searching for one of those puzzle pieces on the map of the United States that Ryan obsessed over. Every new therapy puzzle piece seemed to mean a new state to visit. Maybe we couldn't cure Ryan, but I was convinced he would excel at geography.

Frank and I both liked William's ideas on how to help Ryan. We felt hopeful again with this new expert to help us. Sadly, we were all set to start our in-home ABA program when William was diagnosed with cancer. Fortunately, he did beat the cancer, but not before he could help us or Ryan.

We found the next puzzle piece in New Jersey. William suggested I speak with Scott Wright in Cherry Hill, New Jersey. Scott connected us to another puzzle piece in Chicago, Illinois, named Mindi Fischer.[30] That would have been better news if we really knew William or Scott or Mindi, their credentials, or if they were really any good at this. We called anyway. We didn't know who Mindi was or what we were signing up for, but we had to do something to help Ryan. We put all our eggs and a large sum of money into our latest basket of hope, Mindi. We were going to pay for Mindi's flight, hotel, car, and food in addition to her fee for a two-day ABA training session in our home.

---

30   An interesting side note is that Scott Wright took over as the president and CEO of the Lovaas Institute and LIFE Midwest, Inc., after Dr. Lovaas retired.

CHAPTER 20

MINDI CHANGES THE GAME

If a child cannot learn in the way we teach . . . we must teach in a way the child can learn.

—Dr. O. Ivar Lovaas

A VERY YOUNG girl gave me a big friendly smile when I opened the door to my home. My first thought was, "What is this young *kid* going to teach me?" When I talked to her on the telephone, Mindi sounded so knowledgeable, self-assured, and mature. It's a good thing I didn't know she was only twenty-three when I first spoke with her, or I might have cancelled what was going to be another life-changing event for Ryan.

Since we had already paid for her expenses, and since there was not much left to try, we marched on. What did we have to lose, anyway? *Only more money.* And it was not like we hadn't already pitched bags and bags of it at other autism treatments and interventions that didn't help in the least. We started our home ABA program with Mindi shortly after we began medical treatment with Dr. Harvey.

I packed my living room with people for that first ABA training session. Those in attendance included the director of special education from our school district as well as the district's autism specialist, Shawn. Ryan's potential therapists-in-training were also included. Neither the autism specialist nor our director of special education knew much about ABA. And I had my suspicions they didn't know much about autism, either. I was sure they had never heard of biomedical treatment for autism.

Even so, Shawn seemed like a good person, and I felt he truly cared about helping Ryan. He reminded me of a big, burly teddy bear and was the nicest guy ever. But I never really considered him an expert in autism even though he had several degrees and titles. Shawn began working with Ryan shortly before that training session with Mindi. He couldn't make Ryan comply. When my son didn't want to do something, Shawn just let him not do it. Ryan had Shawn right where he wanted him. Shawn did whatever my kid adamantly demanded. That way there were no confrontations. Sound familiar?

Shawn treated Ryan's autism the same way we originally coped. He enabled and reinforced Ryan's odd behaviors by changing our world to meet Ryan's demands. This attitude helped keep Ryan marooned on Autism Island. Unlike Shawn, Frank and I had realized the futility of this approach even if we hadn't figured out how to do things differently.

Instead of enabling Ryan, Shawn needed to challenge him. Ryan needed to learn he was no longer running the show. We hoped this training session with Mindi would help turn around Shawn's approach. Regretfully, even Mindi couldn't teach our gentle Shawn how to do ABA. He was just too nice. When the weekend training session ended, Shawn came to me and said he wasn't comfortable using these new methods. I understood his apprehension because I wasn't yet convinced either.

Mindi taught us how to use the ABA techniques with Ryan. ABA uses a strict stimulus-response paradigm. It teaches a single behavior and addresses only one behavior at a time. After each new skill Mindi taught us, we practiced by taking turns working with Ryan. She wrote drills and lessons and promoted us to the rank of Chief Drill Sergeants in charge of battling a five-year-old army of one.

This was Mindi's Miracle: there is always an immediate reward for behaving appropriately and always an immediate consequence for behaving inappropriately; mostly we were to *ignore* the behavior completely. It was that simple.

Next, she taught us a second lesson. *Never negotiate* with terrorists, especially if they are named Ryan. She told us not to bargain with Ryan even if that meant he would comply and do what we wanted. No more bribes. We were negotiation experts before Mindi joined our ranks. We'd say to Ryan, "If you do this, I will do that." As in, "If you behave during our trip to the grocery store, I will get you an ice cream cone at Baskin-Robbins." That kind of bribery was *not* allowed in ABA. Our primary method of getting Ryan to comply was now gone.

Mindi counseled us to always act in a confident manner when we worked with Ryan. We couldn't ever let Ryan see insecurity or waffling when it came to our next behavioral strike. We needed to act sure of ourselves even though we soon discovered that wasn't usually the case.

Mindi explained her reasoning: any reaction to Ryan's behavior, whether positive (e.g., praise) or negative (e.g., a disapproving look or sigh) reinforced the probability that he would repeat the very behavior we were trying to eliminate.

We needed to be the ones in charge of the reinforcement schedule—not Ryan.

We were not allowed to roll our eyes or press our lips together when we were exasperated with him. We could not show any negative emotion if he did something wrong. If we screamed at Ryan or smacked his hand, then he was in control because he caused this reaction. His need for sameness was stronger than his need for our approval or disapproval. For us, even this basic ABA rule was extremely challenging in the beginning.

Ryan fought us on every new technique we tried. He hit, bit, and did whatever he could to try and make us stop. He had never been aggressive before we started ABA. But now, he was determined to win and return to the familiarity of Autism Island. It was extremely difficult to be more stubborn than Ryan with this exhausting psychological warfare. Ryan wanted to control everything and everyone in his environment. It was time to turn the tide in this war.

Mindi instructed us to never correct inappropriate behavior, such as biting or scratching, with anger. We were to simply take Ryan by the hand and put him through his ABA paces. Don't show any emotion and do things in a matter-of-fact manner until Ryan complied. In *ABA Speak*, when Ryan did not connect the stimulus to the correct response, his behavior was inappropriate. Our role was to simply facilitate the connection of the stimulus with the correct response. Rinse and repeat the drill over and over again until he learned it. It was called compliance training.

That was the theory. It was easier said than done.

Before ABA, I never really demanded Ryan do things on my terms. Now, his former protector and security guard mother was the "enemy." Was it really any surprise Ryan became aggressive and extremely disagreeable after we started ABA? With ABA, we forced him to follow our rules.

Mindi helped us understand that children with autism want to hold on tightly to their behaviors because it makes their world safe and predictable. A child who never acted violently before often becomes aggressive once you make him do the things expected of any child. In time, if you can outlast them, the meltdowns and outbursts go away.

But she failed to tell us just how long this could take.

Mindi helped alter Ryan's behavior by devising drills specific to what he needed to learn that connected the stimulus (i.e., what we asked him to do) with the correct response (i.e., what he was required to do by us). She told us not to correct too many behaviors at once because Ryan would have difficulty making the correct stimulus-response association and might get the idea he couldn't do anything right.

She strongly advised us to pick one behavior and work on extinguishing only that behavior. She also warned us that any time you try to eliminate an undesirable behavior, the behavior increases before it goes away. This is called an *extinction burst*.

Mindi also emphasized that rewarding a behavior means using a reward that is important to Ryan—not necessarily what is important to us. And she told us to always look for that one thing Ryan did right during the day and reward him for it with something he values. Ignore all the unacceptable things Ryan did. We were to mostly ignore his inappropriate behaviors until it became the targeted behavior we were trying to eliminate. That was the theory. Once again, it was easier said than done. I was stunned when it actually started to work. Newly armed with Mindi's unbreakable rules, lots of telephone support, and a weekend of training, I decided it was time to target a specific behavior and march on until we won the battle.

Ryan's JAWS impression had to go.

Ryan would frequently bite Megan or squeeze her arm until she cried. In the past, I had reacted with angry words, threats, or bribes. Now, I was ready to launch an ABA missile at him. We used our secret weapon.

We called it *The Chair.*

Whenever Ryan bit, squeezed, or scratched anyone, I calmly took him by the hand and sat him in a chair in our playroom. I sat in another chair positioned directly in front of his. I wrapped my legs around his chair to prevent any escape. Next, I demanded that he do what I asked, and I only chose behaviors that I knew he could perform.

I would demand he do something I knew he knew how to do. I might say, "Stand up."

When he did, I praised him for his good behavior, "Good job, Ryan!"

"Touch your head. Good, Ryan!"

When he did two behaviors correctly in a row, I would say, "Okay. Go play." And then let him leave and escape from me and my demands.

If he failed to comply, we kept going (sometimes it felt like forever). He had to follow my directions and do what I asked two times to escape from me and the Chair. Just as Mindi predicted, Ryan's biting and scratching increased when we first introduced this compliance drill. However, it wasn't long before he learned that to be free from our ABA demands, all he had to do was to stop biting and do what we told him to do when we told him to do it.

It sounded so easy, but it wasn't.

There I was, doing laundry, cooking something I didn't want to eat, remembering to talk to Megan, and wondering if Frank would talk to me, when Ryan would do something, and I would have to hit the pause button to do an ABA drill over and over—all day long—every day. I had to do this *immediately* whenever the inappropriate behavior occurred.

I couldn't let Ryan see my uncertainty about using ABA. I knew if I showed any weakness, he would own me. Actually, he already did, and I needed to change that dynamic. It was difficult to remain calm as I lead him to the Chair for what felt like the hundredth time that day And I could only choose one behavior at a time to eliminate.

After the biting was gone, I picked another behavior that needed to go. My success made me want more success. Ryan used to go up to people and grind his chin into their shoulder or another body part. We referred to this as "chinning." I no longer cared that this behavior had a nice, neat, sensory integration explanation that would require a never-ending series of occupational therapy sessions to stop.

The chinning had to go *N-O-W!* It went.

As we became more proficient with basic ABA, we added more complex behavior techniques. We used the *"shaping technique"* to help him learn new things or when we needed him to comply with our commands. If he refused to stand up when requested, I would gently help him stand, and at the same time I would say, "Good!" In shaping, approximations of a target behavior are reinforced.

We always and immediately rewarded any behavior that came close to the behavior we were trying to teach. We shaped his response by allowing a *successive approximation* of the desired behavior we actually wanted from Ryan. This carefully crafted step-by-step process changes behavior. That's the theory, and as with basic ABA, it is easier explained than done.

One day, I tried to show Ryan how to move a game piece around the *Sorry!* gameboard while counting out loud. He just couldn't do it. The motor planning skills he needed were absent. My pre-Mindi interpretation was Ryan was being defiant. My post-Mindi interpretation was that it didn't matter why Ryan did what he did. My son just needed to move that stupid blue plastic piece around the board and do what his mother said.

That was a big learning moment for me. Before, when I believed he was being stubborn and difficult, he really wasn't. Dr. Harvey's scans helped me understand why he acted as he did. Instead of getting mad at him like I so often did, I decided to try a more effective method. This time, I started to encourage and praise him when he barely got close to doing the task correctly. I shaped his behavior by putting my hand on his and helping him count and move the game piece. Anything close to the behavior I was trying to teach him was celebrated.

It took me more than a hundred attempts (no exaggeration) before he demonstrated the behavior of counting while moving the piece from one square to the next. In this situation, behavior shaping worked much better than the constant corrections of old-school ABA. This was a victory for both of us.

If I Knew Then What I Know Now

Mindi only came to our home on two separate occasions. Once for the first two-day training weekend and once for a half-day visit to determine if Ryan's school situation was right. But she was always available by telephone. I called any time I wasn't sure how to tackle a problem behavior or needed to know what skill we needed to teach Ryan next. Mindi was relentless in devising drills that targeted what Ryan needed to learn and she had an unending arsenal of new things to try when what we were doing wasn't effective with Ryan. His new nickname was "Mr. Target." What she taught us in that brief amount of time changed Ryan's life forever.

She really was our Miracle Mindi.

ABA was a game changer. Now we had effective tools to make Ryan comply with what we asked. Now we had our own ABA war chest. We used what Mindi taught us to change Ryan's behavior. In the beginning, Ryan absolutely, totally, and completely did not want to change. He barricaded himself behind a wall of aggressive, combative, and horrible behavior. My son was quite prepared to behave much, much worse in order to stay in the safety of his own world. Initially, it didn't look like we were making progress.

I needed to remember two things as I began to comprehend what was happening. First, even though Ryan seemed somewhat easier to manage before we started ABA, he actually wasn't. He was only easier because we changed our behavior to accommodate his needs. Our behavior was shaped by Ryan to avoid meltdowns. We were like Shawn—loving and ineffective. Second, Mindi had explained to us that behavior often worsens before it goes away and is extinguished. I forgot that important piece of information in the throes of dealing with an out-of-control kid.

Ryan really was getting better. It just didn't look like he was.

Once again, "If you don't feel it, fake it" became my inner mantra as I outwardly remained calm and took Ryan once again to the Chair for the gazillionth time. Inwardly, I felt insecure and unsure of what we were doing. I was bluffing, but my son didn't know that. I had to just keep going with my ABA poker face that showed no emotion until he did what I required. Then I quickly responded with smiles, high fives, and praise that didn't come from my heart.

The double dose of medical intervention to correct his immune issues combined with ABA forced Ryan to interact with us and with the world on our terms, not his. The good news was that as time went on and as this double dose took effect, eliminating and changing Ryan's problem behaviors took a shorter amount of time and less effort. The bad news was there was never a shortage of behaviors to eliminate and change. And we could only do this *one* behavior at a time.

CHAPTER 21

THE DOCTOR WHO SAVED RYAN AND WHY I CANCELLED OUR NEXT APPOINTMENT

They always say time changes things, but you actually have to change them yourself.

—Andy Warhol

WORKING WITH GENIUS can be difficult. Dr. Harvey is a great doctor when he is not yelling at you. But when he thought he was right and was convinced I was wrong, there was no one harder to deal with. Being Dr. H's patient means just that: being patient. As far as I'm concerned, he's the doctor, I'm the mom, and the playing field is level. Not to him. Ours has been a contentious relationship over the decades, but I will always be grateful to him for saving my kid.

Dr. Harvey is very protective of his patients. He also wants parents to follow everything he prescribes to the letter and without question. Sometimes, he yells when he thinks you are experimenting with a non-Harvey-sanctioned cure or anything else he thinks might be harmful to your child. You don't actually have to do either of these things to be the brunt of one of his rants.

His ego often got in the way. If your child is not improving as fast as he would like, then it couldn't be his fault, so it had to be yours. You must not be doing the diet or the rehab correctly. And that's when the yelling would start.

Dr. Harvey's passion to help our children makes him an amazing doctor, but there are times that same passion caused a major doctor-patient communication issue. Over time, I finally realized I did not need to tell him anything he didn't want to hear. After I learned that cookie lesson, things became easier. However, I still question how a doctor can prescribe the right course of treatment when his patients are apprehensive and afraid to tell him the truth.

When I wasn't mad at him, I was in awe over what this amazing doctor did daily. It takes a tremendous amount of stamina to take care of our kids. Dr. H's previous life as a regular pediatrician had to have been easier than treating children with autism. The answers for our children are not obvious. Treatment for children with autism is time and labor intensive and much more difficult than giving an antibiotic for an ear infection. In addition, our children often come with mothers like me. We are a high-maintenance group to work with. I can't imagine how difficult it must be to deal with obsessive, scared, and crazy parents like me all day long.

The medical community is another source of great frustration for Dr. Harvey. After all the research and evidence, some doctors still refuse to accept autism is *medical* and *treatable*. They fail to address or recognize any medical issues that could possibly cause autism, let alone treat them.

Parents must painfully watch as their children slip away while their pediatrician stands by and does nothing. It is not that these physicians don't care; they just don't realize our children can be helped. I'm right there with Dr. Harvey on that one. That makes me want to yell, too.

Dr. Harvey also anguishes over the fact that many of the flavors-of-the-week treatments for autism are often dangerous for our kids. We are vulnerable to any alleged instant cure that comes along. Dealing with autism and seeing your child drift further and further away from you is a horrific way to live.

Some parents, me included, do stupid things in the name of helping our kids. For example, we desperately throw supplements indiscriminately down our children's throat like candy because our pediatricians haven't provided anything else for this "incurable" disease. (While some supplements have helped many children, it is important to tailor the regimen to the individual child's unique makeup.) Recovery can become even more difficult after some of the more invasive or harmful treatments.

One of Dr. H's faults is that he so intensely believes he has the answer that he refuses to believe that his methods might not be working as well as he hoped or that his protocol might not work for all kids.

The upside of Dr. Harvey's strong personality is that it made him fight and work hard for my kid. The downside was his inability to play well with others. We hung in there with Dr. H longer than most families. After one particularly awful disagreement, we stopped seeing Dr. Harvey for Ryan's medical treatment. We were gone for a few years. We turned to our local family practice doctor, whose bedside manner was less confrontational, to continue Ryan's medications.

I was worn out.

If I Knew Then What I Know Now

Dr. H's medical treatment helped many kids recover and get healthier. However, since I'm not a doctor, I don't fully understand why some kids like Ryan recover and other kids do not improve much. Perhaps Dr. Harvey's methods are effective for some subsets of autism, but not for all. This is not yet known and may be better explained after we have categorized different types of autism. This is a very complex disease with a still-emerging protocol. Fortunately, Ryan's type of autism fit what Dr. Harvey did.

Reducing the total load on a child's immune system by the use of antifungal and antiviral medications was a miracle for kids like mine. Whenever I send a family to Dr. H for help, I tell them he is great if your child fits what he does. In the same breath, I warn them that he thinks he knows more about autism than any other human being on the planet. I also suggest that some children may need more interventions than Dr. H offers.

And there might be YELLING!

CHAPTER 22

MEDICAL TREATMENT ALONE WAS NOT ENOUGH

It is our choices that show what we truly are, far more than our abilities.

—Albus Dumbledore, *Harry Potter and the Chamber of Secrets*

by JK Rowling

RYAN'S *ALLERGY SHINERS* were fading, and his *blank stares* abated. That was the medical missile. He responded more to external behavioral control. That was the ABA missile. As Ryan interacted more with the real world, he also became increasingly frustrated with his inability to communicate his wants and needs. Now, he knew what he wanted to say, but he still didn't know how to say it. This caused him to appear worse in the beginning. He had frequent outbursts because now he actually cared about his surroundings and what happened to him. He was getting better, but it just didn't look like it.

How bad were Ryan's communication problems? *Really bad!* At age five and a half, Ryan tested in the third percentile for speech and language. Ninety-seven percent of the children his age comprehended and spoke better than my son. After Mindi and Dr. Harvey came into our lives, Ryan made huge progress. Still, it wasn't until fourth grade that he tested in the eighty-fifth percentile in these areas.

With the dual supports of medical intervention and ABA, Ryan progressed from way below the norm to above the norm for speech and language. Yet during the three percent days, it was often hard for Ryan or for us to believe that dramatic improvement would ever come. It was difficult to see the growth when he still did so many inappropriate things. It was too difficult to look into the future and fight the daily battles at the same time.

Ryan's communication gradually improved. It was so exciting to hear a voice that had been hidden for so long. When he first learned speech using the ABA approach, Ryan's responses were more robotic than conversational. My son didn't have volume control or proper voice inflection. These skills needed to be taught, and his progress wasn't always a steady uphill climb to success.

There were so many times I wanted to quit. This was just taking too long.

Yet, even with these stunning improvements, Ryan was still unfocused, disorganized, and . . . well...weird. His social skills were deficient and a major contributor to his peer isolation despite all the strategies we used to attract other kids. Even when Ryan did start talking in sentences, he spoke about whatever popped into his head. Ryan had no filter, nor did he know how to show interest in anything anyone else said. He said all the things we think but wouldn't ever say out loud. If the lady in the grocery store checkout was overweight, Ryan informed her. If the man next to him had forgotten to take a shower, we were all reminded. I never knew when he would say something that would make most parents want to crawl under a table and hide. And being Ryan's mother cured me of ever being embarrassed again. Good luck trying to embarrass me now.

ABA is a time-intensive, person-intensive, and cost-intensive therapy. As much as I wanted it, no agency could do ABA for us at the level of intensity Ryan required. Most agencies suggest at least forty hours a week of ABA. But we probably did more. Most parents work more than forty hours a week to teach their typical kids all the things they need to know. But it is done naturally, so it doesn't seem like it is work.

Every parent must learn how to work directly with their child, so they can address every behavior and every learning issue as soon as it surfaces, when it surfaces, and every time it surfaces in multiple settings. We must learn the techniques needed to help our kids. And as much as we'd like someone to do this for us, no one is signing up to do our job. This is a job that must and will fall to the parents.

We started ABA with Ryan by holding a training weekend for the people whom I thought would become his therapists. Most of the people involved in the initial training were not the ones we finally ended up with. It isn't enough to want to help a kid with autism; it isn't enough to be nice or patient or kind or loving. You have to be consistent, determined, and relentless in order to be effective with ABA.

When someone didn't have the right personality or the stamina to make Ryan conform to his ABA drills, I let them go. I felt uncomfortable when I fired one of these caring people who just wanted to help my son, but Ryan had to be the first priority. Like Mr. *All-Heart* Shawn, not everyone could deliver ABA in a consistent, effective way. Ryan's antics required a positive attitude, perseverance, and the ability to outlast him. I knew how hard this was because I couldn't always do it myself.

Professionals can help and do provide respite, but parents must be the main ingredient in the teaching process and teach their autistic children wherever they happen to be: at home, in the store, or at the park on the swings. ABA requires the child to connect *stimulus* with desired *response*, and the only way to do this is in a setting outside a therapist's office. The response must be done *immediately* when that teaching moment happens. You must be ready to drop everything else to help the child form that connection each and every time it is needed, no matter the time of day or night.

Medical treatment combined with ABA revolutionized Ryan's world.

Like any child, Ryan learned best when he was healthy. He was getting there. We had always loved Ryan, now we actually liked him, too. When Dr. Harvey and I got tired of fighting about Ryan's diet and that evil cookie I put in my son's lunch, we could always fight about ABA. ABA still remained a major bone of contention between us. I am convinced that every medical protocol needs to be supported by an intense rehabilitation program. Dr. Harvey disagrees and is completely opposed to using ABA.

Dr. Harvey believes normal discipline and teaching are all that is needed to catch our children up on all they missed. He is partially correct. As Ryan became healthier, we were able to we move away from a strict ABA stimulus-response model toward a more natural way of teaching. But **nothing worked before we helped Ryan's immune system function better**—not even ABA.

Dr. Harvey was a big part of saving my child, but he was not the rehabilitation expert he thought he was. He was the medical expert. He needed to stay away from giving behavioral and educational advice and stick to his area of medical expertise. Most of his patients that fully recovered used ABA in one form or another.

One time, after a particularly vicious argument about the merits of ABA, Ryan's doctor jokingly suggested we go to counseling together since we fought like an old married couple. After we laughed about what he said, I realized no one can exasperate me more quickly than he does. Even so, we still share the same mission: to make the medical community understand that our children are *ill*, not *damaged beyond repair*. Where we now differ is in our view of the role of behavioral and educational supports for his medical protocol. Of course, we still fought about the diet. Our cookie argument never really went away.

Everything Ryan missed or lost while he was ill had to be systematically retaught. It was the medical plus ABA combination that opened the door for Ryan's success and learning. Remember, Frank and I desperately tried to teach Ryan for years, and it had been a miserable failure even though we used the ABA techniques we had learned as undergraduates. Children affected by autism need an intensive rehab program until they start to learn like other kids. There are many different types of therapies available in addition to Applied Behavior Analysis (ABA). Speech therapy, occupational therapy, social skills training, Floortime, Relationship Development Intervention® (RDI®), Son-rise, and TEACCH are just a few others. When medical treatment is combined with behavior and educational interventions, that's when recovery becomes possible. So chose the program you like and stick with it. They all work if you can reduce the "total load" on your child's broken immune system.

We used our own version of ABA with a little RDI® thrown in. ABA focuses on reinforcing behaviors you want to increase and ignores the inappropriate ones you are trying to decrease and eliminate. RDI® is an intensive parent training method that guides children in learning how to have a reciprocal relationship. To promote success and learning RDI® uses what our children love and maybe obsess about to motivate them (we did our own version of this even before it was first invented).[31]

I think of these as external therapies because they act upon the child from outside the child's body. It is healing from *without*. Medical interventions act upon the child using the child's internal environment. It is healing from *within*. You need both forms of artillery to win the war.

Medical treatment alone will not correct the autism issue. Initially, our children don't know how to learn on their own. So ABA or whatever focused rehabilitation you like best is also needed. Our family worked all day, every day, intensively supporting Ryan as he learned the things we directly taught him. All children need a supportive family in order to grow and progress, but children with autism need us even more.

I can't explain why some kids don't recover like Ryan. Luck is also a part of the equation. We happened to get the right doctor early enough in Ryan's development to treat him medically. Ryan was lucky that Dr. Harvey's protocol directly addressed his type of autism. Dr. H's treatment plan has helped a great number of children recover, but it doesn't work for all children. Even the Harvey protocol cannot lure every child with autism away from their island. After the medical intervention, the hard part starts. You have to directly teach the children everything they missed.

This is a complex and difficult disease to control, but it is treatable for many. Recovery is possible if a child's immune system is not too compromised by the time they get to a doctor who knows what they are doing. It is also important to note that even if I could have waved a magic wand and made Ryan's immune system normal, he wouldn't have behaved normally. It took years of ABA to develop the speech and appropriate social skills he missed.

---

31 Relationship Development Intervention® (RDI®) is a family-based behavioral treatment developed by Dr. Steven Gutstein, PhD. The goal of RDI® is to fix the social issues that are part of autism by helping children interact positively with family members and others. As children learn to value personal relationships, it becomes easier to use this guided participation to teach them language and social skills.

Usually it takes a typical kid without the immune issues three years to learn speech. In time and with practice, even our children learn to talk naturally with all the slang expressions, confusing idioms, and even a curse word thrown in now and then.

Parents sometimes think their children will begin talking in complete sentences after starting medical treatment, but it doesn't work that way. So, using speech as an indicator that the medical treatment is working is not always a good idea. After we helped Ryan's immune system improve, he then had the capacity to learn speech. We still needed to teach him what he missed. And that wouldn't have happened without some kind of intensive rehab program.

For kids with autism, English is almost like a foreign language.

It took me three years sitting in a Spanish class before I could put together a sentence that wasn't one of the set phrases in the textbook. It is the same with our children on the spectrum.

When you learn another language, first you listen, and then you understand; but you still can't speak the language for some time. I worked with Ryan from morning to night to increase his language and speech.

We did it when we were cruising the supermarket aisles or on the swings in the park. I read to him and watched TV shows with him like *Sesame Street, Mr. Rogers' Neighborhood*, and *Doug*. I provided computer programs by Edmark (everything they do is linguistically based). I wish the iPad and other computer tablets had been around then because they have so many programs that help our kids.

Parents will do anything to help their kids. However, sometimes we don't have the confidence it takes to do so or, maybe more accurately, the stubbornness we need to realize we can do the rehabilitation ourselves with a little training. Many parents believe only trained experts are effective. That is not really true. Nobody does rehabilitation as well as a parent who has that burning desire to help their child recover. What we do wrong in technique is made up for in determination and commitment.

If I Knew Then What I Know Now

I would have paid any amount of money for some respite from the exhausting and full-time job of teaching Ryan everything. I desperately wanted anyone else to do this for me. Fortunately for Ryan, there was no one in Minnesota to pro-vide ABA when we needed it. We had no choice but to learn these methods and do them ourselves. But without knowing it at the time, this turned out to be a blessing in disguise. The fact that our family became proficient using ABA was one of the major factors that helped Ryan recover. He was always learning because we were always teaching him throughout his day.

Unfortunately, any parent embarking on this twenty-four/seven assignment won't have much of a life until their child reaches a certain behavioral level. Frank and I didn't regain any semblance of a social life until Ryan was in fifth grade. For many years before that, it was necessary to sacrifice everything in our own lives to put in the time it took to teach Ryan what he needed to know aca-demically, socially, and behaviorally. The hardest part was giving up everything for years when his future remained uncertain. If I had known he was going to recover, I would have had no trouble keeping the twenty-four/seven pace.

For families, recovering a child is always a balancing act. Often, helping our children becomes our major focus and takes over our lives. When I look back at what it took for Ryan to recover, I was consumed, obsessed, and engulfed by all things autism. Where do you think our kids' obsessive natures come from? The apple doesn't fall far from the tree. I still have difficulty finding a balance. Even though our family escaped from Autism Island, autism still significantly affects every member of our family.

My new challenge is to balance fighting the war against autism for other parents with being a whole person again. I had to write Ryan's story to help others. However, it seemed to take forever for me to write it. There was no work on this book when I helped Megan with her fixer-upper condo or when I helped Ryan find his first apartment. My kids continue to come first before anyone or anything else (even my ever-loving Frank). I'm not sure that is the right thing to do, but it is how I balance my life today.

Sometimes, I feel guilty because Ryan is okay and having a wonderful life. This should be the outcome for all children who are ill with autism. I often question why some of our kids who have amazing parents and do all the right things don't fully recover. Why does it take longer to repair some of our chil-dren's immune issues while others respond immediately and profoundly? Could it be that their children's immune systems are just too compromised? Were their children older by the time they found appropriate medical care, and it took more time to teach them the volumes of things they missed? Or was the doctor working on their child's immune issues not addressing the root of the problem? (In our case, prescription meds were needed, and they still have been needed into adulthood.) And were good therapies done in the wrong order, so the prerequisite building blocks weren't there? As of yet, we don't know the answers to these important questions.

I pray that one day we will know.

CHAPTER 23

THE NOT-SO-FAMOUS "DR. PHIL" TAKES OVER

Everybody should have the opportunity to be everything they can be.

—Dr. Phil McGraw

I TURNED TO our family practice doctor in Minnesota for help after we stopped seeing Dr. Harvey. Dr. Phil Sidell witnessed firsthand how the medications helped Ryan and was willing to continue them. He continued to monitor Ryan's blood work, especially his liver function. Dr. Phil was there when we needed him most. There was a noticeable contrast in the bedside manner of Ryan's two doctors. Sometimes, Dr. Phil had me laughing so hard at Ryan's appointments that I forgot why we were there. We all enjoyed the change.

Around the same time, Ryan's speech teacher, Kathryn Hagen, suddenly and tragically lost her youngest son. Daniel was only twelve (the same age as Ryan) when he died. He had been in the basement watching TV when Kathryn found him.

We all felt the impact and the pain of a death that seemed so unjust. This was Ryan's first experience with death, and his autistic need for order and predictability immediately clashed with the completely unexplained and awful circumstance of Daniel's passing.

Ryan's world suddenly became unpredictable and frightening. My son developed a horrendous fear that what happened to Daniel could happen to him.

Like the rest of us, Ryan struggled to understand Daniel's death. His search for why it occurred expressed itself in repeated and obsessive handwashing. My kid needed to protect himself from the germs he *knew* were responsible for Daniel's death. Maybe it would be safer on Autism Island where no one died while watching television? The repetitive handwashing caused his hands to become raw, and most of our conversations centered on death and dying. Our nerves were soon just as raw.

Even on our worst days with Ryan, we still had a child to hold and love. Kathryn's arms were empty. We all went to the funeral chapel to support Kathryn. When we first walked in, Frank whispered to me that maybe Ryan shouldn't come in because Daniel was in an open casket. However, my child with hypersensitive hearing never missed anything he wasn't supposed to hear.

Ryan immediately responded to Frank's remark by saying, "Too late."

We stayed in the viewing room and waited in line to give Kathryn our condolences. Ryan's teacher hugged him tightly as her son lay in the coffin behind her. Without Ryan saying a word, his beloved Kathryn knew exactly what he was thinking. I will never forget her selfless comment she made to him that day. "Ryan, you know this would never happen to you?"

She ignored her own suffering as she tried to comfort my son. But her sincere words didn't prevent Ryan from becoming consumed with thoughts of dying and germs. When I didn't know what else to do, I called Dr. Phil's office to ask for a referral to a psychiatrist. Dr. Phil told me to bring Ryan into the office instead.

Dr. Phil sat on the examining table next to my son and spent over an hour giving him a crash course in Germs 101. Dr. Phil was a younger version of Marcus Welby, MD. He was like the caring physician on that old television show and spent as much time with his patients as was needed. Dr. Phil treated the whole patient, not just the physical ailment.

Our doctor explained the secret life of germs to Ryan in terms he would understand, adding gross stories and his own version of bathroom humor. Dr. Phil knew of Ryan's restricted interest with anything having to do with airplanes. In a genius move, he linked Ryan's love of airplanes with Daniel's tragic passing.

Dr. Phil asked my son, "How many airplanes out of the thousands in the air all over the country crashed yesterday?" Dr. Phil immediately had Ryan's full attention and was speaking his language. With complete logic, our doctor went on to say that when an airplane crashes, we all hear about it because it happens so infrequently. Dr. Phil informed Ryan that in all his years of being a physician, he never had a kid from his practice die.

And he didn't expect Ryan—a kid in his practice—to die.

That was the beginning of the end of Ryan's handwashing problem. Ryan listened and learned a great lesson. And so did I.

If I Knew Then What I Know Now

I still wonder all these years later if Dr. Phil was talking to me when he helped Ryan understand about death and dying. Maybe my lesson was that autism is kind of like an airplane crash. It is a tragic event, but life goes on. I needed to move on. Maybe I was as obsessed with autism as Ryan had been with handwashing. Ryan searched for germs that did not exist; I searched for cures that did not exist. If that was Dr. Phil's lesson for me, I was still too far in the trenches to hear his voice. I would continue to scrub my hands raw with frustration and anger for many, many years to come. How could I move on and leave Ryan behind to a life in an institution? Still, what Dr. Phil did for Ryan that day was not the first or last time he came to our rescue. I'm not sure I ever really thanked him for all the things he did for us over the years.

But, Dr. Phil, I'm thanking you now.

CHAPTER 24

GENA, BABYSITTER
EXTRAORDINAIRE

When everything goes to hell, the people who stand by you without flinching, they are your family.

—Jim Butcher

DESPERATE PEOPLE DO desperate things. That was me. I approached a stranger in a mall and asked her—almost ordered her—to babysit my kids. I was trying to find shoes for Megan, while Ryan was busy lining up shoeboxes and sniffing the tennis shoes inside. Gena struck up a conversation with Megan and even included Ryan in spite of his limited speech and peculiar olfactory passions. I complimented Gena about her wonderful way with children. Next, I asked if she would ever consider babysitting my kids. We exchanged telephone numbers. Victory was mine. I captured *Gena, Babysitter Extraordinaire*.

Gena soon became part of our ABA family and, in time, our immediate family. She turned out to be the only one from the original ABA training group who could actually do ABA properly. It was a good thing she excelled at ABA because she was going to need it if she was going to be Ryan's babysitter.

Gena unknowingly threw us a life raft. Now, Frank and I could leave Autism Island temporarily. I needed that night out for my sanity and my marriage. And no one else but Gena, Babysitter Extraordinaire, could handle the task.

A babysitter we trusted who used ABA with Ryan while Frank and I escaped to the movies for a short time... *Heaven!*

Gena made Megan and Ryan feel like babysitting them was an invitation to an evening of adventure. Gena earned celebrity status in our house. Frank and I were not usually missed once the doorbell rang announcing Gena's arrival. But even with Gena, things didn't always run smoothly. Somehow we were never fully prepared for what life with Ryan sometimes brought. But living in our unpredictable world made us expect the unexpected.

One evening, when Frank and I left for a much-needed dinner in an adult restaurant with an adult menu, we returned to the kind of crisis and chaos that only comes when a kid with autism lives in your house. Earlier that day, Marie, Megan's beloved goldfish, died. Tommy and Marie were Christmas presents two years before. On that Christmas, she walked right past the elaborate dollhouse I had laboriously decorated for weeks to watch Marie and Tommy swim in and out of their tiny, ugly, plastic fish castle. She never did play with the dollhouse. It became Ryan's present, but the only thing that interested him was the miniature toilet lid, which he opened and closed a billion times.

Earlier that day, we held an afternoon backyard burial ceremony to help Megan mourn Marie's passing, and we tried to cheer her up with the news of Gena's visit that evening. That fish funeral was something to behold. Marie was wrapped in a paper towel shroud and placed in a decorated shoebox. We reverently buried her under the juniper tree and said a few words to send her on her journey across the rainbow bridge to the afterlife. Ryan took a huge interest in all the preparations and tried to figure out what this all meant.

I forgot to explain it to him.

We returned from our evening out to tears of rage streaming down Megan's face. We are lucky Ryan is still alive today because this was one of those times Megan couldn't control herself. She was furious with Ryan. She told us Ryan had deliberately killed Tommy by taking him out of the fish tank.

Tommy was certainly quite dead and lying on his side beside the tank.

Lining up shoeboxes in public, killing a sibling's pet fish, and murderously angry children were reasons why past babysitters never came back. But Gena always did. When we asked Ryan why he took Tommy out of the fish tank, he innocently answered that Tommy wanted to be with Marie. Megan never forgave him for this even though I'm still not sure Ryan was actually responsible for Tommy's demise. If Tommy had been healthy, there is no way Ryan could have caught him and removed him from the tank.

When Gena babysat, she did more than just watch my kids and ensure their safety. It was an intensive therapy session almost the entire evening. Gena used activities and anything Ryan obviously liked as motivation to teach him new things. This concept was one of the important ingredients for success when helping my son. Gena used what he loved (or, more accurately, obsessed about) to reinforce any target behavior we were working on. Using what Ryan loved became our number-one rule when anyone worked with Ryan.

Children who have autism do not find the same things rewarding that a typical child might. It seems obvious to use something that an individual child enjoys to reward behavior, but it is not always easy to identify what those things may be. As parents, we have to stop and think hard about what might work with our children and remember it is different for every child. And remember: all children love hugs and praise even if they don't always show us that is true.

Ryan loved to play hide-and-seek, so Gena used that game and added a new twist to teach him receptive and expressive language. Before anyone found a hiding spot, they had to give a verbal clue that helped the person who was "IT" know where to look. For example, Gena might say, "I'm going to hide where people sleep." That narrowed down the places Ryan had to look. That way, the game didn't go on too long or become frustrating. The bonus was Ryan had to listen carefully and learn receptive language in order to find the Gena he loved.

When it was Ryan's turn to hide, he had to generate a clue of his own (expressive language). He might say in *Ryan Speak*, " . . . where brush teeth." Gena would soon find him in the bathtub hiding behind the shower curtain.

Another mom used this same concept to teach her son speech. One of her son's restricted interests was *Blue's Clues*. She printed paw prints from the Nick Jr. website and hid them all over the house. Next, she would send her son on a mission to find them. When he found one, he was required to tell her where it was located, such as "under the table" or "behind the TV." All of us learn concepts more quickly when we are interested in the subject, motivated, and having fun.

Gena also applied ABA techniques to help Ryan become more flexible. When she played board games such as *Sorry!*, Ryan was no longer always allowed to go first or always use the blue game pieces. This was a huge battle for all of us and a major victory when Ryan finally complied. Strangely enough, when Ryan was an adult and picked his first apartment, it was on First Street, and the building was painted blue. Megan's response after hearing about his new apartment was, "Of course, it is blue and on First Street." All of us still tease Ryan about his old obsessions. In our family, everything we do, good or bad, becomes a source of amusement for the others.

And nothing is ever forgotten.

If I Knew Then What I Know Now

Recruiting, training, and assessing potential ABA therapists for Ryan taught me that too many professionals use their credentials as a substitute for ability. The people equipped with the pedigrees "know" you can't fix kids with autism, so they don't even try. The untrained have not yet been corrupted by dead-end developmental theory. They were usually better ABA therapists for Ryan. They actually believed Ryan could learn and behave, and they expected him to do just that. Do not have anyone on your kid's team who does not believe your child can potentially recover!

I had no references nor knew anything about Gena, but I did know she had the right attitude and personality. I saw how she interacted with Ryan and Megan. Gena was innately positive and set clear limits for Ryan. She had a high school diploma and no advanced degrees. Her main source of income was her position as a salesperson in a department store. But she knew more about how to teach my son than any of those super-credentialed professionals. Gena turned out to be more than I could have anticipated or hoped for.

ABA must be taught methodically, and it works optimally when it is used by everyone in the child's world. Gena helped us appreciate the power of early intervention and made us wish we had started ABA therapy much, much sooner. Extinguishing Ryan's ingrained behaviors, compliance training, and teaching him basic communication and social skills took hours and days and months and years of work. The earlier parents act to help their children, the less reteaching they need to do and the less unwanted behaviors there will be to deal with or extinguish. It just makes sense.

Therapists who come into the child's home are fine, but what they accomplish is easily undone if family members do not continue what the therapists started. For us, ABA was a team effort. The entire family and even the babysitter learned it and applied the ABA techniques consistently throughout Ryan's day.

If that sounds like it was overwhelming . . . it was.

CHAPTER 25

IT TOOK ALL OF US AND THEN SOME TO HELP RYAN

Some of the world's greatest feats were accomplished by people not smart enough to know they were impossible.

—Doug Larson

ABA WAS NOW a family affair. Ryan was our ABA project, and we were in this together. A better Ryan meant a happier family. A happier family meant a happier me. A happier me meant a relieved Frank.

Each of us had a different role in Ryan's therapy and our own set of responsibilities. We worked with Ryan day and night to teach him everything he still needed to learn. Frank was in charge of how to catch a ball and any skills that required physical dexterity. Megan did pretend games, board games, and LEGO toys. Gena was our recreation specialist. She taught him all kinds of things he still needed to learn and at the same time made it fun. All of us incorporated following directions, speech, sequencing, social skills, and compliance in everything we taught Ryan. I filled in wherever I was needed. I also determined what else needed to be taught and suggested possible ways to teach it. But my most important job was making sure everyone was doing what they were supposed to do. That included the management of his home program to incorporate whatever would make Ryan be more successful at school.

Ryan ran his life and our lives by the clock. He liked any game show where events were timed. His favorite was a particular kid's action-adventure TV game show called *Legends of the Hidden Temple*. In this show, different teams competed by performing timed physical stunts and answering general knowledge questions. The show centered on a Mayan temple filled with lost treasures protected by mysterious temple guards. He would watch it over and over again and was fascinated with the time component.

Gena came up with our home version of the game. Ryan used receptive language to follow verbal directions we gave on a house-wide treasure hunt. He needed to answer questions by using expressive language, which allowed him to advance on the Steps of Knowledge just like on his favorite TV show. We asked him questions about sharks, numbers, or one of his other interests. If he answered the question correctly, he would win the right to get closer to the treasure hidden somewhere in our house.

Ryan had to be careful that the evil temple guards, played by Frank and Megan, didn't capture him on the way to the hidden treasure. Sometimes, a temple guard would jump out from a hiding place to get him. Ryan loved playing the game, and he loved being frightened when the temple guards almost got him. On every birthday, part of our family tradition is to share a family memory about the birthday girl or boy. One of Frank's favorite Ryan memories involved this game and the expression on Ryan's face when the temple guards jumped out and tried to get him.

Ryan loved this game, but it was so much more than a game. These activities compelled him to listen and focus on following our directions carefully in order to retrieve the treasure. We started with very simple directions like "Find your car in your bedroom and bring it back to me." When he mastered that skill, we made it harder by involving three-step commands. Eventually, he was able to work up to four-step directions. He thought he was just playing, but our playing had important goals and significant results.

When I wasn't working with him, my husband was. When one of us wasn't teaching him, Megan worked with him. We tag teamed him all day long. Maybe this is why Ryan has such a great work ethic today. Megan taught him how to play like a typical child. Since she was only three years his senior, she was at ease with teaching him how to play, something the rest of us had long forgotten. We paid her a dollar an hour. She was an important part of Ryan's treatment team. Plus, this helped her feel involved and also helped with the fact that Ryan took so much of our time.

Before we could teach Ryan anything, we had to get him to pay attention and to listen. If he didn't, we sometimes used *The Chair* for compliance training. But we mostly made it fun so that he wanted to play. When he didn't do something we asked, or if he did something we were trying to eliminate (like biting his sister), we immediately and calmly led him to The Chair and made him work at something he found mundane. Ryan quickly learned that if he did what was asked, he got to escape from The Chair and *Go Play*. Eventually, he understood that we expected him to listen and comply with whatever we asked him to do even when we weren't playing a game.

After Ryan finally was under control at home, he was still a terror when we went anywhere else.

In public, I didn't have The Chair with me, so he didn't listen to anything I said. He knew I would not make him "Stand up, sit down, and clap your hands" without The Chair. I was lost without my secret weapon, and Ryan knew it.

When I didn't know how to solve this one, I called a mom in Virginia for help. She was the one who first convinced me to give ABA a second look. I was shocked when Cindy said she had been known to do ABA in the middle of the grocery store while everyone was watching. I asked her if she worried about someone calling social services or questioning what she was doing. Cindy solved that dilemma for me as well: she suggested using the restroom. Her message was clear: Focus on the ABA techniques to control Ryan's behavior and gain compliance. Just forget about everyone else, because Ryan's life was at stake.

It didn't take long for Ryan to test me.

Lorene, our family hairdresser (and one of the women I picked for Frank to marry in the event Ryan put me in an early grave) was cutting Ryan's hair when he started another of his classic meltdowns. Haircuts were difficult for Ryan. Lorene was always patient and kind to Ryan, no matter how awful he behaved. That was why I picked her to be one of Frank's possible future brides.

Ryan was sitting on my lap, just like he always did during haircuts. Lorene never used the noisy clippers because Ryan couldn't tolerate the noise they made. She always cut his hair with scissors that gently snipped at his brown locks. I read him his favorite number and letter books to distract him while Lorene set a new Guinness World Record for the fastest haircut ever. At that time, we still used some of the old distraction methods to help Ryan cope. Even though I did everything possible to prevent a meltdown that day, my efforts didn't work.

Ryan tried to fly out of my lap as he began one of his best Linda Blair *Exorcist* impressions. This was clearly an ABA moment, but we were at the salon, and I wasn't armed with my "magic" chair. This time, I wasn't going to wait for Ryan's head to start spinning around. This time, I couldn't make an undignified exit from the mall.

This time, I had to win!

I turned to Lorene and calmly told her we would be right back. Without any emotion or explanation, I took Ryan's hand and led him behind a pillar just outside the salon entrance. Trying to hide behind the pillar didn't work so well. The cement column didn't provide much cover for this battle. Everyone inside and outside the hair salon was staring at us. I did the same routine without the benefit of The Chair. I ended the compliance drill by stating the behavior I expected from him, "Are you going to sit *the right way* and finish getting your haircut?" When his answer was "yes," we went back inside to Lorene's station. That was the last meltdown Ryan had during a haircut. Was it easy to squat behind a pillar and do strange stuff to a child in a public place? No. Everyone stared at me like I was a crazy woman. It should have occurred to me to use the bathroom in the salon, but I didn't think of that.

But it didn't matter. I had put an important notch in my ABA belt.

If ABA was hard for Ryan, it was even harder for me. My personal challenge was to never get mad or show any emotion when we led him to The Chair. Eye rolls, sighs, lips pressed together . . . all my anger outlets were prohibited. Ryan couldn't know he was getting *any* kind of reaction from me. He still craved sameness. He liked a predictable reaction even when it was an angry one. The sameness was more important to Ryan than a positive reward for doing the right thing. I also had to stop feeling sorry for Ryan. I used to rationalize Ryan's behavior by saying he couldn't help doing the things he did. His autism made him act this way. Those kinds of thoughts didn't help.

My feeling sorry for him actually reinforced the behavior I so despised. If Frank had married sweet Lorene, Ryan would have stayed autistic. Frank needed to stay married to me. I just wasn't allowed to die before I completed my mission to fix Ryan. I had to do that not just for Ryan, but because fixing Ryan seemed to be fixing me.

If I Knew Then What I Know Now

Cindy's simple solution to use a restroom and my successful intervention behind a too-small decorative pillar helped me wean myself from my dependence on The Chair. I realized it wasn't about a piece of furniture—it was about the drill—and I needed to stand on my own two ABA feet if I was to really be successful helping Ryan manage his behavior in public places or anywhere else he misbehaved.

Some people who don't understand ABA methods mistakenly think it is a contrived method of teaching that creates robotic responses. During the initial stages of implementing an ABA program, it sometimes looks that way. But when done correctly, ABA facilitates learning. Our favorite and gifted teachers all use these ABA techniques without realizing it.

CHAPTER 26

PAM CHANGED RYAN'S LIFE AND HE CHANGED HERS

It's the little details that are vital. Little things make big things happen.

—John Wooden

PAM WAS RYAN'S private swim instructor and my next potential ABA recruit. Pam was attending the University of Minnesota, and in her spare time she taught swimming lessons. Again, I chose her because I saw how she used ABA principles without even realizing it. Pam set clear limits, positively reinforced desired behaviors, and didn't put up with any of Ryan's crap. That didn't happen with many people. This got me thinking.

When I first approached Pam and asked if she wanted to do ABA with Ryan, she said, "No." I asked Pam several time to reconsider. I think she knew I planned to continue asking. She finally agreed to watch the tape of Mindi teaching us ABA techniques. I'm not sure if she did this to stop my pleading, but it really didn't matter. After watching the tapes, Pam was in!

Pam's strength as an ABA therapist was the same as Gena's. Pam was amazing at identifying and then implementing effective motivators to reinforce and, therefore, to teach new behaviors. She thought of interesting and curious new ways to keep my son's attention to engage him. Pam used Ryan's advanced ability with numbers and maps and his limitless interest in sharks to make him attend to whatever skill she was trying to teach.

Instead of Ryan's restricted interests being a barrier to learning, Pam used them as a bridge to learning. Why was using a restricted interest so important? How many times have we heard our children's teachers complain about the negative impact restricted interests have on the classroom as a whole? How many IEP meetings focus on the nuisance of restricted interests and cite them as a reason to move the child to a more restrictive educational environment or special education classroom?

What so many teachers don't realize is the learning potential those annoying interests hold. Instead of confiscating that book on sharks, instead of forbidding the child from bringing their favorite animal character to school, instead of doing everything they can to rid the classroom of the infestation of restricted interests, teachers need to include our children's interests as an integral part of their education and reinforcement schedule. Both Pam and Gena understood this, and that was why they both were so very effective.

When Pam first came into our lives, my strange and occasionally advanced kid loved to study maps and atlases. He could draw an exact map of Europe to scale, freehand, complete with the capitals of each country. If you wanted to know anything about any kind of shark, just ask Ryan. He could spit out every useless fact about the tiger shark, or any shark for that matter. If you wanted to know anything about Jacques Cousteau, Ryan could tell you. Or if you needed an answer to anything involving math, Ryan was your guy. He was my human calculator and light-years ahead of his peers in math. He used to beg me to go to the teacher supply store to buy him math workbooks. He loved the predictability of workbooks, and his favorite was math probably because the rules were always the same.

Pam designed speech drills about sharks. He loved the computer, so she used it to teach the importance of waiting for his turn. Pam designed physical exercise drills that used his restricted interests to reinforce what she intended to teach him. For Ryan, physical things were the hardest. Occasionally, she used his favorite foods or candy to motivate him for things that were physically challenging and difficult for Ryan.[32] But more often than not, she used his love of numbers instead of the highly motivating but evil cookies and candy. Ryan had to throw a ball into a basket five times. When she put him through an obstacle course to improve his gross motor skills, his favorite computer game was the last thing he had to do at the finish line.

At the beginning of each session, Ryan and Pam would come up with their plan for the day. Ryan chose the first activity because he still always had to be first. Pam ignored this quirkiness for the time being. She saved that battle for later. Pam wrote down his ideas and their plan for the day on the whiteboard. Ryan usually chose to play computer, imaginary play with Fisher Price people sets, board games, Play-Doh, or play *Legends of the Hidden Temple*. Next, it was Pam's turn to pick an activity.

They went back and forth choosing activities until the whiteboard had the entire to-do activities listed for that day's session. Ryan would erase the activity after they completed it. Knowing what to expect was reassuring for Ryan. When it was Pam's turn, she picked a skill or behavior that did not come easily to Ryan. Activity number two might be a fine motor activity such as coloring. At almost six years of age, Ryan only knew how to scribble. To master this skill, Pam colored letters and numbers with Ryan. Sometimes, they did dot-to-dot number pictures because he loved anything that involved numbers or letters. She used every one of his restrictive interests to promote learning.

Every activity that Ryan found difficult was broken down into step-by-step components. First, he would have to outline the number. Second, he would have to color the inside. Third, he would have to choose a different color for each number. Suddenly, coloring was no longer an overwhelming motor planning task. Now there were step-by-step rules he had learned to follow. When Ryan first learned how to write letters and numbers, Pam used dots that he had to connect to write a letter or number. That way, this drill was not so

---

32 In the ABA world things that are intrinsically rewarding like food or candy are called *primary reinforcers*. Primary reinforcers were highly motivating, and we used them with Ryan for behaviors that were difficult for him.

overwhelming. Eventually, these *prompts*[33] were phased out and he could write the numbers and letters without dots to help him.

Eventually, Ryan worked up to coloring larger objects and images, some of which were unrelated to his restricted interests. Having mastered the sequencing skill set, Ryan was now able to relax and be more flexible when they colored. In time, after he experienced success, he even began to enjoy coloring.

Nevertheless, it wasn't always smooth sailing when Pam worked with my son. This was the norm for life with Ryan, and her sessions with him didn't always go as planned. Ryan still needed to conquer one of his personal monsters. He had immense trouble taking turns when playing a game. One day, the two of them sat in the basement in front of the computer screen playing Monopoly. He was upset he couldn't be first, so he didn't want to play anymore.

I listened from upstairs as the battle raged.

Pam remained both calm and consistent during one of the biggest meltdowns Ryan ever had. She made him continue with the Monopoly game over his escalating and piercing shrieks of protest. Pam *made* him comply. I probably would have given in. Pam didn't. She made him take his turn, and then wait while she took hers.

When the session was over, Ryan stayed downstairs as Pam raced up the stairs to escape from my little monster. When she saw me, she burst into tears. I could only hug her as both of us cried. She knew she couldn't let Ryan see that he had gotten to her. That was the only time Ryan pushed her past her limit. Pam was more patient and consistent than anyone else who worked with him, including me.

Ryan had me ready to jump off the ledge on a regular basis even though I tried to never let him know. I was so afraid Pam might not come back to be abused once again by my son that I found myself *calling a florist.*

She came back the very next day at the scheduled time. The flowers had nothing to do with her choice to return. Pam was in it for the long haul. There isn't enough money in the world to compensate Pam for all she did for my son

---

33 The ABA term for any action that makes a desired response more likely to happen.

and our family. She was all about helping kids, and while my Ryan was the first beneficiary of her ABA expertise, he would not be the last.

As it turned out, working with my son influenced what Pam ended up doing for her career. After she graduated from the University of Minnesota, Pam returned to Chicago to work with children who needed ABA.

Along the way, Pam became an RDI® Certified Consultant and worked with parents to empower them to take charge of what to do with their children at school and at home. She still teaches families the techniques necessary to help change outcomes for their child on the spectrum. Pam understands how much autism impacts everyone in the family. She saw our struggle, and she knew that in order to help the child, the entire family has to be part of the solution.

We've stayed in contact with Pam over the years. Whenever Ryan did something extraordinary, or sometimes when he would do something very ordinary that I never dared dream he would do, I would give Pam a call. That is how she first learned about the RDI® school opening up in Los Angeles. She moved from Chicago to take a teaching position there under Dr. Gutstein, the founder of RDI®.

After the school closed, two of her fellow teachers joined forces with Pam to develop the *Engage* classroom program.[34] I know Pam will be instrumental in changing the way our children are taught in our schools because that is what Pam does—she changes lives.

If I Knew Then What I Know Now

Pam proved that ABA can be done effectively without going bankrupt. I didn't pay her nearly enough or even close to what an ABA therapist from an agency would get. Some of those agencies charge ridiculous fees and still don't do ABA correctly. Pam was exactly what Ryan needed and much better than all "the experts" that charge buckets of money for their services. This is just one of the many reasons I think it is important for parents to learn ABA themselves—if only to monitor what the "experts" are doing.

---

34 Pam Smith was my secret weapon when it came to helping Ryan. She still works with kids and their families today. Pam changes lives daily.

Before Pam, I worried Ryan would not get what he needed because no one in Minnesota provided ABA behavior therapists at the time. Not having an agency do ABA with Ryan turned out to be a good thing. I now question if Ryan would have come as far as he has if the ABA experts were running the show. Many parents feel that if an intervention requires a lot of money it is better. It is more important to use the right intervention instead of those that cost a fortune.

How much ABA is enough ABA? We did about ten hours a week of Pam formally working with Ryan. However, since we were all trained in ABA, we used ABA techniques all throughout his waking hours. If you count up the ABA hours in Ryan's day, we probably did more than the forty hours per week often recommended.[35] Yet it didn't seem that way to Ryan or us because we were *playing*. We taught him each skill as soon as we saw the need.

Whenever we went anywhere, we just did what parents should do naturally with kids but with a little ABA thrown in. Most times, Ryan had no idea we were teaching him or that we did everything with specific goals in mind. ABA was implemented in the most natural settings using games and Ryan's interests to keep him focused and working.[36]

---

35 Research has shown that forty hours per week of ABA is the optimal amount for children with autism. But regional centers, insurance companies and school districts typically do not fund that many hours. There is little time left for school, and other therapies like OT and speech with that much ABA.

36 Some books we used to learn how to do ABA and other books we found helpful are listed in references section.

Part 5

Conquering the New World

CHAPTER 27

SCHOOL, IEP MEETINGS, AND OTHER CHALLENGES

Hell! There ain't no rules around here. We're trying to accomplish something!

—Thomas Alva Edison

CHILDREN LIVE IN two worlds: home and school. Children with autism excel at failing in both of them. At home, Ryan always had me and the rest of his family to guide and protect him. But I worried about who would do that for him at school. Ryan's hover mother couldn't pack herself next to that cookie in his lunchbox to make sure he was safe, understood, and getting what he needed. I think Individualized Education Programs (IEPs) were created because teachers didn't want us moms coming to school with our children.

The purpose of the IEP meeting is to bring qualified professionals together with you to decide what services your child should receive in order to meet their unique needs. Parents often don't realize their child is entitled to free services immediately after the school district identifies that a need exists—even before starting elementary school.[37]

---

37 Check with your local school district and/or early intervention program to see at what age services may begin. The Individuals with Disabilities Education Act (IDEA) says that all children with disabilities have available to them a "free appropriate public education" (FAPE) to meet their unique needs.

If you want to be a successful advocate for your child, you have to know about IEPs. The IEP process is somewhat difficult to explain and understand, so I want to apologize in advance for that. However, it is something you need to know about. The only thing worse than reading about IEP meetings is preparing for or going to one. But if you understand how things work, the IEP process becomes much easier to navigate.

Is this whole process overwhelming and terribly intimidating? You bet it is!

But don't get too overwhelmed by the thought of IEPs. They are one of those things you have to figure out as you go, kind of like parenting. And the process is a whole lot easier to figure out than our kids. In the beginning, everyone needs someone to help them learn the IEP process. At first, Jackie Rains (our old psychologist) went with us to these meetings. Once we got our sea legs, Frank and I did the meetings on our own. Other parents with older special needs children were also a great resource. They had names for advocates and attorneys who specialize in IEPs.

At the beginning of the IEP process, we didn't have a clue as to what we needed to do. It was difficult to even know what services to ask for. The purpose of this chapter is to help you avoid the same mistakes we made. I hope it saves you time so that your child can receive the services they need as soon as possible. For help getting an IEP started, contact the special education department of your school district. Then request an IEP meeting. If you live in a location with something like the California network of regional centers, then you can also ask your regional center for assistance.

To the teachers involved, your IEP meeting is simply another meeting. To you, your child's entire educational life is at stake. There is the official IEP process of rules and regulations, and there is also the unofficial process that occurs when a team works a little bit harder and goes that extra mile because they genuinely care about you and your child. "You catch more flies with honey" was a phrase that served us well during the IEP process.

After I understood how things worked, IEP planning became my homework. I had to do this while raising a family, becoming a behavioral expert, keeping a house clean, cooking specialty meals, and managing medication issues. I learned how to schmooze the staff, develop personal relationships, and exercise my authority as Ryan's parent. I had to be a diplomat, a crusader, an advocate, and, occasionally, a witch. And sometimes a witch spelled with a "B."

Most of the school personnel who worked with Ryan put his needs first. That being said, there were times I wanted to do bodily harm to a few people in the room during an IEP meeting when they didn't understand my child, what he needed, and what he was entitled to receive. Frank was known to kick me under the table to keep me in check. Most times this worked and kept me from saying things I shouldn't but wanted to very, very badly.

Here are a few things I learned about the IEP process.

Early Intervention Is Critical

Autism doesn't get better without intervention, and each day not doing anything is another day lost to autism. How do you know if your child even needs an IEP? You don't, until you start the process. There are the kids with autism that have an IEP longer than the IRS tax code and some that have only a few interventions. Just like autism, there is a whole spectrum when it comes to IEPs. If your child is struggling with language acquisition, fails behaviorally, or is socially atypical, then it is time to contact your school district and discuss the IEP process. An IEP may help parents obtain the resources to teach their children, especially if what they are doing is not working.

Document Everything

I was lucky to learn to document everything early in the game. Ryan was still in preschool when Gay Pirri taught me one of the most important things I ever learned. Gay was in charge of the speech department for our school district. When no one else was around, she quietly advised me to put *ALL* requests for services *in writing*. Now I understand why Gay said this, but back then I was clueless. When things are put in writing, there are no questions about what you asked for or what is needed to help your child.

The educators involved in your child's IEP are expected to plan wonderful programs for hundreds of kids, fill out piles and piles of paperwork, and actually try to teach your child something in between. They really do want to help your kid, but you need to make it easier for them, so they can. Gay's advice to document everything made us become a more integrated part of the team. Gay realized how hard we were working to help Ryan, so she wanted to help us be as effective as possible.

When things are in writing and documented, it usually prevents misunderstandings about what "is necessary to meet your child's unique educational needs." Remember that phrase. It is an important signal to the IEP team that you know your rights and will take legal action if they do not provide what is requested. I know this all sounds very confrontational. But these meetings really weren't.

Before each IEP meeting, I would send the entire team a note about what Frank and I thought Ryan needed in order to be successful at school. With this advance communication, the team had time to think through the ideas we proposed. They were never caught off guard. Before the meeting, they had time to check to see if what we asked for was even a possibility. This also saved the IEP team time by doing some of the grunt work and communication for them, and in the process we helped Ryan.

The notes I sent before an IEP meeting helped everyone on our IEP team think outside the box. The members of our team came to our meetings prepared and armed with constructive ideas to help my son. At times, we asked the team to do things differently than the district had ever done before.

For example, when Ryan needed adaptive physical education, we asked if these services could be delivered before school. These skills were taught the morning of or the day before they were presented during the regular physical education period to all the children in his class. To be able to participate in the regular PE class, the skills my son didn't know had to be pre-taught in Ryan's adaptive program.

Another reason we never had Ryan pulled out for services was because children with autism have trouble with transitions. I didn't want Ryan to have any services interrupt his school day.

Most times, we never had to be confrontational or get in anyone's face, probably because the staff knew we would if that's what was necessary. And they actually appreciated the fact that I spent a considerable amount of time writing some of the IEP goals so they didn't have to.

As I said before, you always catch more flies with honey. To every IEP meeting, I brought treats; there were cookies and soft drinks for all who attended. This helped make the atmosphere of the meeting lighter. And as a result, I believe we received more cooperation and help from everyone involved in Ryan's IEP.

The IEP is a document that should evolve as your child changes. For us, it never really mattered what the IEP said as long as the people who were helping Ryan did what was needed to address his deficits. But goals in writing become extremely important if your child is not getting the previously agreed upon interventions. These written goals create a paper trail as to what was decided at the IEP meeting and which corresponding services should be happening in the school setting.

Documentation is priceless, so save all the reams of paperwork you accumulate even if you eventually decide to close your child's IEP file. If you have a child who might one day need extra time when he takes the SAT or ACT tests, you will need documentation from the very beginning of his diagnosis or IEP assessments to support your request. This advice might seem like a ridiculously distant possibility when your child is four years old, nonverbal, and having hourly melt-downs, but it turned out to be essential for Ryan to get accommodations on his SAT and ACT college exams.

Of course, parents are so busy managing their kid's autism that their documentation piles tend to look a lot like messy laundry piles. And that just might be the easiest way to impose some order to these mounds of paperwork. Buy a large plastic tub and throw all the documents in there, facedown, using year dividers to separate layers. The layers might be untidy, but at least they will be chronological.

Understand Your Child's Label

The autism label isn't what it used to be. At the time Ryan was diagnosed and receiving school services, an autism spectrum disorder diagnosis came packaged with many different kinds of labels. Today, the DSM-V (that big manual used to define mental disorders) has simplified the diagnosis to "autism spectrum disorder." You either have it, or you don't. However, it still doesn't work that way in IEP meetings.

Sometimes, there is reluctance to use the term "autism" because of the devastation it brings to families and the stigma it assigns to children. When my four-year-old was first diagnosed, I was in denial. I did not want to believe Ryan had autism, and I didn't want anyone to ever say or even think he did. In my mind, the doctors had to be wrong, and he wasn't really autistic at all. Pervasive developmental disorder (PDD) sounded so much better to me than autism.

Mostly, I didn't want my child labeled at all. That was a big mistake on my part. While autism is a hopelessly out-of-date and inaccurate term to describe what our kids suffer from, it is still the only word that opens the door to get the services your child needs. Things like occupational therapy, speech therapy, social skills training, sensory integration therapy, or any other substantial educational services won't happen without the autism label. The terms "NIDS, PDD, or sensory processing disorder" won't do it. Informed parents know what their children really suffer from is autoimmune encephalitis, but it still needs to be called "autism" on the IEP paperwork.

In reality, what I was doing by not using the term "autism" was hurting my son and limiting the services he could obtain to overcome it. It took me some time to realize that I needed to use the A-word so Ryan qualified for services from the school district. With an autism label, he was eligible for an aide in the classroom, more speech and language instruction, and all the other things that would not have happened with any other label. The autism label was necessary to obtain services, but at the same time, unimportant to how we helped him. Saying he had autism shouldn't have bothered me so much because we still remediated Ryan's issues the same way no matter what label we attached to it.

Consider Requesting an Aide

In my opinion, every classroom needs an aide. This is true of classrooms with or without special needs kids. This is especially necessary in the early grades when children are still learning so much about how school works and the behavior expected there. Aides are great at handling the details and problems that occur in classrooms, so teachers can actually teach.

Aides are specifically assigned to your child or assigned to the classroom. I requested that Ryan's aide be introduced as the aide for the entire class even though technically, it was Ryan's label that paid her salary. Ryan's aide helped everyone in his classroom. Ryan never knew that he was the reason for the aide. We didn't want Ryan to become too dependent on anyone. There are aides, and then there are *aides*. Make sure your child doesn't have an aide who does everything, including breathing, for them. Don't ever let the aide sit next to your kid's desk to constantly hover. I know that's almost funny coming from Ryan's mother.

Our school used Ryan's aide in a very efficient manner that helped more children than just my son. Ethan, a boy who struggled with academics all through elementary school, was always placed in Ryan's class. Although Ethan was behind academically, he was not far enough behind to qualify for an aide or any other assistance. In our district, you had to test at least two years behind to qualify for any extra help. In the process of helping Ryan, our IEP team helped other kids like Ethan. Without Ryan, Ethan would have been left alone to struggle. Sometimes having a kid with autism in your class can be a good thing.

Although Ryan rarely needed help with academic instruction, the aide was there to correct him when he was socially inappropriate. When he made a mistake socially, she was immediately there to teach him what was acceptable or the right way to do things. The aide was also there to redirect Ryan when he had trouble attending to the teacher. When he lost his papers and couldn't remember where he put anything, she helped him with organizational skills. The aide also addressed his self-confidence problem by creating situations for him to interact more appropriately. She often had him tutor other kids in math or help them with other academics.

Having autism doesn't automatically entitle your child to an aide, but I believe Ryan's aide was a huge part of helping him learn what he needed to know. Don't be afraid to push the issue of an aide with the IEP team. Remember, you are a key member of the team and know your child better than any of the experts at these meetings. Don't be intimidated by their knowledge or degrees. Ask questions.

If the school says it can't afford an aide, that's not necessarily true. Or if they say your kid doesn't need one, don't believe they know what is best for your child. The list of excuses not to meet your unique child's educational needs can be endless. Excuses might include things like speech is too good, behavior is too bad, kid is too smart or too social, and so on. They might use any excuse to avoid providing additional services.

You have to hold your ground on the important issues. Hire a private psychologist to advocate or to validate that your child needs an aide if that's what you have to do to get one. It will be money well spent. Also, make sure the assigned aide is effective. And never let a lack of credentials make you disqualify a potential aide; sometimes no credentials can actually be a plus. No credentials means there aren't any preconceived ideas about what your kid can't learn or can accomplish.

Summer School Options and Thinking Outside the Box

The idea of summer school does not instill confidence in anyone. No one puffs their chest and boasts, "My son is going to summer school." Nevertheless, summer school or an *extended school year* can be a wonderful option for your child, a big contribution to your sanity, and provide the opportunity to spend one-on-one time with your child's sibling.

When Ryan was in elementary school, the only summer service offered was summer school where all the children on the spectrum were thrown in together in a six-week class. That wouldn't have helped Ryan much, so we declined. Instead, we asked if Ryan's speech therapy could be continued over the summer months in our home for that six-week period. The school district had never done this before, probably because no one had ever asked.

Speech therapy was offered twice a week for only forty-five minutes. That wouldn't have been enough to correct the enormous deficits in Ryan's speech and language. So, we did things a different way. On the other five days Pam or I did forty-five minutes of speech with Ryan. When the speech teacher came to our house, I watched and learned from her. I used her knowledge and expertise to determine what area of speech we needed to tackle next. Her guidance in the beginning years was invaluable until I had the confidence and knowledge to do this on my own.

Our speech therapists also loaned us the costly speech materials we needed. I showed Pam the next area to work on with Ryan. Summers and vacations were the time we worked the hardest since there was no school to interfere with our home program. There is no vacation when you have autism. But we did make the lessons fun for Ryan. We always remembered our number one rule: Use what your kid loves or obsesses about to motivate them. Make learning fun so they want more.

Accepting or Rejecting the IEP Is Not an All or Nothing Proposition

The school district must comply with the law that guarantees a *free and appropriate public education (FAPE) for all students*. Remember, you don't have to accept the entire IEP proposal. It is okay to consent to parts of the IEP and reject other sections. You can do this by adding an additional page to the end of the IEP after the signature page. There, simply list the items you accept followed by the page number where it appears in the IEP. If you consent to most of the IEP, make that additional page about what you will not accept. Then provide the team with three possible dates you are available to meet again to discuss the IEP document. Doing that shows the team that you are cooperating.

Don't Mess with Ryan or His Mother

This is something the IEP team learned from me. I was never afraid to ask for someone else to work with my son when I saw that the person assigned to Ryan was not effective. Our preschool caseworker was the best, but the one in elementary school was awful. She would fight me at every turn and did not offer any real solutions for Ryan.

She should have known better than to take on Ryan's mother.

I had no qualms going over her head to the director of special education and asking for a replacement. They eventually gave us someone who was part of the district staff but not assigned to our particular school. Remember, sometimes thinking outside the box can make good things happen for your child.

Ryan was lucky because he had a mother with chutzpah who trusted her gut. I never waited for someone else to do or plan his program or what he needed. There are many children whose parents lack the confidence or drive to speak up. Remember, you are the expert on your child and know them best. Yes, these people have all the degrees and credentials, but that doesn't mean they know what works for your kid! And don't wait for them to tell you about any programs that might help your child. Some districts purposely withhold information, so they don't have to pay for what your child needs.

If I Knew Then What I Know Now

It took some time before we fully understood that parents have the most important (and final) vote when the IEP team decides on how to meet your child's educational needs. Don't feel that you are required to sign the IEP document at the meeting. Sometimes it is a good idea to take time to think things over. *Remember, no changes to your child's IEP program can be made without your approval.* Just tell the team you need a little more time to discuss things, and you will get back to them in a few days.

There is a fine line you need to walk. You must appear that you are cooperating while at the same time send the message that you will not settle when it comes to the important things for your child. If there is a service you need, but it is denied, you can ask the team to please respond to your request in writing and to please reference the policy that prevents them from granting what you asked for. Sometimes, their objections suddenly disappear with this technique. If they actually give you their objections in writing, and they haven't done things correctly, you have a tremendous amount of leverage.

The Individuals with Disabilities Education Act (IDEA) entitles our children to a "free appropriate public education" (FAPE). But sometimes, we still need to fight to get what our children need. Some think that the fight is even worse now than in years past when I was doing this because now there are so many more options to help our kids. For example, many auditory training therapies are expensive, and schools might try to say there isn't data to justify their paying for them.

To make things worse, there is, of course, an epidemic increase in autism, which has resulted in an increased demand for services. There are not nearly enough resources to meet the growing demand. And parents who are lucky enough to know about a variety of therapeutic programs often have to fight for their children to gain access to them.

A special education attorney once suggested to me that I should record every IEP meeting. Most smartphones now have recording capabilities on them that makes this easier. However, I never taped these meetings because I felt it appeared too confrontational. Our school district was very cooperative, and we usually got the important things we needed for Ryan. However, you may need to consider recording IEP meetings if your school district won't work with you. If you need to enlist the services of an attorney, then there will be a record of what has transpired.

I also made the mistake of thinking all the teachers and IEP team members had to understand Ryan's medical treatment and the ABA behavioral interventions we were using in Ryan's home program. It took me a while to realize that when I spoke about these interventions, all the eyes in the room glazed over. It was almost the same as the look on Ryan's face when he tuned me out. The district personnel had never seen ABA in action nor had any idea that autism could be treated medically back then.

These well-meaning educators didn't believe my kid could actually recover. At that time, I wasn't so sure either. My saying so didn't make them think it. To them, I was just another delusional mom who couldn't accept or deal with my child's diagnosis. What they thought was unimportant as long as Ryan got the services he needed. However, I must admit it felt good when their opinions changed as my child got better. In time, they realized my kid was different from the other children they worked with who hadn't had medical treatment or an intensive rehab program. Later, some even asked about the medical things we did so they could help their other students.

CHAPTER 28

EVERYTHING RYAN NEEDED TO KNOW HE DIDN'T LEARN IN KINDERGARTEN

The greatest pleasure in life is doing what people say you cannot do.

—Walter Bagehot

MOST PARENTS FEEL excited and happy about the first day of kindergarten...*not* us.

This is just one more way life is different for parents in the A-Club. Ryan wasn't even close to being ready to start kindergarten. We had been doing the medical and ABA interventions for almost a year, Ryan had gained skills, but there was still so much he didn't know. We already knew our son didn't learn like other kids, and he was definitely behind developmentally. For him, everything had to be broken down into step-by-step instructions if he were going to be able to learn anything. Other kids just seemed to know what to do and what was expected. Not ours.

Ryan was the oldest kid in his class, and we celebrated Ryan's sixth birthday two weeks after he started kindergarten. Academically, Ryan knew his stuff. He had his letters and numbers down cold. However, his speech, social skills, and maturity level were light-years behind the other kindergarteners. It didn't matter that we worked all day every day on this stuff; following simple directions and staying on task were skills he still hadn't yet mastered.

How would he survive at school without having me there to explain why he did what he did? No one would comprehend his odd way of communicating. Nor would they understand what he wanted or needed. Ryan was only in the third percentile for speech back then. But we couldn't wait any longer for him to start. We couldn't have a kindergartener who had to shave before going to school.

I was scared out of my mind about the approaching school year. Frank was apprehensive, but he was probably more annoyed with me and my neurotic fears about kindergarten. I needed to talk about which school my son should attend and which teacher to choose over and over again. We even talked about what kind of backpack he should take. This was my way of coping. When I didn't know what to do, I had to talk about all the possibilities.

Mr. I Need to Know Everything Before It Happens, aka Ryan, required a trial run the day before kindergarten started. Frank and I showed him where the bus stop and his classroom were located. We explained what his first day would look like. We weren't sure he actually understood the things we were telling him, but we did it anyway. He never acknowledged that he even heard what we said. Our prekindergarten adventure ended with all of us climbing on the playground equipment and playing in the schoolyard. Trusting that a bus ride would appeal to him because of his interest in mechanics, we hoped we had prepared him.

We felt totally unprepared.

Ryan was picked up by the *short bus* (the bus for special education students) right on schedule. Frank and I jumped in the car, video camera in hand. We raced to school to beat the bus, so we could capture Ryan's first day of kindergarten on film. We could have taken our time because there was no bus and no Ryan. We waited and waited. Our thoughts of celebration soon gave way to apprehension and next to panic. Nearly an hour later, his bus finally showed up. The driver had taken Ryan to the wrong school.

This happened to be one of those rare occurrences when our children's stubbornness can be a good thing. When the driver tried to drop off Ryan at a different school, Ryan refused to get off the bus. He knew it wasn't the same school we had shown him the day before. This victory for Ryan was quickly replaced by the certainty that kindergarten was going to be hard and that almost every day would be a struggle. He might have mastered the bus, but he couldn't master circle time.

At the time Ryan started kindergarten, there were still morning and afternoon half-day sessions. We chose the afternoon program for Ryan, an option that might not be available today since most schools have moved to all-day kindergarten. There's nothing easy about getting a kid with autism dressed and ready for school. But being in the afternoon class gave Ryan (and me) more time to get him out the door. During these years, we were still knee-deep in his hour-long dressing and eating rituals. My son, who still is not a morning person, was less difficult when he was not rushed. Even if we had enrolled in the morning program, he couldn't have gotten there until the afternoon.

I asked that Ryan be allowed to attend Concord Elementary School instead of our assigned school. Ms. Donna Erstad, Megan's former kindergarten teacher, now worked at Concord. She was a great teacher! My grand plan for Ryan was that he be assigned to Ms. Erstad's kindergarten class. I made an appointment to observe her classroom to reassure myself that this was the right place for Ryan. It didn't take long for me to see that, although Ms. Erstad was perfect for Megan, she was not a good fit for Ryan. Donna's classroom was a creative, constantly changing wonderland with a hundred different activities going on at once. Megan thrived in this kind of creative, controlled chaos. Ryan never could have survived it. He needed a quieter, highly structured environment that minimized distractions.

So, here we were scheduled to go to Concord because of Donna Erstad's remarkable teaching ability, but she wasn't the right teacher for my son. I quickly instituted Plan B: teacher shopping. The May before Ryan was scheduled to start school, I observed every kindergarten teacher at Concord in action. All of them were extremely qualified, but no one had all the qualities Ryan needed for success. If the teacher was kind and loving, her classroom moved too quickly for my son.

The teacher I ultimately picked for Ryan was Sherry Paul. Although she was young, Sherry Paul reminded me of an old schoolmarm. She didn't put up with any nonsense from her students and ran a very controlled classroom—quiet, structured, organized, and predictable. Although Ms. Paul seemed very capable, she was not overly warm and fuzzy like the other kindergarten teachers. That worried me since Ryan rarely connected with anyone outside our family other than Pam and Gena.

Although it wasn't really possible to describe Ryan or how he worked to anyone, I sent Ms. Paul a note I hoped would help her understand my son. The following letter was way too long and had too much information:

Dear Ms. Paul,

We feel funny writing this letter. We really aren't neurotic parents (well maybe just a little). Everyone at Concord already has helped so much, and we want to make sure we don't lose any time at the beginning of the year. Sometimes, it takes a while to figure out just how capable Ryan is and that you have to demand that he perform.

This is a list of the things Ryan still needs to learn. Currently, we are working on many of these at home and hope you can tackle some of them at school. This list will hopefully give you some insight, so you know when he is not doing something on purpose or if he truly doesn't understand how to do it. Some things that should be easy for him at his age, he hasn't mastered yet. So, here is the list:

- *Sustain prolonged eye contact with people he's talking to. (This has become very consistent with us at home, but it needs work with people he does not know well or when he is placed in a new or stressful situation.)*
- *Follow directions the first time they are given.*
- *Have more natural conversation instead of asking questions to talk to others. He has learned to engage people by asking questions rather than relate what has happened. We have worked on WH-questions involving conversation (who, what, when, where, why). Maybe this is part of the reason he does this instead of using a more typical way of conversing with others.*
- *Don't interrupt or talk when others are talking.*

- *Talk about other things instead of the learned scripts (we tend to have the same conversations over and over about computers or sharks). He only talks about what he is interested in.*
- *Initiate play with friends.*
- *Expand his experiences to play games that are not the same, familiar ones.*
- *Read nonverbal social cues.*
- *Not touch his friends in a way that makes them uncomfortable (no poking kids over and over again to get their attention).*
- *Learn how to express his feelings and say things like "I don't want to get dressed!" instead of saying "What if I put all my clothes down the drain so I don't have to get dressed?"*
- *Play ball and physical activities.*
- *Run without arm-flapping.*
- *Stop picking at his nails and other parts of his body.*
- *Answer the telephone when it rings without being afraid to talk to someone on the other end.*
- *Go to a friend's door, knock, and ask them to play.*
- *Expand his interest areas and toys he wants to play with.*
- *Learn how to wave and blow out candles on a cake.*
- *Ryan is just starting to watch TV. I want us all to be able to go to the movies together.*
- *Learn to color in the lines as well as draw stick people, houses, flowers, etc.*
- *Parts of language are missing. I realized the other day he didn't know the meaning of the words "eyebrow" and "eyelash."*
- *Eating with a spoon and a fork need work.*
- *Sit at the kitchen table with his legs down instead of one leg in a bent position.*
- *He's starting to tell us about past events, but this area needs real work. He can't come up with any of these ideas on his own but can only*

answer sometimes when we ask him direct questions about what he did today.

- *Flexibility when things do not go according to plan, e.g., the road is blocked, and we need to drive to the park a different way. This would be unsettling for him. He wants to sit in the same seat in the car, the one behind mom.*

- *Appropriate voice intonation and volume. His voice is often flat, and sometimes he speaks way too loud or too soft.*

- *Don't squeeze his friends or poke them when he gets excited about something or just wants their attention.*

- *Learn to ask again if someone doesn't hear him or do what he asks. Instead, he gives up after his initial attempt and walks away.*

- *Ryan can tell me what he wants for breakfast if he is given choices. But if I ask, "What do you want for breakfast?" then he can't answer that question.*

- *Although dressing is improving, he needs to be able to choose clothing and then dress without step-by-step instructions.*

- *Cross the street safely without help.*

- *When playing a game, he needs to accept when he loses. Also, he must learn he can't always be the blue game piece or the first to play.*

- *Wear a coat when it is cold without objecting.*

- *Learn to say "please" and "thank you" without reminders.*

(This was my list for Ryan's kindergarten teacher. But please feel free to plagiarize anything I wrote in my letters to teachers that will help your child.)

I can't believe I actually sent pages and pages of instructions to Ms. Paul. She must have been worried before she ever set eyes on my son. Still, Ms. Paul turned out to be a good choice for Ryan. She was strict, all business, and her rules were clear. The most important thing about Ms. Paul was she treated Ryan exactly the same as the other children. She expected my son to behave, and if he didn't, there were consequences. When he misbehaved, Ryan had a time-out at the table. As a result, Ryan did not often test the limits with Ms. Paul.

Ryan's kindergarten teacher used positive reinforcement as the main way of shaping all the children's behavior (although she was never formally trained in ABA). She spoke slowly and gave clear, specific directions to the class. This was imperative since Ryan's receptive and expressive language was poor and his social skills and ability to follow directions were still quite delayed.

Even though I liked Ms. Paul, Ms. Paul didn't like me. I think the problem started with the letter I sent her. After reading it, she knew Ryan was going to be a lot of extra work, but it was probably me that concerned her more than Ryan. I was a hover mother. Surely, one of the worst she ever met. I really didn't want to be a pain, but I had no choice. Ryan wasn't going to make it if I didn't help him. Ryan was a kid with autism who was way out of his depth in a mainstream classroom even with the capable Sherry Paul.

We threw him in anyway.

Not surprisingly, Ryan didn't fit at school. He was too smart for a special class but did not have enough language or maturity for a typical class. Chronologically and academically, he was a kindergarten student. Developmentally, he was struggling way below the preschool level. What Ryan needed was a classroom that taught kindergarten academics and preschool social skills run by a teacher who was ABA-certified plus a structured, organized disciplinarian with a big red phone on her desk with a direct line to me.

There was no such thing.

I told his teachers my goal was to get Ryan to the point where he was somewhat similar to his peers even though he had a long way to get there. I said this to convince myself almost as much as them; otherwise, it would have been impossible for me face each new problem that arose in kindergarten as the year wore on. I secretly doubted his survival there was even possible.

Kindergarten was a struggle almost every day. We decided to not interrupt Ryan's school day by pulling him out for services. We also didn't want him to appear different. Kids notice this kind of stuff. Extra services like speech were done at home or sometimes before and after school. We worked the poor kid morning 'til night.

Weekends and vacation time were big crunch times for us. It was easier to teach him when he wasn't tired after a long school day. When other kids were losing skills during the summer months, Ryan was gaining. Social skills were taught by the school social worker with a small group of kids during the lunch period or after school in our home by me. This no *pull-out* kind of program had never been done before in our district for kids with autism. Transitions are difficult for children with autism, so my reasoning was to not make my son deal with any more of them than he had to. School would be harder if Ryan had to leave and then reenter the learning environment,

The worst part of kindergarten was when it was my turn to be the classroom helper. Those days were usually followed by a good cry. That's when it hit me right between the eyes how different Ryan really was. My son was not comfortable at school. When Ryan became stressed, which was the norm for him at school, he retreated into his weird autistic coping behaviors that managed to shut out the world and also drew negative attention from his classmates. My kid was Mr. Wizard at connecting electrical cords, but he desperately needed help connecting with his classmates.

Barbara Wiley, his aide that year, was also a certified teacher. She was a brand spanking new teacher, the warm and fuzzy kind. Ryan had the perfect combination of teachers: one made him feel loved, and one took no prisoners. I asked Barbara to share the names of children he liked so I could invite them over to play. A one-on-one interaction was much easier than the group dynamics Ryan had to deal with at school.

The kids who came to play didn't always have the most attentive parents. I picked them because their parents never seemed to notice how strange Ryan acted or asked any questions about my kid. These parents never worried about my child's influence on their children's actions or if his autism symptoms were catching. They loved the fact that I picked up their kid from school and delivered him back to their home when the play date was over. I used the excuse that transportation was no problem since I didn't work. What they never knew was that Ryan was the toughest full-time job I ever had.

Sam, a kid Ryan semi-connected with at school, was a good match. I needed Sam to teach Ryan kid rules and social skills. I was willing to be free daycare for his parents to facilitate my son's learning. My kid was never invited to Sam's house to play. I paid for everything, but that was okay. Sam's services were actually cheap if you considered the cost of professional social skills therapy.

Joey was another potential friend who spent a lot of time with us. We chose activities that didn't require a lot of talking. We walked to the park, played on the swing set, bounced on the trampoline, or played in the treehouse. Some days, we'd go to Goodwill to buy old radios or other electronics. Ryan and his new friends loved to take apart and reconstruct gadgets. It takes quite a bit of cooperation and conversational skills for two kids to accomplish this.

One of Ryan's favorite playmates was a little girl named Savannah. Ryan followed her around like a lovesick puppy. Ryan did whatever she wanted. Savannah insisted that Ryan answer her questions. When he failed to do so, she would loudly demand, *"Did ya HEAR me?"* At home, we adopted Savannah's same words and intonation to make Ryan answer our questions, too. It became a family joke regarding what we did when he didn't answer us.

Play dates were always at our house. That way I was there to help when Ryan needed me to do so. I facilitated the interactions to make sure the kids had fun and would want to return. The other reason I facilitated these interactions was so Ryan could experience success socially. When I saw he was handling things on his own, I faded into the background. However, this hover mother usually hovered close by so that I could jump in if Ryan needed help making things work. I never seemed to be needed when he played video games or computer with his friends. Somehow our kids don't require assistance when technology is involved.

At first, we had only one child over at a time. We'd take turns choosing what to play. We worked to make Ryan more flexible. He needed to learn he couldn't always go first in a game or demand to use the cherished blue game piece. When it was Ryan's turn to pick the activity, he usually chose to go outside or to play with the computer, LEGO toys, or Play-Doh. Next, his friend had a turn to pick. When I picked, I'd choose something that didn't come easily to Ryan, like taking turns in a game of Chutes and Ladders. We often played board games because the rules were clear and predictable. The day before a play date, we role-played and practiced what we would do and say with his friends the next day.

Sometimes, we played the games I planned to use. Success always involved pre-teaching back then. And Ryan and I took turns pretending to be Joey or Sam the day before.

Other parents had no idea of what I was up to. I was simply a stay-at-home mom who cooked, cleaned a little, ate bonbons, and watched soap operas. It was almost like I had a secret life. Some of the other moms probably thought I was too involved with my kids and way too overprotective. But I knew raising both my kids was the most important job I would ever have. This all would have been easier if I had known that someday my son would be okay. But the constant worry about my son's future was always present. I could never just go with the flow or enjoy the moment. It would have been nice, just for one day, to be a soap-opera-watching, bonbon-eating sex siren.

If I Knew Then What I Know Now

Our request to put Ryan at Concord Elementary School turned out to be another life-changing event. If Ryan had gone to our assigned school, I'm not convinced he would have had the same outcome. Concord was staffed with exceptional teachers and a principal who was willing to work with us. That was a critical piece of my son's recovery.

Ryan wasn't ready for kindergarten, but I sent him anyway. In preschool, Ryan attended a *hand-in-hand* classroom run by the school district. Hand-in-hand meant half the kids were supposed to be typical and half were special needs. In reality, most of the kids in this class had issues. Not many parents of typical kids want their child placed in a special-needs classroom, and so any attempt at this sort of structured inclusion usually didn't achieve the desired objective. There are too many special-needs kids and not enough general-education kids. Ryan was clearly one of the special-needs kids. As a matter of fact, he was the worst behaved and most severely affected student in his preschool class.

The preschool teachers provided and facilitated a great learning environment. However, on those rare occasions when Ryan was appropriate and asked another child a question, the other child sometimes failed to respond. There were too few children modeling appropriate behavior for real social skills immersion learning to take place. His class had plenty of examples of how not to behave at school. And my son already excelled at every one of them. But at the time, there was really no other choice since Ryan was so severely affected. I'm not sure the teachers from a regular preschool could have handled him. The mistake I made was in thinking that somehow, one year later, Ryan would be able to make the enormous leap from a special education preschool class to a typical kindergarten class.

My decision to place Ryan in a typically developing class, even with a highly qualified teacher and a highly qualified aide, was asking Ryan to cope with a lot. I set him up for stress and failure and went home crying each time I witnessed that failure enacted in his daily classroom experiences. But I'm not sure what else I could have done. Ryan didn't fit in special education and he definitely didn't fit in a mainstream classroom. So, I did the next best thing. I asked for an aide and, ready or not, I threw him in. As a result, we had to teach him all the skills most kindergarteners already know every day after school, almost like a whole other day of kindergarten.

My list to Ms. Paul was overwhelmingly long and confused the goals of academic education with the goals of behavioral therapy. How would I have felt if she had sent home a long list of what she wanted me to work on as a mother? I probably just needed to trust Ms. Paul since she was the best possible teacher for Ryan. But I didn't trust anyone with my son. Instead, we asked Ryan to rise to the occasion. Eventually he did, but not during that kindergarten year. That was a tough year for him, his teachers, and his family.

The right teacher is essential for a child with autism. If you need to make a choice, pick the strict one with definite rules over the nice one without the needed structure. Pick one with clear speech patterns. The right teacher was critical to Ryan's success. If you don't know what your child needs (and it can be really hard to know), then it is imperative to ask for guidance from the IEP team and other professionals.

My decision to keep Ryan in the classroom and not pull him out for anything eventually worked for him, but that isn't the right decision for all kids. I asked a lot of Ryan. Some children with autism require a 365-day approach to the school year. Summer vacation for us consisted of more pre-teaching and reteaching. Our teaching included days at the pool, the park, or McDonald's PlayPlace, where I taught him the things he needed to know at the same time he had fun. It wasn't fun for me; it was hard work.

Facilitating Ryan's school friendships was probably my smartest move. Many moms of children with autism recognize the trade-off of doing all the work to organize and implement a play date in order for it to happen. Kids who are under-parented, kids who have emotional issues, and kids whose parents are divorcing seem to be our child's most likely playmates because the parents as well as their kids are struggling. These children needed us as much as we needed them.

CHAPTER 29

SOMETIMES IT'S BETTER TO KEEP YOUR MOUTH SHUT

The real art of conversation is not only to say the right thing at the right place, but to leave unsaid the wrong thing at the tempting moment.

—Dorothy Nevill

"KIDS LEARN TO do things at different times." Donna Erstad, my daughter's kindergarten teacher, shared these words of wisdom when I had expressed my concern about Megan not reading yet. To some degree, it doesn't matter what age our children learn to do something—just that they do. Do our children really need to be one of the first readers in their class? Is it really important at exactly what age our children take their first steps? After they grow up, no one asks when they started to walk or read.

I repeat Donna's wise words to parents with kids on the spectrum. It's critical that our children learn to communicate. They must develop appropriate behavior and social skills. Even if these skills come later to our kids, it is okay as long as these important skills eventually do develop.

Words of wisdom usually come from experience and quiet reflection. There's not much time for that when you are fighting a war against autism. That's why I have to say **kids do things at different times** over and over to parents who have children on the spectrum. These parents have a hard time hearing it, a harder time believing it, and an even harder time applying it to their own situation. I was no exception.

At the beginning of every school year, I sent Ryan's new teacher an updated version of "The List." It was never quite as long as the first one I sent Sherry Paul. But it did include all the age-appropriate things he hadn't mastered yet. I'm not sure if this list helped his teachers or was just annoying to them, but it turned out to be extremely important for me. As I updated the list each school year, I was always surprised by the number of now-mastered skills I could cross off. Many times, I didn't realize how much Ryan had progressed until I saw it in black and white on that list.

As parents, we never fail to notice our children's lack of speech or when they do something weird, but sometimes we forget to notice what they have accomplished. Nobody can miss a child with autism with their noises, arm flapping, and tantrums. We are so focused on getting rid of those behaviors that we fail to recognize the things they are doing right. However, Ryan eventually did learn not to poke his friends to get attention from them. And sometime during the kindergarten year, he started to learn how to color within the lines and wait his turn.

We used a communication notebook that went back and forth daily between home and school. Ryan's aide was in charge of the communication log book that was so instrumental in helping us know what we still needed to teach at home, so he could survive at school. The book was just a spiral notebook filled with blank pages. But it was the information his aide wrote on those pages that was imperative to Ryan's success at school. Barbara entered the date and sent us notes about what Ryan didn't know how to do. We set up situations at home to teach these skills he still needed to learn. We used ABA behavioral techniques and anything else that worked.

In the early days, it was depressing to read the entries. There was so much he didn't know. Ryan went to kindergarten during the day and relearned kindergarten every night. As you can tell by the entry below, anything that required coordinated physical movements was a challenge for my son:

September 2

Barbara wrote: During our opening, we did Mickey Mousercise. It is a movement activity. I think Ryan was overwhelmed with it and had difficulty doing some of the movements.

I asked for a copy of the Mousercise tape so we could practice it at home. In the beginning, Ryan learned most things at home first so that he could participate at school. We had to pre-teach things like Mousercise, the hokey pokey, and every physical education skill. Anything we thought he might struggle with at school was learned in advance at home.

September 3

I wrote back to Barbara: I appreciate your sending the song and book list. We will teach him "If You're Happy and You Know It" and "Mr. Sun." However, he's on his own for the other two. They are not in my singing repertoire.

Ryan surprised me one day when he started singing a song that I hadn't taught him. He learned it without any pre-teaching just like the other kids. That was a major cause for celebration. Any big accomplishment and a lot of minor ones were my excuse not to cook. We went out to eat to celebrate. The good days kept us going. Positive reinforcement worked on us, too.

The next big problem to solve was Ryan's behavior in circle time. Ryan didn't think he needed to sit or pay attention to anything the teacher said. He didn't listen or follow directions. Circle time was complicated. It involved multiple behaviors and skills we had to break down into smaller, easier steps. So at home, we played school. I was the pretend teacher, while Ryan, Megan, Shannon (Megan's friend and our extra daughter), Frank, and the dog played the kids in our school at home.

My husband's job was to behave exactly like Ryan did in circle time at school. Frank would call out answers, demand attention from the teacher, be outrageously inattentive, and walk around aimlessly. For someone who had always been one of the good kids at school, Frank excelled at being bad. He was also a great source of amusement. Megan and Shannon laughed at his outrageous antics. Ryan observed his father intently but remained mostly quiet. Frank was a perfect replica of Ryan at school. In time, Ryan made the connection that Frank got in trouble for the same things he did at school.

When Frank did something wrong at our pretend school, there were immediate consequences. He'd have to sit at the table with his head down or do something else Ms. Paul used as discipline at school. Ryan enjoyed being the good kid who did things correctly in the at-home classroom.

Whenever anyone in our pretend class raised their hand, there was big praise and reinforcement. Ryan never raised his hand at school. We needed to shape this behavior. We didn't expect him to be perfect, but any movement toward appropriate circle time behavior was rewarded and encouraged. Shannon and Megan were great at role-playing how kids should act. They sometimes bluntly told Frank when he was doing things wrong to depict what the kids at school did with Ryan. We tackled Ryan's circle time issues one behavior at a time. It took way too much time, but the light finally came on for Ryan. We thought that problem was solved.

But it really wasn't. It was never that easy with Ryan.

The newest complaint in the communication book was that he was disruptive in the library when the librarian read a story to the class. Ryan never made the connection or generalized any rule he learned until he was much older. Children with autism have trouble with *generalization*.

Ryan didn't realize that the rules for story time in the library and circle time in his classroom were the same. Although the library rules were simply circle time in another room, he needed to be directly taught that lesson. So, we played library at home. Sometimes the targeted behavior your child needs to learn must be taught in several settings.

I pretended to be Ms. Bales, our favorite librarian, while Megan, Shannon, and the dog listened to the story I read. As you might have guessed, Frank didn't listen at all and was inappropriate once again. He interrupted while I read the story and did anything else he could think of that Ryan might do wrong during story time. Frank was removed from the reading circle and had to sit with his head down in shame at our library table. With less time than it took for circle time, Ryan mastered what was expected in the library.

I used the communication book to positively reinforce his teacher's behavior and encourage them to use techniques we knew worked with Ryan. However, when offering advice, we had to be very careful so our ideas were not inadvertently taken as criticism. We didn't want his teachers to think we thought they were incompetent or that we knew how to teach him better. In reality, we were not usually critical of their methods. We just had more experience and time to understand Ryan. As a result, we sometimes, but not always, knew which methods worked best and which ones didn't work at all.

We often had to switch gears to keep things working. Sometimes, something would work for a while and then was no longer effective. Often, we gave Ryan stickers to reinforce behaviors we wanted to see. Ryan loved stickers, so we used them. We put a sticker next to the current entry in the communication book when he had a great day. This worked for a while, but we stopped giving stickers after the following entry in the communication book:

> *September 30*
> *Barbara wrote: Group time was just okay today. Ryan did a lot of yelling out to answer questions without raising his hand. Sherry and I are trying to ignore this, but it is hard. I noticed almost every day Ryan has started yelling during work time, "What are you writing in my book?"*

Ryan had learned when Barbara wrote in the book, he might get a sticker that day. Ryan liked stickers more than doing things correctly. That caused him to concentrate on what Barbara did rather than doing the things the teachers expected. All he thought he had to do was act in a way and Barbara would write in the book. And just maybe, then a beloved sticker would follow. He didn't make the right connection for the behavior/response in this instance. He also didn't understand what having a good day meant. We changed the association to a much clearer one: "When Barbara writes in the book *because you did something good*, then there will be a sticker." Ryan needed immediate and clear rewards.

October 27

Marcia wrote: I'm glad yesterday went so well. I got a little teary-eyed when I read Barbara's note because I was so happy. I know that with Ryan it isn't always steady upward movement. We usually take one step back after three steps forward. But yesterday was definitely ten steps forward, thanks to both of you! He is making amazing progress. We so appreciate all you do. Next, we are working to bake chocolate chip cookies. How do you guys feel about eating those? Thanks for the detailed note. It really helps me know what I need to teach at home. Volunteering in the classroom helped a lot also. Now I better understand how things are done. I know my "thank you" isn't as good as cookies or cake, but don't worry—we will be baking brownies to reward his appropriate behavior. I will be sending them to his fabulous teachers soon.

ABA techniques worked on the teachers, too. When I wrote in the communication book, I praised the actions I wanted to see his teachers repeat. I ignored the things that I didn't agree with and instead talked about the things they were doing right. Positive reinforcement made everyone do the things I wanted to see happen more often. But finding the thing teachers or kids do right is not always easy.

November 15

Barbara wrote: Ryan had a difficult time counting the days left of school with the class in the morning circle time. I can't figure out why. I know he knows everything when it comes to numbers.

Ryan craved attention—even negative attention. We had certainly learned that lesson in our pre-ABA years of parenting. At times, he'd revisit the old behaviors that had successfully controlled his parents for so long. The challenge was to help his teachers realize that fact, rather than assume he couldn't do what they asked of him. In this scenario, Barbara didn't comprehend that when she would talk to Ryan daily about why he was not counting, her attention became reinforcing for Ryan. She tried to be kind and handle the problem in a way that worked for most kids.

But Ryan definitely wasn't most kids.

The more Ryan didn't count, the more one-on-one time he got with his beloved aide. He loved Barbara, and he loved it when she talked to him each day about why he wasn't counting. This gave him the extra attention he craved. If Barbara had ignored his behavior and hadn't mentioned anything to him, it would have worked better.

Barbara assumed Ryan understood the words she was saying. However, he didn't understand how classrooms worked and never mastered the implicit meaning[38] of her request. Ryan was adrift in a room full of strangers doing strange things. That was kindergarten to him.[39] Ryan liked having Barbara all to himself. That was comforting. It was almost like having his mom there, before mom got smart. We had to be careful how we solved this problem. We didn't want Barbara to think we were critical of her methods. So, we did what we do with Ryan. We ignored what Barbara was doing wrong and praised what she did right.

Even though Mindi instructed us not to negotiate with terrorists, I still used some of our old methods when it was an emergency, such as counting at school. I told Ryan if he counted with the kids at morning meeting all week, then we would make a chocolate cake when he got home from school on Friday. Ryan loved to cook—and still does. Licking the sugary batter from the big bowl was an equally important part of the reward to him. We used a preset consequence and this type of positive reinforcement to help him do what he should be doing. It worked, and I sent two huge pieces of cake for his teachers to enjoy on Monday. We did a lot of cooking and baking that year.

This all sounds logical and easy. It wasn't.

---

38   He didn't perceive kindergarten as a group to which he was supposed to belong. A child with autism will have difficulty shifting his attention from what he is thinking about to what he needs to be doing as part of the group. He may not understand the *implicit* behavioral sequence he needs to do in order to do what a teacher requests.

39   Parents often assume a child with autism *knows* what school is because they go there every day. It can come as a surprise to find that even middle-school children with autism may not actually know why they go to school beyond it being a part of their routine.

If I Knew Then What I Know Now

Progress for Ryan meant an attitude adjustment for me. Sometimes, after reading the entries in the communication notebook, it seemed like Ryan couldn't do anything right. Although this book was an important tool, it was also a source of great frustration because the reports sometimes seemed so negative.

Barbara was simply trying to tell us what we needed to work on, which is what I had asked her to do. But what I actually wanted was a book full of blank pages or, better yet, one filled with accolades. That way, I would know Ryan was okay. After a rough school day, I wished I could throw the communication book in the trash. Not knowing what the future would bring for my son was always the worst thing to deal with. I was his mom and took every entry way too personally.

Frank was right when he suggested I sometimes saw negativity where there was none, and this negativity stemmed from my continual fear for Ryan's dismal future so clearly predicted by the experts we had consulted. My fears made it hard to see things clearly. I often assumed the teachers hated my kid because he took so much more time than the others. Or if they did seem to like Ryan, I decided it was *me* they hated because of all the extra work I created for them.

Many parents of children with autism are held hostage by developmental milestones. We read books on ages and stages of typical kids and begin to worry when our atypical child doesn't seem to fit anyplace. Panic sets in if/when our child loses developmental gains. The bigger picture needs to be that any forward progress is always good. We need to do anything to help our children become more successful at home and at school. Keep it simple. The more complicated behaviors are mastered only when you put all the smaller gains together.

We used whatever worked to help Ryan progress. Sometimes that meant combining ABA with other methods. Mindi's warning on negotiating with terrorists was sometimes placed on the back burner, and nothing terrible happened. In fact, something good occurred: Ryan began counting in a group. How could this be? A modified version of ABA worked even better for my son. The explanation was that in this situation we had moved from the ABA model to a model most parents have some familiarity with. If you do *this*, you will get *that*.

The first rule of ABA is that you provide an immediate consequence for a behavior. In this situation, we were providing a delayed consequence. We said to Ryan, "If you count with the kids at morning meeting all week, we will make a chocolate cake when you get home from school on Friday."

By this time, Ryan didn't always need only immediate rewards. Ryan learned to perform this behavior all week. After much ABA, Ryan was ready to transition to a more typical kid teaching strategy. But he wasn't totally better. When faced with the power of a restricted interest like stickers, Ryan still needed the nonstop, immediate ABA reinforcement missile to control his behavior.

Communication books are only as good as the people doing the communicating. Ryan's teacher and aide were both highly effective. They put time and effort into letting us know what Ryan still needed to learn. They created a bridge for learning between Ryan's home life and Ryan's school life. But beware: not all educators are created equal.

I was careful not to use the autism label with Ryan's kindergarten teachers or anyone else who worked with him. In my mind, the A-word immediately lowered expectations to somewhere below ground level. Instead, I explained that Ryan was very ill with immune issues when he was younger and needed all of us working together to catch up on what he missed. Back then, no one thought kids with autism could get better and lead normal lives (sometimes not even me).

His teachers probably knew about the autism label even though I tried so hard to keep it from them. It would have been all over his IEP as his qualifying category, and his teachers were directly responsible for implementing his IEP. In reality, I just thought I was hiding it.

Teachers talk even though now there are confidentiality laws that supposedly stop that from happening. I know they share even though they are supposed to keep certain things private. When I taught school, kids' issues were openly discussed in the lunchroom among staff. Most times, it was not to gossip, but rather in hope of finding solutions for problem behavior or a troubled child. I'm sure Ryan's teachers were told he had autism even though I requested that the special education department not use that label.

I didn't know if Ryan's kindergarten teachers ever believed Ryan could get better, but it didn't matter as long as they did what he needed. On more than one occasion, Ms. Paul chastised me for calling too much and taking too much of her time. I will never forget the time she said, "You know, I have thirty-nine other parents with both my morning and afternoon kindergarten classes, and I need to talk to all of them, too. You are not the only parent I have."

As a teacher, I never would have said that to a parent no matter how difficult they made my life. But I said nothing, even though the frustration my son caused left me primed and ready to come out swinging. I knew any confrontation with Ryan's teacher was not in his best interest. She was essential for Ryan's progress in kindergarten. I needed to keep my mouth shut, and we had to get along.

CHAPTER 30

ISN'T FIRST GRADE SUPPOSED TO BE FUN?

The only thing that gets in the way of my learning is my education.

—Albert Einstein

WHILE RYAN WAS trying to understand kindergarten, I was trying to understand how the school system worked. We both felt the struggle. However, when Michelle Sanders was assigned as Ryan's first grade teacher, we both had a major victory. Michelle was warm, kind, and an extremely gifted teacher. She was understanding, had clear rules, and *expected* him to act like the other kids. If there was one thing Ryan needed, it was clear rules and high expectations.

Ms. Sanders grew up with parents who were deaf. As a result, Michelle spoke slowly and deliberately so her parents could read her lips. How she naturally communicated helped Ryan with his speech issues. At this time, he didn't converse much, and his functional speech was way behind his peers. Ryan continued to have deficits in his vocabulary that would remain for many years to come.

The school district didn't allow teacher shopping, but I did it anyway. I observed the first-grade teachers in action near the end of Ryan's kindergarten year. This time, the decision of who would be the best first grade teacher was clear. I sent my request directly to the principal because, as a previous teacher, I knew she was the ultimate decision-maker when it came to the final makeup of the classrooms. The principal listened to my requests even though teacher shopping was against the rules. I didn't tell anyone that I did this, not even his current teachers. My requests wouldn't have been granted if other parents started to do the same. That would have made the principal's life impossible. I wrote the following letter to Dr. Davis, the principal at that time. I thought this was the best way to get what Ryan needed:

Letter to the Principal
March 10, 1995

Dear Dr. Davis,

We wanted to thank you for the dedicated professionals that have helped Ryan grow so much this year. Ryan's improvement and success in kindergarten was a direct result of Sherry Paul and Barbara Wiley's enthusiasm, hard work, and dedication. Besides being gifted at teaching, they have done so much that is above and beyond to help Ryan.

We want you to know that we have every confidence in your ability to get Ryan where he needs to be. So, please take this as nothing more than helpful hints we have learned along the way that will ensure Ryan succeeds at school. We would like to request that Ryan be placed in Michelle Sanders's first grade class. Ms. Sanders would be an excellent teacher for any child, but for Ryan she is essential.

Ms. Sanders gives very clear and specific directions to her class. In addition to speaking slowly and distinctly, she uses visual cues when speaking. Ryan needs a classroom like Ms. Sanders's that is extremely structured, organized, and predictable. She sets clear limits and uses positive reinforcement as the main way of shaping behavior. Research and the Lovaas method [early ABA] we use at home support that this is the way children with autism learn best.

In addition, when you are making the class lists, we would like to request that you consider placing one of Ryan's friends in the same class. Social skills are an area of weakness for Ryan and having a friend already in place would help facilitate growth in this area. Even with his kindergarten teacher's diligent efforts in this area, it was not until the end of February that we started to see more typical interactions with a few select peers.

We appreciate the opportunity to provide our input. Sometimes he may do things that are puzzling. We're just trying to save time when you are trying to figure him out and best meet his educational needs. Thank you for your time and consideration.

Sincerely,
Frank and Marcia Hinds

The thing that concerned me most about first grade was Ryan's aide—he didn't have one yet. I solved the problem by finding the aide myself. After Gena, our babysitter extraordinaire, was no longer with us, we found *Anything Amy* to be our new babysitter. Amy could get Ryan to do almost anything and understood basic ABA principles. I finagled things so Amy was hired by the school district to be Ryan's aide. Clearly an outside-the-box move. I found new ways to work around how things were done at school if it helped Ryan.

It wasn't too hard to get Amy hired by the school district as Ryan's aide. Schools want trained aides and competent people. The problem is sometimes they can't find them with the salaries they offer. And if they can find good people, they usually don't have the funds to train them properly. Amy was more than any administrator could ask for in an aide. She was great with kids and was highly trained after we taught her how to deal with Ryan.

Most of Ryan's first grade behavioral issues resulted from an absence of language, poor social skills, and lack of organization. Amy needed to correct Ryan's frequent social blunders as soon as they occurred. Social skills are hard to teach since they usually involve multiple steps. Any teaching must address the current social environment, which is never the same as thirty seconds ago. Since it is difficult to pre-teach or think of every social situation Ryan might encounter, the real reason for an aide was to teach, reteach, and remediate these important skills as soon as any issue developed. Instruction must be *immediate*. Amy knew that, and this was the reason she was so effective.

Amy provided direct, immediate, ABA-based instruction to address Ryan's social missteps. All the kids in the class benefitted from having Amy there. She could easily handle any problem that arose. As a result, the classroom ran much more smoothly. She made it so Michelle could actually teach and didn't have to deal with the small issues that happen in every classroom. Ryan progressed at a record pace that year. Michelle and Amy got along famously. The best part was that I didn't have to explain anything to either teacher. They both understood how capable Ryan was and maintained high expectations.

Before first grade, Ryan was frequently sick with strep throat and ear infections. These repeated infections that resulted in repeated courses of antibiotics were a huge stress on his immune system. We made the decision to have his tonsils and adenoids removed on the recommendation of Ryan's ENT (ear, nose, and throat) doctor and against Dr. Harvey's strong and vocal objections. After the surgery, his health greatly improved, and it was easier for him to learn. Ryan's future wife doesn't know it yet, but she will be happy we lost the tonsils and adenoids. Before the surgery, his snoring was louder than a freight train and could be heard from any corner in our home. Is it possible that removing Ryan's tonsils and adenoids help with a sleep apnea issue that children with autism sometimes have?

Ryan made rapid gains in development and speech after the surgery. He bombarded the other first graders with his extensive vocabulary and knowledge of his beloved sharks and computers. Oddly, though, he still struggled with the meanings of simple words he should know. An example was the word "hood." He had no clue what a hood was even though we wore hooded coats daily in Minnesota winters. The things he didn't know still surprised me.

Organization and sequencing continued to be a major issue for my son. His desk and locker looked like they had been in the path of a Minnesota tornado, and Ryan seemed genuinely confused about how to keep them tidy. But Amy had a plan. She created a checklist to help him zero in on what he needed to learn. Her checklist kept Ryan and all of us focused. It quickly replaced the communication book because it was easier and faster to use. The following checklist contains several sample checkmarks and entries from Amy, whose comments are in italics. They demonstrate how we used the checklist to accomplish the arrival, recess, and lunch transition skills that Ryan so badly needed:

DAILY CHECKLIST FOR PROGRESS

Arrival Goals:

- ☐ Hangs up coat, snow pants, mittens, and hat.
- ☐ Remembers to take homework folder to the turn-in basket with math message.
- ☐ Greets teachers/classmates. (If time, converses with other kids.)

Comments

Ryan did it all today. Put his snow gear away and hung up his coat. He forgot about putting his homework in the basket, but quickly remembered when I caught his eye and pointed at the basket.

Learning Time Goals:

- ☐ Eyes on teacher while she is talking.
- ☐ Does work carefully and correctly (does not rush).
- ☐ Holds pencil correctly.
- ☐ Puts papers in proper folders.
- ☐ General organization (puts things away and straightens desk).

Comments

Snack Time Goals:

- ☐ Initiates and responds appropriately to conversation.
- ☐ Cleans up after himself.

Comments

Recess Goals:

- ☐ Takes a reasonable amount of time to dress for the weather (puts on sweatshirt and warm enough clothes).
- ☐ Demonstrates flexibility in choosing friends for play. If one is not available, he tries another. *See Comment*
- ☐ Initiates/joins appropriate activity with fewer clues.

- Please keep Marcia informed about some of the school activities here. That way she can talk about them at home. This allows for reinforcement of appropriate behavior and gives her great topics for conversation.

Comments

Before recess, Ryan had a concern about him and Anna being excluded on the equipment. However, recess went well and he handled it on his own. Ryan and Nat ran out together and did not separate! Nat is really excited to have Ryan for a friend and says he can't wait to go to your house to play today. He played well with Claudia, Stephanie O., and Anna on the playground equipment. What progress!

Lunch Time Goals:

- Initiates and responds appropriately to conversations with group.
- Answers everyone, not just the kids he is more comfortable with.

Comments

Ryan had some trouble at lunch in line. It might have been because I was right there with him. He knows what to do, but instead relied more on me than usual. He sometimes says he is scared to have lunch—getting there, standing in line, and finding a seat at the class table sometimes seems like too much. It is very busy and noisy in there. Once he realized Nat was saving a place for him things were better. Nat actually asked Ryan to sit with him first.

But that "awful" lunch lady actually put beans on his tray without asking. She puts them on everyone's plate. Remind him even though they are there he doesn't need to eat them.

During lunch, Ryan and Joseph had a deep discussion about God before he quickly changed the topic back to sharks and computers.

Dismissal Goals:

- Remembers to put papers and books for homework in backpack.
- Initiates saying goodbye to teachers/classmates.

Comments

Physical Education Goals:

- ☐ Eyes on teacher while she is talking.
- ☐ Improve physical skills. (Provide info about what we need work on at home, what is coming up next so we can preteach the skills needed for the activity.)
- ☐ Increase confidence level.

Comments

Art, Music, Computer, and Library Goals:

- ☐ Attends to central activity.
- ☐ Eyes on teacher while she is talking.
- ☐ Raises hand, volunteers, and answers questions. (No yelling out answers.)
- ☐ Initiates and responds appropriately to conversation.
- ☐ Continue to reinforce self-esteem and boost confidence by making him a helper and sending other children to him for assistance.
- ☐ Bring library book home on Fridays and return it the following Friday.

Comments

Strengths, Areas to work on, and General Comments on Behavior

Amy didn't comment on every item of the checklist every day, just the things we needed to know. She knew Ryan craved sweets since they were mostly absent from his diet. Amy rewarded Ryan with a small hard candy at the end of each day if his locker and desk looked like they weren't a complete wreck. She positively reinforced anything that even slightly resembled improvement, shaping his behavior one organizational step at a time.

The problems that resulted from his lack of organization continued for many years even though we constantly worked on this. Ryan completed all assignments, but he forgot to put them in the basket. He forgot everything and never put anything where it belonged. Coats, books, and belongings were often lost. Sometimes I went with him to search for them in the lost-and-found. Most of the time, we didn't bother to look because it took too much of the precious time we needed to teach Ryan what he still needed to learn. It was the same at home. No matter how many times I said, "If you put things away after you use them, then you won't lose them," his stuff was still misplaced. My nagging didn't seem to make a difference. It was so difficult to ignore these things and concentrate on the positive.

The list of things Ryan needed to learn was getting shorter, but it was still daunting. Attending to the teacher and what was happening with group activities remained a central concern. We continued to focus on better eye contact. He needed to initiate and sustain conversations with others. Since he did not look at people, Ryan often missed the important nonverbal communication that went on in the classroom.

Every behavior had to be broken down into step-by-step directions. Sometimes, I had to break things down for myself, too, so I wouldn't become overwhelmed by all the things Ryan still needed to learn. I had to teach him one behavior at a time. But there were days when that didn't work. It was difficult to cope. That's when I would concentrate on putting one foot in front of the other. I could only think about the current behavior we needed to master and how to accomplish that. Looking too far ahead was not helpful in the least if I were to survive the daily torment that was part of helping Ryan.

Ryan's progress was very up and down. Just when I thought he had mastered something at school and started to feel better about how things were going, a note would come home that pointed out just how erratic his behavior was. Even after he mastered a big-ticket item, there were still ten thousand other things he didn't know how to do—things he needed to know *today* and things he should have learned *yesterday*! Some days he was brilliant, and then a small thing would set off a meltdown. At those times, I thought he would never get better.

It seemed like Ryan needed someone giving him direct instruction all day, every day. All of us were up on the tightrope with him. The anxiety this created was overwhelming. If something happened that Ryan couldn't anticipate, it was very easy for him and us to lose our balance. We never knew what would cause a meltdown or send us falling from the tightrope we lived on.

Although the social piece slowly started to come, Ryan still couldn't tell us anything about what happened at school. When I asked about his day, the answer was from his usual script, "School was fine." He offered no details and didn't understand that I wanted him to give me an account of at least one event that had happened.

In time, I learned to ask more specific questions, "What did you do today at recess?" or "Who did you sit next to at lunch?" It was more than a decade before Ryan learned the art of small talk, but it took less time to notice the nonverbal clues that give meaning to every social situation.

Physical education continued to be a huge issue. Ryan was uncoordinated and tired easily. It wasn't until after Dr. Harvey started the antiviral medication (for Ryan, at age ten) that this actually improved.[40] We pre-taught the skills for kickball or whatever they were learning in gym. And yet with all the pre-teaching, he still couldn't do it. Ryan had adaptive PE two days a week. He needed help with PE because of his lack of motor planning. Mr. Bender, his regular PE teacher, was also certified to teach adaptive PE. He met with Ryan on Tuesdays and Thursdays for a half hour before school to pre-teach what his physical education class would learn later that day.

The pre-teaching once again helped, but it was not enough.

He wasn't much better at running than talking. He had trouble keeping up with the boys on the playground. When they played kickball or soccer, he just couldn't do it; eventually he stopped trying. I sometimes stalked Ryan from outside the school fence where he couldn't see me. My heart broke as I checked on him. He was sad and alone. Ryan wanted friends; he just didn't have the communication and physical skills to make that happen.

For Ryan, recess and lunch proved to be the most difficult part of his school day. After I figured this out, I suggested Amy take her lunch break at

---

40 Starting an antiviral medication was one of the *first* things our autism specialist usually prescribed, but it didn't happen that way with Ryan. It was approximately five years after we initially started with Dr. H that the antiviral was implemented. I sometimes wonder if Ryan would have gotten better sooner, if he had been put on an antiviral earlier in his treatment.

an alternate time. That way she would be there to facilitate social interaction with other kids during lunch and recess. When Ryan had to deal with multiple kids talking and ten million activities going on at the same time, he had trouble.

All the students in his first-grade class loved Amy and couldn't wait to be part of anything she did. Amy excelled at making Ryan become a part of any group. When she did that, he never realized that she was addressing his issues. She would start a game with a few kids and then nonchalantly invite Ryan to join them. She chose activities like four square, tag, the jungle gym, or anything else that didn't require conversation. She was truly gifted at not letting Ryan or any of the kids know all of this was orchestrated for my son's benefit. This was especially important in promoting his independence and acceptance by other kids. I worried about his social skills the most. They were the hardest to teach, and without these important skills, he would never have the things in life that mattered most: love, acceptance, and belonging.

Ryan and his friend, Joey, decided they wanted to perform in the school talent show in first grade. I worried my son would fail in front of the entire school. But Ryan was about to teach me a lesson about just how capable he could be. To my astonishment, the boys came up with their own joke-telling act. They wouldn't even give me a preview.

I helped them with costumes, and they looked like a couple of comedians. Ryan was dressed in a black and silver sequined shirt with a funny hat perched on top of his tousled hair, and Joey had on a red too-shiny tuxedo.

Joey opened the act when he said in a loud voice:

"Now for our *first* joke, why do hummingbirds hum?"

Ryan said, "I don't know, why *DO* hummingbirds hum?"

Joey answered with his slight adorable lisp, "Because they *don't* know the words."

They made it seem like they might be up there for the better part of eternity and would tell a barrel of jokes, but everyone laughed when Ryan next announced, "Now for our *last* joke . . . "

Joey asked, "*Why* do birds fly south for the winter?"

"Because it's *too far* to walk," Ryan giggled.

The audience was clapping and cheering. The boys were up there only for an instant, the jokes were corny, but they were a big hit. I watched in stunned silence. Ryan and Joey had everyone laughing. They were so cute, and their delivery was perfect. This reaction from the audience was even more than I thought possible. Tears were streaming down my face as I watched them take their bows.

Ryan's ability to perform surprised me. Who would have ever thought my kid could be up there in front of the entire school and be a star? This was the same kid who had trouble having a one-on-one conversation with a friend. Ryan wasn't even nervous in front of the large crowd that filled the auditorium. Ryan actually looked *cool* instead of *weird*. In front of the audience, he knew what to say because his lines were scripted. He didn't have to come up with the topic of conversation on his own. For a moment I even forgot he was the same kid who often didn't look at anyone, only talked about what he wanted, and never bothered to listen to anything anyone else said. It was a good day. We celebrated with dinner out, but after dinner, we went right back to work.

If I Knew Then What I Know Now

I thought my idea of Amy helping Ryan during lunch and recess was brilliant. That way she would be there to help Ryan learn the skills needed to navigate these unstructured times. I was so focused on Ryan that I didn't realize this great idea was a huge mistake on my part.

My request for Amy to assist Ryan during recess and lunch made Amy and Ms. Sanders resent me. They couldn't have lunch together or get the grown-up time we all so desperately need. I thought everything was fine since Ryan was doing so well, but it really wasn't. It wasn't until it was time to pick his teacher for the following year that I learned I had demanded too much.

Ryan's poor organizational skills continued to be a problem. Sometimes those old struggles surface occasionally. It still makes my blood boil if I see him searching for something he lost or misplaced because it reminds me of his past issues. The difference now is he no longer loses everything. Now the lost articles mostly involve his keys, wallet, or phone. Still, I can't complain since I have a similar issue. All of us have to compensate for our deficiencies.

Where do you think our kids get this forgetfulness from? Just yesterday, I forgot to bring in the groceries from the car. Those were expensive steaks I had to toss. More often it's my purse that goes missing. I compensate by calling my phone to locate my purse. However, that trick only works if I remember to put my cell phone back in my purse and have the sound turned on.

One time when Ryan was home visiting from college, he placed his phone and keys on top of the car after a day of surfing. He forgot they were there as he put his surfboard away. The next morning, Frank and I drove that car to the bank. When we parked at the bank, Frank heard the thump of Ryan's wallet hitting the pavement. Fortunately, Ryan's smartphone was still on the roof of the car.

Frank was furious. We overreact, and our blood pressure rises when we have to deal with old issues we thought were gone. Frank wanted to keep Ryan's phone and wallet and make him suffer when he searched for them. But I just couldn't do it since I am also absentminded. As a result, I can't complain about him when he does these kinds of things.

Recently, Ryan lost his ID from work. As a result, entering and leaving work became extremely difficult for him. He had to walk several extra blocks to enter the aerospace facility's front entrance. I didn't say a word. These natural consequences finally helped him locate his missing ID at the grocery store where he left it. The funny part was when he found it he told me, "Mom, I love you, but I hate that I inherited your *forgetting* gene."

CHAPTER 31

THINGS DIDN'T TURN OUT LIKE WE PLANNED IN LIFE OR SECOND GRADE

Obstacles don't have to stop you. If you run into a wall, don't turn around and give up. Figure out how to climb it, go through it, or work around it.
—Michael Jordan

JUST AS RYAN didn't read the classroom social context correctly, I didn't always read the IEP team context correctly. I thought the Michelle and Amy tag team was the solution to all that Ryan needed. I didn't realize they were not happy dealing with my constant new and evolving ideas to help my son. When Ms. Sanders decided to move up to second grade for the next school year, I was thrilled. I assumed Ryan would continue with Michelle and Amy for another amazing year. The bonus for me was that I wouldn't have to explain how my son worked to his second-grade teacher. I was also relieved that this year I wouldn't have to write another letter to a teacher about what he still needed to learn.

That's what I thought, but that's not what happened.

Without informing me, Ryan was reassigned to Ms. Johnson's class for his second-grade placement. Michelle and Amy didn't want to continue as Ryan's *dynamic duo* for another year. I don't think Michelle and Amy ditched us because they thought dealing with my son was too difficult. They loved him and even his quirky ways of doing things. What I suspect happened was that they didn't want to deal with Ryan's *mother* for another year. I was driven to fix

Ryan's autism. My intense focus sometimes made me less than sensitive to any needs the teachers might have that were not centered on my son. My world revolved around recovering my son, and I assumed they shared my passion.

They did—just not as much.

Ryan was quietly switched at the last minute and only a few days before the start of second grade. I tried to rationalize that maybe the IEP team knew more about what Ryan needed than I did. A wiser me now knows this was done as part of the master plan to circumvent Ryan's overbearing mother.

Ryan's new placement was presented as a win for us. Ms. Johnson had a special education credential and a special needs child of her own. The principal and Ryan's case manager tried to sell this new classroom assignment by saying Ryan could improve more quickly with a more qualified teacher. Wouldn't Ms. Johnson with all her credentials and experience be a better choice for Ryan? But that wasn't true.

No one was better than Michelle and Amy.

Past experience had taught me that great credentials didn't guarantee a person would know how to work with my son. For Ryan, paper qualifications had never been the best predictor of success. I went with the flow when I shouldn't have. I told myself I had to choose my battles carefully and not fight this last-minute change. There really wasn't much I could do about it, anyway. The IEP team knew it looked good on paper in the event of any dispute. I could have refused to sign off on it, but I felt cornered.

Although Ms. Johnson was very kind to Ryan and didn't do any significant or long-lasting damage during his second-grade experience, he didn't make much progress that year. She just wanted him to be the *best little autistic boy* he could be. She had no expectation for him to act like typical kids. She had all the training to "know" kids with autism couldn't get better.

Michelle and Amy not wanting Ryan—or more likely, me—left me emotionally distraught. In the past, I never cared much what people thought. Someone could badmouth me all over town and that didn't matter, but getting fired from the Michelle and Amy team really got to me. I loved these two women and all they had done to help my son. I thought together we were an excellent team. Wasn't Ryan the entire reason Amy had been hired by the school district in the first place? But for families with autism, you and your child that are the only team that you can count on to be there.

The new plan from the IEP team was made without any input from us, Ryan's parents. That was technically against the law. After Ryan was given a different second grade teacher, he was assigned two different aides. Two aides are better than one, right? How could I possibly object? The multiple-aides idea was a bad one. You don't give a child who has a significant need for structure and sameness two different aides unless they are clones. I questioned what happened to the notion that parents are members of the IEP team. Shouldn't team decisions include parent participation?

Remembering my rule of documenting everything, I jumped over the IEP team the same way they jumped over me and responded with a terse letter to the director of special education services. I didn't even try to maintain any semblance of diplomacy.

Letter to Dr. Carthaus, Director of Special Education
August 22, 1996

Dear Dr. Carthaus:

I was very concerned about the conversation we had August 19, 1996, and wanted to follow-up with this letter to prevent any future misunderstandings. After the problem we had with Beth [Ryan's case manager] and Ryan's teacher selection for this school year, I was assured by both you and the assistant director of special education that Beth would no longer be in charge of his program.

Laws were broken when everyone on the IEP team except Frank and I knew about the change concerning Ryan's teacher for second grade. Beth was responsible for this. We are members of the team and legally have the right to be involved in the decisions that affect his educational needs. Decisions were made that greatly affect Ryan and without our knowledge or consent. When we last spoke, you told me that Beth said two aides were needed so that no one would experience "burnout."

I resent the statement that my son causes burnout. Ryan is just not that tough. Ryan needs the consistency that one aide would provide. Having two different people at two different times in the classroom is just not a viable option for a child who needs consistency and stability. This just reinforces my belief that Beth knows nothing about Ryan, what works best, and what he needs.

In the past, you decided on Ryan's aide. I hope we are not limited to one school location to find the person who will meet Ryan's needs. I trust your judgment and know you will look at all the possibilities in the district to ensure that an appropriate aide will be found. However, I must insist that Beth not be involved in this decision or any future decisions concerning Ryan.

Once again, I do not want the aide to know that Ryan has autism. A lack of knowledge concerning autism makes some believe that children afflicted with it are weird and incapable of learning. A prime example is Beth's burnout statement.

People cannot assume Ryan can't do things. He must not experience the stigma associated with the A-word. Also, with the growth Ryan has had socially this summer, I would like to start the year without an aide at recess. If he is not successful, we can reevaluate this decision.

I hope we will be able to work this out. We have always had a good working relationship built on trust. I know our usual method of open and honest communication will continue in the future and ensure that Ryan's educational needs will be met. Thank you for your assistance with this matter. I look forward to hearing from you.

Sincerely,
Marcia Hinds

I was hurt, and I was angry about the actions of the IEP team. To make things worse, they were not doing what was best for my son. I never said, "Be careful or I will sue your ass," but my intent was clear, and they got the message. They backed down from their two-aide plan.

I later found out the real reason a two-aide plan developed. One of the aides they tried to assign to my son was incompetent and worthless. I didn't want this inept woman anywhere near Ryan. Unfortunately, this unprofessional, lazy, and untrained aide was allowed to continue to work with kids whose parents never questioned things. We were given a different aide who eventually continued with Ryan all the way through fifth grade. Ms. Sutton was great, and we loved her even though she never had any formal ABA training.

If I Knew Then What I Know Now

Second grade was the only year Ryan didn't significantly improve. This shows just how important teacher and aide selection are for our children's success in school. Ms. Johnson had all the credentials in the world and was a very nice person. But she was not the right choice for Ryan. Ryan needed a teacher who would challenge him, make him work hard, and make him feel good about himself at the same time. He needed Michelle Sanders. Teachers with all the training, like Ms. Johnson, know enough to falsely believe our kids can never recover. That was not the kind of understanding of autism I wanted for my child.

IEP team meetings are frequently hard and emotionally draining for everyone. Parents cry, teachers feel frustrated, administrators squirm. It is crucial to understand your child's rights and your rights as the whole team struggles toward a plan that works for your child and realistic in terms of the resources available to help your child. And never ask for something you don't actually need or can provide yourself. That takes services away from other children.

A history of confrontation will gut the IEP and staff relationships you spent years carefully crafting. But also remember IEP teams don't always follow the rules. This works both ways. In this situation, the IEP team made decisions without our input. This was legally wrong and undermined any spirit of collaboration. However, sometimes an IEP team may quietly arrange for your child to receive services above and beyond what they legally need to provide. This can be done by saying one thing on paper and doing another in the classroom. I tried to promote collaboration and made the meetings more relaxed by saying I didn't really care what the IEP said as long as Ryan got what he needed. An IEP meeting is a dance, and the experience is much better when you know and trust your dance partner.

Know when to *collaborate* and know when to *confront*.

I worried far too much about the teachers and the IEP team liking Ryan and me. What I needed to do was to stop worrying about their personal feelings and thoughts, learn to tread softly, and carry a big legal, documented stick. Although, the school personnel liked me for the most part, I think they were a little afraid of me, too. Fear can be a good thing to help you get what your kid needs as long as in the process you don't make anyone too angry. Most times it was never necessary to carry a stick because the team genuinely cared about helping my son. Frank usually accompanied me to these meetings. We had our own rendition of good cop, bad cop. I know I don't have to spell out what Frank's roll was—everyone always loves Frank. That was not always the case with me.

Frank and I used to refer to this stick-and-carrot IEP management tactic as *"getting loud."* It's kind of like when you are complaining in a store about a problem. When you increase the volume, other customers hear what you are saying, so management does whatever you ask in order to shut you up. Most times we never had to get *loud* because they knew I would. Nobody wanted to take on Ryan's mother.

Whenever I had to attend an IEP meeting without Frank, his first question to me was, "Did you have to get *loud* to make sure Ryan got what he needed?" I always tried the nice way first. But if that didn't work, then I *got loud*. Most times I didn't have to since they knew I would. And I could get *very, very LOUD*.[41]

---

41   Check out the book by Dr. Vaughn Lauer called, *When the School Says No...How to Get the Yes!* This book has important info about IEPs and how to get the services your child needs.

CHAPTER 32

ALMOST NORMAL, BUT NOT NORMAL ENOUGH

You won't realize the distance you've walked until you take a look around and realize how far you've come.

—Author Unknown

THE ONLY THING Ryan remembers about second grade is getting into trouble for working ahead in his math journal. Ms. Johnson, his credentialed and experienced special needs teacher, couldn't understand why he did this, nor was she happy about it. Instead of explaining what she expected, Ms. Johnson took away his completed math workbook and replaced it with a blank one for him to stare at. Ryan had to complete the same math workbook all over again, but this time with the rest of the class. She never understood my son. Ryan just wanted her to know he was smart. This teacher didn't want smart—she wanted compliant. I know compliance is essential in a classroom, but Ms. Johnson never treated my son like he was at all capable.

At school, there were not many areas where Ryan experienced success. Math happened to be one of them. He was scary smart when it came to numbers. My little human calculator loved everything about them. I assumed this was because numbers are orderly and predictable—unlike people. Sadly, Ms. Johnson became another unpredictable adult. Instead of getting the praise he expected for completing his work perfectly and ahead of schedule, she punished him. She became the anti-ABA teacher and insisted he do the entire workbook all over again. She failed to reinforce his efforts. My son only wanted to show his teacher that he was capable and smart. Ms. Johnson never considered that he worked ahead because math was an area that made him feel good about himself.

I totally understood her wanting him to conform and work along with the rest of the class, but couldn't she find another way to make him feel good about himself? A little praise for his extraordinary math skills would have encouraged him to keep at it. Couldn't she have given him extra worksheets or some other way for him to shine? Sadly, in her class, everyone had to be doing the same thing at the same time. There was no differentiated instruction to meet the needs of different students working at different levels.

For a teacher with a master's in special education, she didn't understand how children learn best. No matter how many times I tried, I couldn't make her get it. She ignored me and my requests. That worked about as well on me as it did with Ryan. When a behavior is not encouraged or rewarded it fades away, or goes extinct. In *ABA Speak*, Ms. Johnson put me on "extinction" and got rid of my unwanted behavior. After a while, I gave up trying.

Ms. Johnson was a good teacher for most kids, just not Ryan. She was like most people who didn't get it. Her assumption that Ryan's strange behaviors like making noises, poking kids, and repeating the same topics of conversation over and over meant my son was as behind intellectually as he was in the area of social skills. She never realized how capable Ryan truly was or that she needed to let him shine where he excelled. She never recognized there was an intelligent kid *in there* who needed her to believe in him.

Instead, she gave him way too much help and reinforced the negative behaviors we worked so hard to eliminate. Ryan knew the fastest way to get extra attention from Ms. Johnson was to act like he wasn't capable. This also helped to reinforce Ms. Johnson's belief that my son was incompetent.

It was quite discouraging that, after two years of concentrated effort, we were right back to Ryan's old behaviors of seeking negative attention. Ms. Johnson was the only teacher I did not handpick during the elementary school years. She was Ryan's only teacher who had a background in special education. With all her special credentials, she did not realize my son just needed high expectations and positive reinforcement. She shouldn't have given him so much help with the things he already knew how to do, which is what Barbara had done with counting in kindergarten. Ms. Johnson needed to force my son to join the rest of the world by discovering and reinforcing his strengths.

Ms. Jarvis was a big relief after second grade. We had too many things to learn to spend time with anyone who didn't move the train forward. Ryan entered Ms. Jarvis's classroom a developmental and social mess. He was a basket of contradictions. He reluctantly played soccer and basketball, but he refused to watch these sports on TV. He watched football and baseball, but never wanted to play them. Ryan hated playing any sport and needed his dad's constant encouragement to keep trying. So, Frank was the coach of whatever Ryan happened to be trying to play at the time.

He was different from other kids and did not share many of their interests. Ryan only read nonfiction books because they contained facts and information presented in a predictable way. Fiction books had too many implied meanings. Most kids don't find nonfiction topics as interesting, but for my son, they were much easier to understand. I didn't care what he was reading as long as he read. His struggle with reading comprehension skills followed him past elementary school and into middle school.

At times I didn't realize how Ryan's developmental deficits impacted his behavior. Motor planning issues and lack of stamina caused his difficulties in sports. His restricted interest in numbers fueled his super math ability. His struggle to write imaginary stories was because he lacked the ability to imagine much of anything. And his issues with order and sequencing caused a whole host of other problems. Without the basic foundation for these developmental skills, Ryan's social skills didn't have a chance to develop.

Except, his social skills weren't as bad at home.

We continued to see a big difference between *Home Ryan* and *School Ryan*. The less safe he felt at school, the more he shut down and the more autistic he acted. When he didn't know what to do, he simply retreated to Autism Island. It was hard to understand the disconnect. I know his teachers thought I was embellishing or maybe just delusional when I told them about the things he did at home. Ryan mastered new things at home long before he did them at school. The reasons for this were not complicated. Home was where felt accepted, safe, and loved. There were also fewer things happening at the same time at home; so, life was easier to navigate there. In school Ryan had to work in groups, and he was not comfortable in groups. When the numbers of children in a small group increased or when Ryan was not sure of what to do, we would see more weird behaviors. That's when his classmates would see hand-flapping or hear strange elevator noises. And who would want to be with someone who acted like that?

Thankfully, a few girls did, perhaps because they were more accepting and encouraging.

I came up with endless theories about why he preferred to play with girls rather than boys. Maybe girls didn't play as rough as boys. Perhaps they had better social skills than the boys; maybe they were being maternal. Or was it because Ryan understood *Girl Speak* better because of his sister? All I knew was that Ryan wanted to have friends. He didn't care about gender. He just didn't know how to connect, make small talk, or interact in the right way. Social skills deficits are a huge part of defining autism. I was starting to appreciate just how profound an impact a social skills deficit could have on his school experience and quality of life.

Ms. Jarvis helped him move in the right direction again by focusing on two areas: self-confidence and social skills. My son had experienced way too much failure in his young life. Ryan thought he couldn't do anything right and was too afraid to try. Sometimes, he would stand paralyzed in the middle of the classroom with that blank and dazed expression just waiting for anyone to tell him what to do next.

Whenever possible, Ms. Jarvis placed Ryan in situations where he was the leader or special helper. Since he excelled at math and computers, she had him help other children in these areas. This became part of the solution for his lack-of-confidence issue. She didn't stop there. She had actually read and implemented most of the suggestions that we sent in the following letter at the beginning of the year:

Dear Ms. Jarvis,

Since this is such a group effort, we wanted to communicate what we feel are the most important skills and goals that need to be emphasized with Ryan. The areas of concern that we want to address are confidence/social skills, attentiveness/compliance, and academics.

Ryan is strong in almost all academic areas, except writing stories. Since language came late to him, this continues to be an area of concern. Most of his difficulties come from nonattentiveness (missing or misunderstanding directions, not picking up nonverbal communication, and thinking he already knows what to do and, therefore, doesn't pay attention).

He needs to be encouraged to ask about things he doesn't know. Although he has an extensive vocabulary, occasionally he does not know the meaning of very simple words. Kathryn Hagen [Ryan's speech teacher] picked up on this right away in testing Ryan. She not only understood his speech deficits, but she also quickly figured out how Ryan works. We were a little upset that something that had taken us nine years to understand only took her a couple of hours.

In addition, Ryan needs work in expressive areas that require him to use his imagination. He can write a paragraph on how to make a peanut butter and jelly sandwich, but he has trouble with an imaginary story. In art, he can draw the street where he lives, but drawing something he has never seen would be difficult for him.

There are still large holes in Ryan's language. There are many figurative or slang expressions that he takes literally. For example, when his next-door neighbor asked Ryan who his closest friend was, Ryan answered, "You are, Greg, you live right next door." Fortunately, this time Ryan had the right answer either way.

The difficulties Ryan has with social interaction come from three things: a lack of confidence, a fear of failure, and an unwillingness to compromise. At home, where he is sure of himself, Ryan is successful at having friends. Our house is always filled with all his neighborhood friends, but somehow this has not generalized to school.

Please don't feel sorry for him or think he can't do something. That is the most detrimental thing that could happen to him. It is crucial that there be high expectations for Ryan. It is a difficult balancing act between helping Ryan and promoting his independence. Please only help him the same way you would any other child. Please use the same discipline/consequences you would for any child. In the past, people have assumed Ryan is not intelligent and can't do anything. He was given too much help with the best of intentions. Ryan will try to convince you that he can't do something to get that extra attention. If it is very clear in the beginning that he must comply, be organized, and attentive, then he will do it.

Thanks so much for taking the time to read this and let us ramble on too long about our kid. We know with you as his teacher, this will be a great year. And please believe we are only a little neurotic.

Sincerely,
Marcia Hinds

Ms. Jarvis assigned Ryan the lead role in the class play, *The Shoemaker and the Elves*. He did a great job as Hans, the shoemaker. Ironically, at the same time he played the part of the shoemaker, he still had an unending hatred of all shoes, except for his slip-on sneakers and boat shoes. Those shoes would have worked if we had lived in sunny California. But if you've never lived in cold country or through a Minnesota winter, you can't fully understand just how ridiculous it was to wear those kinds of shoes instead of snow boots.

Ryan was wonderful at pretending to be Hans, but not so wonderful pretending to be a regular student. Back in the classroom war zone, Ryan avoided eye contact and tried not to answer questions his teachers or peers asked. This was a big source of his problems. Ryan listened, but he usually wasn't watching when the teacher gave a lesson in front of the class. He stared out the window or concentrated on the hands moving around the clock. He missed a lot of the nonverbal cues needed to comprehend what was actually happening in a classroom.

I once asked an adult that was affected by autism to explain why people on the spectrum have trouble making eye contact. He explained that the reason he didn't look at people was because there were too many things going on at once. It was hard for him to listen, understand what someone was saying, and still look at the person talking all at the same time. If he left out eye contact, then it was easier for him to focus on what was being said. But, just like with Ryan, this caused him to miss the nonverbal cues we all use to effectively communicate.

Ms. Jarvis's style of teaching and classroom management were big factors in the solution to this issue. She used teaching techniques that required Ryan (and every child) to look at her and focus. She demanded that Ryan maintain eye contact and attend to nonverbal cues by not talking to him until he was looking at her. She simply ignored what was not appropriate. After the initial adjustment period, Ryan became very attentive to Ms. Jarvis because she expected that and insisted on it.

Whenever the class discussed current events, Ms. Jarvis randomly picked a stick out of a coffee can with a child's name on it. That student would have to summarize what was just talked about in class. This was perfect for Ryan. He had to attend because he might be called on. Before Ms. Jarvis, he often missed classroom instructions as well as information the teacher pointed to or wrote on the board. However, it is interesting to note that when a student teacher took over Ms. Jarvis's classroom, Ryan's inattention to nonverbal cues returned. He did only what was expected and demanded of him.

Ryan also developed an excellent coping mechanism. If he missed the initial instructions the teacher gave, then he would watch what the other students were doing during transitions. Then he would copy what they did. Sometimes, the child sitting next to him would help him with what he needed to be doing when they saw he was off-track. Ms. Jarvis surrounded him with the nice kids. The atmosphere of the classroom Ms. Jarvis created was almost like that of a family. They helped each other succeed and helped those who needed it even more.

Home support remained an essential part of his school success. We continued to pre-teach and reteach. Ms. Sutton, his aide, kept us informed via the communication book. I know giving this feedback was a lot to ask, but this school-to-home communication was critical. It was difficult for Ryan when a lesson contained something that hadn't been practiced at home. Writing stories was an example of this. But Ms. Jarvis and Ms. Sutton were on top of it. When Ryan wrote a story at school, one of them would stroll by his desk and casually encourage him to write more than the minimum. He wasn't allowed to just write one sentence or take the easy way out. It helped that he adored them both and wanted to please them. They also expected that he complete all assignments and not just the ones he was interested in.

Nothing was ever an easy fix with Ryan. These teachers required that he had to sometimes redo a messy assignment or a story that was not his best effort. At first, his handwriting was too large. Later, after we showed him what he was doing wrong, Ryan overcompensated by writing too small. With practice, his handwriting improved, but even now he sometimes writes too small.

We continued to set up situations at home to practice the skills he needed to master. On one particular day, I signed up to be the mom helper during the Friday morning meeting time. Friday was joke day. Ryan came up with an original joke that really bombed. After telling jokes at the talent show, I thought I could cross this off the to-do list. I didn't understand that Ryan was okay when it came to reading a scripted joke, but creating one was entirely different. That skill had not yet been mastered.

Ryan didn't get it. What was hilarious to him didn't make sense to his peers. I explained that kids sometimes learn jokes from books. We bought a joke book and practiced. He did a wonderful, memorized performance the following Friday. It took years before he acquired his father's sense of humor. Spontaneous joke telling didn't develop until sometime during the college years.

Even with Ms. Jarvis's direct intervention in social skills plus all the work at home, Ryan remained on the outside looking in socially. We worked hard on anything we could do to make him more accepted by other kids. He had haircuts and clothes that were the latest style. Megan became the clothes police because Ryan's mother had no clue as to what looked fashionable. Looking cute and cool helped peers sometimes overlook weird behavior. Although kids were rarely mean to him, he was not usually included in activities at lunch or recess.

He was left out because getting him to answer questions or talk about something that was not one of his restricted interests took too much effort for anyone—sometimes even his family who loved him.

Mr. Beverage, Ryan's fourth grade—and first male—teacher, was another gem. He was the perfect choice to address Ryan's self-confidence and social skills issues. Ryan immediately connected with him. But the ever-present social issues were still there. Even though my son now tested in the eighty-eighth percentile for language on the standardized Iowa Tests, reading comprehension continued to be an issue. He still had odd behaviors that made him seem different from the other kids, but they were becoming less noticeable. More importantly, my son was starting to have the beginnings of a few friendships.

Ben, a classmate of Ryan's, won a miniature golfing trip at the school carnival. The golf excursion was with Ryan's kindergarten teacher, Ms. Paul. Ben picked Ryan as the friend he wanted to take with him. Sherry Paul called me after they went golfing. She complimented Ryan on what a wonderful boy he had grown up to be. According to Ms. Paul, he had the best manners and was a delight. I think this was her way of apologizing for all the crap she gave me when he was in her kindergarten class. But the way she treated me back then was unimportant. She was essential for Ryan's progress in kindergarten. She provided the structure and discipline he needed at that time.

The unstructured times of his school day continued to be the most difficult for my son. He still struggled during lunch and recess even though he had a few *almost friends* like Ben. But Ben liked to talk with lots of kids during lunch and was always playing ball at recess. Neither of those was a strong suit for Ryan.

In fourth grade, Kari Pederson, the school social worker, joined our team. Kari invited Ryan to pick a small group of kids to meet in her office twice a week during the dreaded lunch period. There they played board games and did other activities. This gave Ryan a more structured way to connect with other kids in his class. All the kids wanted to go with him to Ms. Pederson's room for all the fun.

Before I really knew Kari, I wasn't sure she could help Ryan. I'm embarrassed to admit my own prejudice got in the way when we first met. Kari was born with cerebral palsy. She walked with a limp, and one of her hands was turned in. I mistakenly assumed that her disability affected her teaching ability. I judged her in the very same way others did Ryan. I was as ignorant about Kari's condition as most people were about Ryan's autism. Later, she became a top candidate on Frank's list of future brides. I loved this woman and all the wonderful things she did for my son.

Kari and Sarah (Ryan's speech specialist) became what Frank and I referred to as the *Kari and Sarah Show*. They came into Ryan's classroom and effectively taught social skills lessons to his entire class. They covered topics like how to make friends and what it takes to keep a friend. All the children in his class benefitted from what they taught. Kari correctly assumed if these lessons in communication skills were presented to all the kids, then maybe Ryan wouldn't feel like we were trying to fix him or that he wasn't good enough. That was a huge problem for my son at the time. He withdrew whenever he surmised that's what we were doing.

Even with the *Kari and Sarah Show*, Ryan's self-confidence remained fragile. When Ryan was younger, he often exploded with anger, but now his anger transitioned to bouts of sadness. The good news was that the medical interventions plus school and home therapies were helping him become more engaged with the real world. The bad news was that now he was recovered enough to realize he wasn't included. He didn't really fit in this new world. The worst news was that he still had trouble with the complex social skills required for real friendships and connecting with most kids.

When I had to watch Ryan cry because he was never invited to play or didn't have anyone who wanted to sit with him at lunch, I cried, too. I remember thinking I would be the happiest woman in the world if Ryan was just invited to a birthday party. That was my wish-bone wish every Thanksgiving and the same one I made every year when I blew out my birthday candles.

I would have traded all the things he excelled at academically for one good friend at school. It was increasingly obvious that my child was not having much success socially anywhere. Friends weren't happening at school and were barely happening at home during play dates. He was lonely; his parents and sister were his only friends, except we weren't really his friends—we were his family. Ryan had *no* real friends.

All I could do was to keep creating social skills opportunities at school and keep them happening at home with play dates. One morning, I found Ryan crying. When I asked why, he told me he didn't have any friends. As our conversation continued, he confessed that he was afraid to talk to me about this because he knew I wanted him to have friends more than anything.

We were discussing one kid, the son of a family friend, who didn't treat Ryan kindly. That's when Ryan said to me, "You mean you wouldn't rather have James as a son because he has so many friends?" It broke my heart that Ryan didn't realize he was, and continues to be, the best thing that ever happened to me.

Although he tried to reach out to kids, Ryan's methods usually resulted in rejection. Instead of asking someone to play, Ryan sometimes regressed to poking them. Next, he asked questions about restricted interests that had nothing to do with what was happening at the time or weren't anywhere close to age-appropriate. After the many inevitable rejections, he stopped trying to connect with other kids and just withdrew.

At home with his family, things were different. Ryan had no fear of rejection from us. We didn't shut him down when he started talking about sharks. We listened and acted fascinated when we heard the same thing for the hundredth time. We tried to engage him and expand his limited topics of conversation. It was easy to see why kids didn't want to work that hard to have a playmate. Even his family who loved him grew tired of his antics.

At school, he didn't act like the sweet kid who felt so safe and loved at home. If it had been possible for him to stop worrying so much and just be himself, he'd have all the friends he could ever want. Since he didn't know how to successfully approach other kids, he would do anything to get noticed. His old friend Mr. Negative Attention was better than no attention at all. Trying to break into social situations can be difficult for any of us. Imagine trying to break into a group when you don't know the right thing to say or any of the social customs.

On those rare occasions when Ryan had someone to play with at school, the weirdness went away because he felt good about himself. We tried to help these social successes become more common by having kids from his class over. We facilitated friendships at home and hoped they would transfer to school. Home was familiar. There he didn't have to navigate thirty different kids doing thirty different things on a noisy playground full of a million nonverbal cues he didn't understand.

We looked for other ways to help Ryan. We put him in an after-school chess club with kids from his class. Ryan loved to play chess. He was good at it. Ryan regularly thumped his dad at chess, not to mention poker, blackjack, backgammon, and video games. We even thought that our Ryan could possibly be the reincarnation of Bobby Fischer, whom some consider the best chess player of all time.

Although he didn't hang out at the track yet, Ryan had been known to make the games more interesting with a friendly wager. We bet on anything and everything back then (and still do). Once my kids bet on the date I would finally admit the dog we were fostering was ours for life.

The stakes were varied. It ranged from the coins in his father's pockets to who had to make Ryan's bed in the morning. I think Ryan's grand plan at that time might have been to attend Scripps Institute of Oceanography, become the next Jacques Cousteau, and pay for all of this out of his winnings. He just wouldn't have any friends to invite to the celebration.

On the first day of fifth grade, his new teacher Ms. Dahlquist wore a Monopoly dress. Ms. D's enthusiasm for Monopoly rivaled Ryan's passion for sharks. The Monopoly theme went on for weeks, and we were all involved with her obsession. She even displayed a picture of each student on giant Monopoly properties and hung them from the ceiling of the classroom. On the bottom of each property was written *"VALUE: PRICELESS!"* That pretty much summed up how she felt about kids. She put in an incredible amount of time and effort to ensure each child experienced success, success, and more success. Our kids need teachers like Ms. Dahlquist in their lives: teachers who help them feel good about themselves and make school fun and engaging.

Ryan loved Ms. D. and the *All About ME* book he had to write that year. He said this about her and fifth grade in that book: "Ms. Dahlquist always thinks of her students before herself. She gives up her lunch time to help us with subjects that we are having trouble with and teaches us things like how to cross-stitch. But the most important thing Ms. Dahlquist taught me is how to be a good person. I wish I could get 'Fs' and flunk fifth grade, just so I could have another year with Ms. Dahlquist. After that year, I'd have to flunk again and again, so my whole life would be in Ms. Dahlquist's room. I'm going to *really* miss her. But I *won't* miss her homework. She gives way too much!"

Ms. D. later became a principal in our school district. When Ryan was in middle school, she would occasionally stop by our house to invite Ryan to go on walks with her and her own children on the nature trails across the street from our house. When we took a short trip to Las Vegas, we took a picture of Ryan in the Monopoly-themed restaurant we just had to visit. Ms. D. loved that picture of Ryan.

The high caliber of teachers and staff Ryan had in elementary school were a huge part of his recovery. It had to be more than coincidence that he had so many wonderful people in his life.

If I Knew Then What I Know Now

We sometimes forget what a war zone school is for children with autism. The one hidden social rule for school is this: do not act autistic. Autistic behaviors make our kids highly visible. Their oddness encourages criticism, discourages social interaction, sets them up as targets for bullies, and puts them at risk of being reassigned to a more restrictive special education classroom.

The book *Social Skills Activities for Special Children* by Darlene Mannix helped us teach Ryan how to behave at school. This activity book helped my son recognize that his social skills had to change depending if he was at school, at home, or at a friend's house. You won't be disappointed if you take the time to check out Darlene's books. All her books are great for teaching these kinds of important lessons.

Ryan loved the special time snuggling with mom each night to do one of the activities listed in the book. Together each evening, we solved a small part of why other people behaved so inconsistently. We followed the book's lesson plan orally rather than in writing. I really can't pinpoint the exact moment when Ryan started learning like other children. The timing varied for the different skills. But it finally started to happen, and over time he no longer needed to be pre-taught every new skill. He was starting to learn without my direct instruction. Yet there seemed to always be something else we needed to tackle.

Once Ryan learned what was expected or a new rule, he followed it religiously without question. You would never catch him riding in a car without his seatbelt because that was a rule. At school, kids weren't supposed to talk during work time. Since that was a rule, Ryan never talked to the kids who sat next to him at school. When he came home one day with news that he'd gotten in trouble for talking in class, I secretly cheered. That meant he was being social and cared more about having friends than following the rules.

CHAPTER 33

THE SOCIAL SKILLS ARE THE LAST TO COME

What would happen if the autism gene was eliminated from the gene pool? You would have a bunch of people standing around in a cave, chatting and socializing and not getting anything done.

—Temple Grandin

TEACHING SOCIAL SKILLS is a long, grueling process. It takes a lifetime to learn all of them and only a moment to break one of the rules. Each of us remembers our mistakes more clearly and with more uncomfortable intensity than all the times we were successful socially. We are often described by our social abilities: Joe is a warm person; Susan is a cold fish. Children with autism are quickly classified by their peers and excluded because of their atypical and confusing social missteps.

There are life social skills and there are school social skills. Not being proficient in these skills interfered with my son's success everywhere. It was hard for Ryan to understand why you were allowed to do some things at home, but these same things couldn't be done at school. Ryan usually didn't understand what was expected of him. At our house, no one closed the door when they used the bathroom, but at school that behavior is always unacceptable. There are so many social rules, and each one changes depending on where you are. Even though Ryan was starting to catch up, we still had to teach him each rule for every situation and setting.

I started deliberately encouraging social interaction by play dates in our home when Ryan was around five. That was about four and a half years too late. We had been too busy pretending nothing was wrong. Teaching social skills to a child with what I call "social dyslexia" is overwhelming. I didn't know how to teach these skills because I didn't have any idea of how I had learned them myself.

It is much easier in the short-run for parents to put on a video and let their children veg away the afternoon. It is easier to watch *Star Wars* for the fiftieth time than to try and teach a simple social skill like saying "please" over and over again. However, we knew that if we didn't teach Ryan these important skills, he wasn't going to learn them on his own. How was I going to get Ryan to excel at complex multistep behaviors when I couldn't even get him to say "Hi" or look at anyone when he walked into a room?

While he had some language, it was not functional language. Ryan didn't understand how to communicate effectively within any of the tons of social situations that occur every day. I had wrongly assumed that if he just started to talk more, everything would be okay. I didn't realize words were not enough. Ryan needed to be able to use language in an effective way to make friends and engage others. But my son spoke from the same script over and over again.

Ryan never talked about events that happened in his daily life, his fears, or his dreams for the future. When he started elementary school, Ryan began to participate in small talk with teachers and friends. But he only used the predictable scripts we practiced at home. Spontaneous language didn't come until many years later. Ryan only asked the questions we taught him to ask when he first tried to engage friends in conversation. His speech was scripted from our practice sessions at home and seemed almost robotic at times. Ryan was often too busy planning what he would say next to be a good listener.[42]

---

42   When Ryan was in middle school, I came across the book *Teach Me Language* by Sabrina Freeman. Too bad I didn't find it when he was still learning about the back-and-forth conversation skills; it would have been great resource for higher-level language and social skills. But this book is not for beginning language. It contains advanced lessons in communication and social skills. See the References section for more information.

Ryan didn't have conversations that anyone else found interesting. The kids at school valued the ability to play capture the flag and dodgeball way more than an exceptional aptitude for math. They didn't want to only talk about technology or sharks. My son was excelling in the wrong areas. When a boy from his classroom had a birthday, sometimes he was the only one not included. Ryan was invited to only one birthday party during all of elementary school.

Autism doesn't have a monopoly on social skills issues (no pun intended, Ms. Dahlquist). Social skills instruction for the entire class benefits more than just the child with autism. Beyond the classroom, the whole world could use lessons in kindness and compassion. But kids with autism require a comprehensive social skills curriculum. They need this almost as much as they need oxygen.

Teaching Ryan social skills was a step-by-step process. I realized early on that these were the most important things I needed to teach my son. If he didn't know how to interact, he wouldn't have any of the most worthwhile things in life. But I didn't know where to start. In hindsight, it might look like I knew what I was doing. But that really wasn't the case. I did not have a plan. I had no idea if any of the things I tried would help his future outcome. I made many mistakes and was mostly flying by the seat of my pants. I was just trying to get through each day. And sometimes our survival was minute-by-minute.

I still fantasized that Ryan would grow up to be like Jacques Cousteau, Albert Einstein, or Thomas Edison, who were successful and brilliant even if different. Ryan and I still read stories together about these men. I wasn't sure if this was for his sake or mine. These stories kept me going so I wouldn't think about my fear of my son ending up in a group home all alone.

Helping Ryan was all I did. I was a mom on a mission. I couldn't give up because there wasn't anyone else who wanted to save him. Parents seem to be the only ones equipped with the stamina to do this job. And I didn't have much else but my gut to guide me. It seems like I shouldn't have felt so alone when I had such a warm and supportive husband and family. But I felt all alone and isolated on Autism Island with Ryan.

I started my quest for Ryan to be social and have friendships by borrowing kids from my friends in our neighborhood. I had to force Ryan to interact because he didn't know how. And at first he didn't want to. I told him having friends over was mandatory and either he could pick who was coming for a play date or I would. When I first began mandatory human interaction, I was the one who played with the other kids while Ryan hid in the back of the house.

When he finally did venture out, he quickly proved that playing with him was not fun. To compensate, I made my house the place every kid wanted to be. I had the best toys and the best treats. We even built a Gucci playhouse, got a trampoline, video games, and anything else that would be a kid-attractor. These children liked the one-on-one attention they got from me. I used anything and everything to make them want to come back.

We took turns when we had friends over and picked activities where the rules for social interaction were simple. Ryan and his play buddy jumped on the trampoline, went sledding, and played board, computer, or video games. There was no pretend play or any activity that required a higher level of conversation or much social ability. Going to the park or the movies were our field trips. Playing on the equipment at the park or sitting in a movie didn't take advanced language or social skills. It took quite some time before my son joined in and years before he could fly solo.

At first, play dates did not last long because I wanted Ryan to experience success. But one of the reasons they were short was so the kids we invited would not have to witness one of Ryan's inevitable meltdowns. We increased the playtime only after Ryan became more comfortable. We started with one child once a week. After Ryan could handle the interaction with one kid, we did it more often. In time, we tried two kids and eventually small groups several times a week.

The further he progressed in social skills, the more challenging I made the play dates. Ryan loved to cook and do science experiments. We practiced and role-played doing these activities solo before attempting them with anyone else. Our activities had a script and were predictable. When he was ready, we added another child to the mix. It took a long time before we attempted small groups of children. We used his interests to teach following directions, cooperation, and how to wait your turn.

Shawn, our gentle autism "expert" from the school district, was supposed to teach Ryan social skills at our home as part of Ryan's IEP. However, most times it ended up with me teaching Shawn how to teach my son.

At first, I was happy to have an extra pair of hands, but sometimes Shawn made life harder for me. After he came for a play session with Ryan, it looked like a tornado had hit the premises. Shawn never made Ryan put anything away. But worse than the mess, I was left to deal with Ryan after Shawn's forty-five minutes of therapy. Ryan controlled Shawn. A soft-spoken style and kind way of doing business, which may have been perfect for some kids, didn't work with my son. Ryan needed direct, constant, and repeated in-your-face behavioral shaping. Shawn should have fit the therapy to the kid—not the other way around.

My responsibility when Shawn came for a session was to have another child at our house ready to play. All Shawn had to do was show up and facilitate these social interactions. He was wonderful with my son as long as he didn't ask Ryan to do anything Ryan didn't want to do. Instead of teaching Ryan how to take turns, he avoided any confrontation by letting Ryan be first and use the blue game piece every time. If I had let this continue, Ryan would learn to expect the world to revolve around him and his wants for the rest of his life; so, I began to intervene.

If there was a problem like crying, a meltdown, or hitting when Ryan didn't get what he wanted, I would calmly take Ryan to the back of the house so Ryan's playmate wouldn't witness what I did next. I put Ryan through his ABA paces just like I did behind the post at the mall or any other place he misbehaved. Shawn was left to entertain his playmate while I convinced Ryan to comply. Ryan had to do what I asked. After he did two things like touch his head or clap his hands, he was allowed to escape. It didn't really matter what I asked my son to do—*only that he did it*. Afterwards, I would ask him, "Are you ready to go back and play properly now?" If the answer was "Yes," then I sent him back to play. Otherwise, I kept going. I made him continue doing whatever I told him to do until I won the battle. I knew Shawn wasn't really helping Ryan, but he was a nice man who truly cared about my son. I didn't want to hurt Shawn's feelings, so we continued these social skill sessions, and I made Ryan comply.

Ryan had a killer smile when he wasn't frowning or in the middle of a meltdown. Most times, he looked like he had a permanent scowl plastered on his face. His expression seemed to say he was mad at the world even when he wasn't. I had to teach him how to look friendly and approachable. So, we practiced and learned how to do that. When we were in the waiting room at the doctor's office or before the meal at a restaurant, we discussed the things that made some people look nice and how they looked when they had a frown on their face.

I would ask Ryan to point out people he thought looked friendly and easy to be friends with. We searched restaurants before our food arrived to find people who would be fun to talk to. Next, I would ask him, "Why would you rather be friends with them instead of the guy across the room who looks kind of mean? What made them look friendly and fun? Was it their smiling eyes? Or was it the big grin plastered on their face?" After months of doing this, Ryan started to smile more often. This game helped with everyone's attitude and acceptance, especially mine.

I used other children to model appropriate social interaction. Shannon, Megan's best girlfriend from the neighborhood, was a constant fixture at our house. Their play exemplified typical interactions for Ryan to model. Shannon loved Ryan. She was part of our family, and Megan only occasionally minded when her annoying little brother was present. Usually he simply ignored them, but sometimes I caught him watching and learning from what they did.

Greg, who lived next door, was the closet person Ryan had to a friend. Although Greg was almost a year younger, he proved to be a perfect role model. Ryan learned a lot about social skills and social interaction from Greg. They both loved figuring out how things worked. Trips to the Goodwill store for old mechanical objects were trips to discover some treasure they could take apart and examine. I would give them each a screwdriver, and soon they were busy playing alongside each other and talking about electronics.

I thought his mother, Jill, and I were friends. But after she witnessed some of Ryan's odd behaviors, she seemed wary of him. As a nurse, you would think she should know that autism wasn't contagious, but that is not how she treated my son. Although we had Greg over constantly, she never included Ryan—ever. One day, Jill decided to take a group of neighborhood kids on a long bike ride.

I was both surprised and thrilled when Ryan ran inside to ask if he could go. He quickly dashed out to join the rest of the neighborhood gang.

A minute later, he was back... and in tears.

Jill told Ryan he couldn't go because he was too slow to keep up with the group. It took all my control to not go outside and confront her. I hated her for the way she hurt my son that day, but I desperately needed Greg to teach my son social skills. And I still loved Greg. It wasn't his fault that Jill was his mother.

Please don't get the impression that I am a nice person, especially after someone messes with one of my kids. I'm not. And it wasn't until years later that I finally got even with Jill for what she did to my son that day. Ryan's mother never forgets.

On a trip back to Minnesota after we'd moved to California, I stopped by Jill's house to *visit*. I was really quite awful that day. I told story after story of what Megan and Ryan had both accomplished. I made sure Jill knew Ryan had a scholarship for college and Megan was doing great. I also bragged about Megan and all her accomplishments. (I would never have done that with anyone else.)

I did feel better and somehow vindicated after I showed her that my son, whom she thought was defective, accomplished more than most kids who don't have to overcome autism or having a crappy mother like Jill. Even today, when I ask my son who his favorite mom is, instead of giving me a hug like I want, he still answers, "Jill," and then laughs.

On the days that Jill didn't need someone to watch her children, she wouldn't let Greg come over to play. On those days, I picked girls for our play dates. Girls are natural speech therapists. They usually talk more than boys. The girls we picked were motherly and kind. They also seemed more tolerant of my son's weirdness. The girls I liked best were the bossy ones. They made Ryan do all kinds of things he'd never do for me. Maybe one day he will find one to marry.

Emily was his favorite playmate when he was younger. I had to travel across town to get her, but *Engaging Emily* was worth the extra drive. She would dress Ryan up, make him dance, even hold pretend wedding ceremonies. He wanted to talk to her, so he began to talk to her. He was in love.

And then one day this perfect friendship ended.

Emily came over for a fun adventure of sledding in a nearby park. Snooper, our dog, would chase both kids down the hill and try to jump on their snow donuts. The day was perfect, until it was time for the fun to end. I was just starting to feel more confident with our social skill instruction as we pulled into Emily's driveway. That's when Ryan started screaming at the top of his lungs right in Emily's ear. He didn't want her to leave or for the fun to be over. He wanted everything to stay the same. Since he couldn't find the words to use, he just screamed. My kid, who looked so very typical just fifteen minutes earlier, had one of his worst meltdowns ever. After that incident, Emily didn't want to come back.

At first, I wasn't going to tell Ryan that Emily wouldn't be back. I wanted to shield him from the reality and the consequences of his actions. But that wouldn't have helped Ryan learn anything. I had to fight my instincts to protect Ryan's feelings. If I wasn't careful, I could become my son's worst enemy.

I explained that Emily wouldn't be coming over to play anymore because he screamed and acted badly when it was time for her to go home. It was because of his actions that she didn't want to play with him anymore. After that talk, he and I both cried together. That discussion was a turning point for us. It was a big "aha!" moment for me. I still had to protect Ryan from the world, but I learned it was critical to let him feel the consequences of his bad behavior.

Even though our ABA expert, Mindi, lived far away in Chicago, she was often whispering in my ear about how to do things with my son. I knew as long as Ryan was still little and cute, people would excuse his strange behavior. I also knew that as Ryan got older, this would no longer be the case. One day I wouldn't be there anymore to help my son. If he were ever going to live independently, he would have to learn the difference between acceptable versus unacceptable behavior.

When all the neighborhood kids went somewhere together, Ryan was usually not included. On one rare occasion, a very kind neighbor offered to take Ryan swimming at the community pool with the rest of the gang. One thing I learned from this was if you get that precious invitation, remember not to frighten other parents with too much information.

I didn't know that yet, so that's what I did. I screwed it up for Ryan.

I went into great detail about all the things Kim needed to avoid to make sure Ryan wouldn't freak out. Ryan was still very sound sensitive at age seven. This was before the antiviral medications were added at age ten and before the medical intervention addressed this issue. I worried if there was a loud noise, he might start screaming. I didn't want him to go ballistic or have a meltdown at any time, but I especially didn't want him to do that with someone who wouldn't know how to handle it.

After I finished my long and vivid explanation of how to deal with Ryan, Kim had a look on her face that told me she wouldn't be doing this again. It wasn't Ryan that was stopping her, but his hover mother who worried too much about every little thing. I should have kept my mouth shut and let her figure it out. Then if he didn't get invited back, I would know it was the result of his actions and not mine.

When Ryan was finally invited to a birthday party, I was so happy. My son was going to Joey Todd's birthday party! But the more I thought about it, the more frightened I became. What if Ryan started to make noises or act weird at the party? What if the only things he wanted to talk about were sharks and computers? What if he had one of his larger-than-life meltdowns when he didn't know what to do or how to act? Ryan was now eight and it had been sometime since his last epic one with Emily. But Ryan was still unpredictable.

I had prayed and prayed for anyone to invite him over, but now that my birthday and Thanksgiving wishes finally came true, I was afraid to let him go. I was your typical mother who is never happy. It was like the story of the mom who buys her kid two shirts: when he wears one she says, "So... you didn't like the *other* one?" I was and still am that same mom.

Ryan understood school routine and rules and would act relatively normal there. But at Joey's party, he wouldn't know what was coming next or understand anything else that was expected. I wanted to accompany him to the party, but kids in the third grade do not bring their hover mother along. Instead, he went armed with a little bit of sugary magic.

For school parties, I often sent a treat that was okay for Ryan's diet. This time, I realized just how important it was for Ryan not to appear or feel different. Although Dr. Harvey insisted Ryan should never deviate from the diet, I went with my gut and did what I knew was best for my son. I told Ryan we had a new rule. At birthday parties he was to eat the same things the other kids did: cake, ice cream, and pizza. He smiled and nodded his head in agreement. Since that was one of the few birthday parties he ever went to, these diet deviations didn't happen too often. He did go to that party without his mother, but I never did find out how he did at Joey's party since he still didn't have the language to tell me.

But I was the first mom there at pick-up time.

We all suffered the next day after the birthday bash when Ryan was allowed to have his cake and eat it, too. At the beginning of medical treatment, Ryan's behavior disintegrated with even the smallest amount of dairy. I learned over time if he ate an offending food, the adverse reaction would go away faster if I increased his water intake and exercise. Swimming seemed to work best for my son. After many years of helping him regain his health, he eventually hit the point when his system wasn't quite so fragile and didn't react to foods as much.

If I Knew Then What I Know Now

In the short run, it would have been much easier to let my son do what he wanted, stay autistic, and not force him to play with other children. It would have been easier to let him wander the house plugging that portable radio into every outlet in the house. And it would have been easier not to have confrontations when I expected him to do something he didn't want to do. However, if I had given in, he never would have learned the right way to behave with other children. And that was simply not an option.[43]

By middle school, Ryan had gained the basics of social skills. He had a few friends. When Velin, Nathan, or Jonathan came over to our house, things seemed relatively normal. Yet he still hadn't put all these social skills into practice at school. Although he excelled at home with friends, his social success was less frequent at school. During middle school a new problem arose—bullying.

---

43   Michelle, Lonnie *How Kids Make Friends*. Evanston: Freedom, 1995. This paperback was not written especially for children affected by autism, but it has very important information all children need to know about how to make friends.

CHAPTER 34

MIDDLE SCHOOL WAS BULLYING AT ITS WORST

You know there is a problem with the education system when you realize
that out of the 3 R's only one begins with an R.

—Dennis Miller

A CROWD OF boys surrounded Ryan. They circled him and shoved him back
and forth to taunts of "gay" and "retard." None of the other thirty-two students
in the classroom tried to stop them. If they had, they could have been next.

Ryan suffered this *circle of pain* once or twice a week.

The science teacher didn't stop it. Ironically, she was stationed down the hall
to prevent this kind of behavior and bullying from happening there. This was
the middle school lunatic asylum, and my child was the perfect victim for every
bully. In elementary school, Ryan didn't always fit in or have many friends, but
no one had been openly, actively cruel. He was just left out. In middle school,
Ryan was the go-to guy for bullying.

I worried nonstop before he started middle school. There were so many
things that could go wrong. I knew middle school is hard for many children. I
was one of those kids who didn't really fit, either. I also knew that for children
who are socially and behaviorally different, middle school can be hell. Kids with
autism are just some of the many kids harassed and teased there. Since our kids

lack social awareness and have few friends to protect them, they become easy targets for bullies. And Ryan was no exception.

I remember being bullied like it happened yesterday. The hurt stays with us. I was laughed at when I couldn't climb the rope in gym and was the last one picked for every sports team. I was the fat kid, and that sometimes made me the subject of ridicule. Most of us put bullying behind us and even become stronger as a result. But what if bullying occurred every week or every day? Would it be as easy to overcome? Ryan still carries the scars of what happened during those painful middle school years.

I never realized the extent of the bullying problem because Ryan never shared what happened during his day. When he came home, I gave him a hug and asked how school went.

The answer was always the same, "School was fine."

I should have recognized the signs. Every morning when it was time to get ready, the panic started, and he didn't want to go. He dragged his feet. It took forever to get him out the door. As we got closer and closer to school, he got weirder and weirder. Sometimes, he refused to get out of the car. But we were late again, and I was so tired of his antics. I was annoyed and yelled at him to get out of the car. I just wanted him anywhere far away from me. I should have realized this apprehension was not part of his autism or his fear of new situations. Something was terribly wrong.

I knew Ryan was often not accepted at school, but I had no knowledge of the daily torment he endured. As extraordinary as it seems, this hover mother didn't have a clue. I attributed his behavior to his autism: He was difficult *because he had autism*. He was being obstinate *because he had autism*. He had trouble making the transition from home to school because he *had autism*. Wrong!

I now realize he was afraid to tell me about the harassment. In his mind, he thought I would get mad and blame him for being the cause of the bullying. I'm ashamed to admit that he might have been right. I was often critical of him. I told him the reason kids didn't accept him was because he didn't act like other kids. Then I'd ask him to watch how other kids acted and to try to act more like they did. Unfortunately, *they* were the bullies. I put more pressure on him, when he was already struggling with a horrific situation. He still sometimes reminds me how wrong I was to make these kinds of comments.

Even with his above-average intelligence and his extensive vocabulary, Ryan still had trouble communicating in middle school. His social communication was far less developed than his vocabulary. I made the mistake of thinking since he sounded smart, he was socially smart. But Ryan couldn't even tell me about what happened at school unless I asked him specific questions. To glean any information at all, I'd ask about a math test or if anyone got in trouble again in science class. But for Ryan to come home and give me chapter and verse about what went on at school just didn't happen. It didn't happen because it *couldn't* happen. He wasn't there yet.

Before middle school started, I had Ryan's special education file sealed. I wanted him to be treated like everyone else and not be singled out for anything. That didn't really work. Ryan stuck out like a sore thumb. Although he'd advanced a great deal, he was not even close to the other kids socially.

Ryan still didn't fit in.

Middle school is also a time when parents are encouraged to let kids become more independent and handle things on their own. I wanted Ryan to be ready to do things on his own. I thought he was ready, and I wanted him to have the same consequences for behavior that other kids did. But Ryan wasn't ready. His teachers had no knowledge of his past history since I had his special education file sealed. He looked like a disorganized kid who often left his assignments at home and had to call his mommy to bring them.

If his teachers had known about his past, they probably would have been impressed with all he had accomplished. They may have been more watchful and willing to help protect him. Even though I picked the best team of teachers for Ryan and even though I worked hard to help Ryan with his organizational issues, there was no longer one person in charge of watching out for him or helping him when he got into trouble socially. I had no control over what occurred in the classroom anymore, and now he had six different teachers with completely different classrooms to navigate.

I wanted Ryan to make it by himself even as I was concurrently searching for ways to make school better for him. My husband didn't agree with all I did.

Frank thought I was too hands-on and should back off. Although Frank and I still argued about Ryan, once we had a plan, he was always in Ryan's corner fighting for what was best for him.

Frank continued to question my agenda for Ryan to make sure I was doing the right thing for our son. Most men would have given up arguing about it a long time ago. That would have left me to do what I wanted, but Frank hung in there as the voice of reason. When Ryan's mommy was way too protective, Frank was there to make Ryan stronger and independent. He often kept me from doing the things that weren't best for our son.

When Ryan became disorganized and forgetful, he called home in a panic. That's when he begged me to drop everything I was doing and bring him the homework or permission slip he had left at home. I did. It was Frank who suggested that I start the clock and keep track of the time it took me to do this recurring chore. When Ryan arrived home after school, he had to pay back the same length of time it took me to bring the thing he forgot. Ryan had to shovel the snow off the driveway for that amount of time or some other physical chore he hated. That was also Frank's suggestion, and he was right. The problem with it was that my mommy gene was always in high gear. I just wanted to put my arms around Ryan and protect him. This included everything from bringing him his homework to helping him learn everything he still needed to know.

I was so worried about catching him up and helping his organizational skills that I was unaware of the bullying. I was focused on academics. His weakness in reading comprehension was my main concern. I knew this skill was part of every middle school subject. Throughout elementary school, Ryan struggled with reading comprehension. When he brought home his first reading assignment from his sixth grade English class, we sat down to muddle through together. I said, "Let's read these pages silently to ourselves, and when we are both finished reading, I will ask you a few questions about the section we just read." To my surprise, he finished light-years ahead of me. At first, I thought he hadn't read it thoroughly.

So I asked, "Did you *really* read all of that?" He insisted he did. So I grilled him on what he read. He knew all the answers. When I moved on to the more complex questions where the answers weren't obvious but inferred, he knew those too. Ryan answered every question I asked him—even the ones that needed complex interpretation of what happened in the story. Somewhere along the way, without my help and when I wasn't looking, Ryan mastered reading comprehension. It probably resulted from all the time he spent reading things on the computer. Without pre-teaching, he started to learn like other kids. That was the last time I helped him with his reading assignments.

As a previous teacher, I knew reading comprehension was mostly practice, but I was surprised when he finally mastered this skill all on his own. I guess those years spent surfing the internet had the side benefit of making him read at warp speed as well as learn the important reading comprehension skills. We should have celebrated more, but his reports and English compositions still needed work. We immediately turned our attention to those areas.

Academically he did well, but Ryan's lack of social skills continued to be an issue through all of middle school and even into high school. Ryan never had true friends until college. He still worries too much if people like him. And the *circle of pain* was not the only bullying he had to endure.

Although I was unaware of the depth and viciousness of the bullying, I did try to support Ryan socially at school. I encouraged (or maybe forced) Ryan to audition for school plays. My thinking was that acting in front of an audience would help with his self-confidence, and a more confident Ryan would be a Ryan more likely to make and keep friends. What a long string of assumptions. At first, Ryan didn't want to choose any activity, but I insisted, and he remembered the rule of "either you pick, or I will." Sports seemed like a significantly greater torture, so he chose theater.

Theater was the sometimes the secret home of special-needs kids like Ryan. The theater kids accepted Ryan and everyone—no exceptions. Many of them viewed being different as a badge of honor. They looked out for Ryan and tried to protect him during the long, terrifying school day. Being part of the theater group gave Ryan a place to belong. I had already established myself as the costume lady for the school when Megan was in theater. This created the perfect opportunity for me to keep a close eye on Ryan without him or anyone else realizing what I was up to. I still needed to know what he needed to learn next.

Ms. Lora Hemminger, the drama teacher, gave Ryan the role of Mr. Bundles in the musical *Annie*. It was a small part, but it was a part for which she had huge plans. Ms. Hemminger not only put on a good show, but she changed lives in the process. She helped each child grow into their role on stage. Sometimes, she would pick the last kid I would ever have chosen for a part. However, she was never wrong.

Ryan's part was small, but he stole the show. He looked directly at the audience every time he spoke and that made everyone laugh. I cried as I watched him perform. My kid, who had trouble talking one-on-one, had no fear standing in front of hundreds of people. I thought my plan had worked. Of course, the reality was that on stage, Ryan never had to come up with topics of conversation or navigate the complex social skills needed to communicate effectively with others. *Annie* was just a more complex performance of Friday Joke Day and the talent show.

Onstage, Ryan was a success. Offstage, not so much.

The contrast was heart-wrenching. Offstage Ryan was bullied, afraid of rejection, self-isolating, and only had a few friends. What he could do onstage did not generalize or occur in his offstage life. It didn't help that Nerdy was Ryan's middle name. Ryan was more interested in academics than in TV, music, pop culture, or any of the usual topics of middle school social life. Ryan loved to discuss politics, and he still does. This was not the focus of most kids his age. They didn't care much about what was happening in the Capitol and certainly didn't want to hear about it constantly.

Ryan hated class projects because it meant he needed to find a partner or group. Nobody picked him to be in their group, and he was too afraid to ask anyone to be his partner. The teacher usually assigned him to someone or some group. That didn't help his popularity, either. Nobody wanted the teacher telling them whom they had to work with, and nobody wanted to work with nerdy Ryan. To make things worse, Ryan spent a lot of time talking to his teachers. They were kind and accepting, and he didn't have many kids who talked to him. This made him appear to be a suck-up. Being super smart and being a bit of a know-it-all didn't help his cause, either. He was still on Autism Island, with lots of sharks right offshore.

To make things worse, his social rejection happened every day, in almost every class, and for most of the time. It wasn't until partway through sixth grade that he met the terrific trio of Velin, Nathan, and Jonathan. His new three best friends were smart like him, but they were of foreign descent. One was Bulgarian, one Romanian, and the other Russian. Ryan's buddies also didn't quite fit. These wonderful kids often didn't understand the subtle social cues and slang of a second language and culture. They were perfect friends for my son.

Their last names and accents also kept them out of the popular crowd. But they didn't care about the cool kids and never wanted to be part of that group. They were much more confident than Ryan; as a result, they were never targets for the bullies. They accepted Ryan unconditionally and spent a lot of time together. I was thrilled that Ryan was no longer eating lunch alone. Unfortunately, lunch was only thirty-five minutes long. That meant the rest of the day was still open season on my son.

Being rejected and bullied caused Ryan to channel his energy away from social interaction and into academic achievement. If bullies were going to call him a nerd, he may as well be the best nerd ever. Academics became his focus and how he survived at school. He thought getting an A was the only acceptable grade. He didn't know how to get a B. If he earned a B on anything, he was devastated. He brought home all A's on his report card with virtually no assistance except for my help with writing assignments. Since language came late to my son, this area still needed work.

At home, his beloved computer took the place of the friends he should have had. My son was constantly studying and surfing the internet to learn as much as he could about any topic that interested him, and surfing the net provided the escape he needed from the stress of school. What I didn't understand was how much he *needed* that time and how precious it was to him.

Although I never limited his computer time, his computer time created a problem for the rest of the family. Way back then, computers were more expensive, and most families shared one. None of us could ever use the computer when Ryan was in the house. Ryan believed the family computer was his and disregarded the user rules we had established. Ryan thought it would be interesting and fun to experiment with everything a computer could do. He inadvertently did horrible things to our family computer without asking or checking with us first. This resulted in a Guinness World Record for most reformats of a hard drive.

Frank and Ryan had frequent arguments about our computer that sounded something like this . . . Ryan tried to excuse what he did to the computer by saying, "Dad, I didn't mean to do it." Next he said, "What's the use of having a computer, if you can't do stuff with it?" Followed by, "Maybe, it wasn't my fault. It could have been a virus from Mom's friends." Finally Ryan admitted, "I *really* needed to download those games from the internet!"

After every reformat, his father could be heard yelling, "Didn't I tell you not to download anything without asking me *first*?"

That's when Ryan said, "I just *had to*, Dad."

The upside of these aggravating situations was that our boy genius eventually learned how to fix anything that could go wrong with a computer. No more extended warranties for us. We had the *extended warranty* living with us.

His new skill even came in handy. Right before my deadline for a project to further autism research, our computer crashed. After two hours on the phone with Dell technical support, I was told that the problem couldn't be fixed, and I would probably have to wipe the hard drive clean. That would have been as bad as it sounded. Fearing that or another reformat, I called the middle school. I told them Ryan got a last-minute doctor's appointment. I raced to the school to pick up my boy wonder. Ryan fixed the computer and was out of the house within five minutes. He arrived back at school without even missing lunch.

He loved everything computer, and I used that to help me control his behavior. Remember that old adage to use what they love to teach and motivate them? Ryan had reached the point where I started to parent the same as you do for most kids. When he did something wrong, I took away his computer for a half hour. Loss of computer time was my big hammer. If he didn't do what I asked or was disrespectful, then he lost computer time. If the behavior continued, then I'd up the punishment. When Ryan was off the computer for an entire day, you knew that kid had done something seriously wrong. At those times, I was sometimes punished too. When I took away his beloved computer, he sometimes got so mad he'd hit me.

Hitting was our dirty little secret. I never told anyone except Frank about this aggressive behavior. I was embarrassed he acted this way and that, initially, I couldn't control him. But I was the only one he ever hit. And it happened way too often. When he got really frustrated, I was the one who was a safe outlet for his anger. He knew no matter what he did, I would still be in his corner and love him. I suspect the hitting resulted from the bullying he had to endure at school. Or maybe it was the frustration he felt because I took away one of his few friends—his computer. Or maybe it was a little of both.

The hitting stopped after I became more stubborn than my son and became more serious about enforcing consequences. In short, I stood up to him. No matter how much he didn't want to do something, I insisted he was going to do it. Disrespect from either of my kids was my hot button. He finally learned the consequence of his behavior was the loss of more computer time. When he was older and I was trying to help another mom in a similar situation, I asked him why he stopped hitting me. He said it was because I took away his beloved computer and wouldn't give it back until he behaved the right way.

There was no safe place for Ryan at school. He was the perfect target for kids—even the shrimpy ones. One day after costuming some kids, I went to Ryan's locker to find him. I saw Ryan cowering as this kid, who was at least a foot shorter, got in Ryan's face. I was too far away to hear what that boy said, but from Ryan's body language, I knew he was terrified.

As I approached the lockers, the kid ran off. Ryan looked relieved, but he wouldn't tell me what had happened. It was difficult for me to understand why Ryan was afraid of that kid. Ryan had a brown belt in karate and could have easily taken him out without much effort.

I often assumed these incidents were his fault so maybe that's why my son didn't tell me about the bullying. Or it could have been he didn't have the communication skills yet to do so. When he was younger, I told him he needed to act more like other kids. And whenever he did anything wrong, my usual tactic would be to role-play what he could say or do to prevent it from happening again. I'm still not sure what else I could have done. However, I shouldn't have blamed him. I thought I understood what he was going through. But I didn't have a clue. We were both stuck in the same place. We both felt powerless to change our circumstances and didn't know how to change anything.

In my mind, Ryan needed to stand up and not show any fear. But for his own protection, Ryan isolated himself even more. That didn't work. The bullies even followed Ryan home after school to our house, where he should have been safe. Ryan got crank calls. Kids hung up without saying anything. The look on his face after this type of incident was awful. There wasn't any place left for him to go where he could escape their daily torment.

One time, I called the parents of some of the culprits. I cried as I explained what their children were doing. Those particular kids stopped, but there were always others to take their place. I began to answer the telephone before I handed it to Ryan. Bullying Ryan was an all-day sport for these children.

The bullying at his school was out of control. Even during class time with the teacher present, it was open season on my son. One afternoon in front of the entire class, a boy jumped on the table in front of Ryan and simulated humping his face in biology class. The teacher did nothing. I only heard about this incident when a theater kid quietly told me what everyone else in the school was talking about. When I asked Ryan about it, he started to cry.

My goal for my son changed. Suddenly, I really didn't care if Ryan was acting the right way at all. Somehow, the bullying had to stop. I marched into the principal's office to ask what he planned to do and when he was going to fire this worthless teacher. He reassured me he would look into it and showed me the door. But this principal usually went down the path of least resistance. Instead of interrogating the tormentor, who already had a terrible reputation for trouble, he called Ryan into his office for a talk. Ryan was mortified, embarrassed, and worried about further victimization if he was labeled a tattletale. He lied and told the principal he couldn't remember what happened.

The entire biology class witnessed what happened. Still, the principal did nothing and intended to do nothing. It was easier for him to confront my kid than the bully. Instead of dealing with the bullying problem that permeated his school, he chose to ignore it and blame the weird kid for his own victimization.

The bullies had taken over and were running the asylum. The school culture needed to be fixed—and not just for my kid.

Ryan desperately wanted to escape. He continually asked if we could move to California. His sister was already there in college. He knew how much we missed her, and he begged us to move. Ryan said if we moved we'd be closer to Megan and the rest of our extended family.

I attended PTA meetings and did other things to bring attention to the bullying problem. I researched and found comprehensive programs for the school that would empower all the children to stop the bullying. But the school never even considered using them. Instead, they wanted to hide the problem. But, as I suspected, Ryan was not the only one suffering. I heard plenty of horror stories from other parents who called me after they read my articles in the school newspaper and told me stories of the torment their children had to endure.

The bullying continued as I continued to try to change the caustic atmosphere permeating our school. My efforts were not enough. If I had it to do over again, I would have sued their butts. The settlement would have been used to put into action the anti-bullying programs I begged them to institute.

After the bullies were done with Ryan, they moved on to someone else. Their next victim was picked on by a few of the worst offenders, a mean group of eighth-grade boys who decided they would enhance their power and position by picking on anyone weaker. These bullies harassed anyone who could not fight back. This poor kid committed suicide. After that and without any discussion, Frank and I agreed *"we're out of here!"* We no longer tried to fix the problem; our sole focus became to protect our child.

At about the same time, I found out our middle school principal was to be promoted to the high school, which was the very same school Ryan was supposed to attend the following year. That cemented our decision to escape to California. Ryan would not and could not be at a school where the principal failed to protect children, especially those who were not capable of protecting themselves. My son would never again attend a school where the absence of any administrative backbone further endangered kids who needed bodyguards to get through a school day. Although we were afraid to leave this award-winning school district, we did. It didn't matter that California schools ranked way behind Minnesota schools or that California was close to the bottom of the list. Ryan's safety came before everything else.

This ended up being one of the best things we ever did for Ryan. It gave him the opportunity to start all over and leave behind the painful memories of middle school. He could be anyone he wanted to be in California—and that changed his life.

If I Knew Then What I Know Now

When Ryan was younger and he didn't like something he'd say, "There should be a law against that." That is how I feel about middle school. Maybe we should have a law that kids don't have to attend middle school . . . ever. It is awful for many kids, but for children who are socially and behaviorally different, it is unbearable. Ryan was painfully aware that he was different from the other kids. He wanted more friends, but he was too scared of rejection to approach anyone else.

We are blessed Ryan is still with us after the torment he had to endure. But how could I solve a problem when I didn't really understand all that was happening to my son? Sometimes it's what you don't see that can be most dangerous.

Middle school kids take the act of being self-conscious to a new level. They worry way too much about who is cool and who is not. This self-centered way of looking at the world is typical for kids their age, but it gives the bullies too much power. Those in the popular group decided who was "in" and who was "out," and their power came from putting others down.

At Ryan's school, there were no anti-bullying programs to teach kids how to defuse these power brokers. Those programs should be mandatory at all schools. That is the only way to truly stop the bullies who prey on vulnerable children.

I wanted to do that, but I couldn't make it happen.

The bullies ran the show. Their cruelty infected the social environment and hurt the academic achievement of all children there. Bullying must never be tolerated. It leaves permanent scars on the victim, the witnesses, and even the bully. Too often, schools and parents accept it as an inevitable part of childhood. They couldn't be more wrong.

After we moved to California, I tutored a student in math who was on the spectrum. His mother saved him from the bullies by home-schooling him during the middle school years. He returned to the school setting for high school. I wish I had done that for Ryan. I mistakenly thought Ryan couldn't improve his social skills if I removed him from the school setting. What I didn't realize, that this mother did, was I could put him in all kinds of activities and home school groups to address the social-skill deficit.

With all things bad, usually something good comes. In spite of how difficult the bullying was to endure in middle school, it helped instill important values in Ryan. He will never stand by when someone needs help. My son always treats others with the respect and dignity they deserve, no matter how different they are. Ryan is always there to help anyone in need. I used to wish I could erase these terrible bullying incidents from his memory. I know these painful experiences will always be with him. But without them, I'm not sure if he would be the same wonderful and caring person he is today.

CHAPTER 35

THE NEW AND IMPROVED RYAN IN HIGH SCHOOL

Whether you think you can or think you can't . . . you are right.

—Henry Ford

THE ONLY THING that saved the life of the woman turning left in front of us was me frantically waving and screaming, "STOP!" Ryan pulled into the driveway totally clueless about the woman or the mailbox he almost demolished or the two cars that nearly lost their side mirrors. He had a huge smile on his face. Driving lesson one was finally over.

Ryan got his driving permit after we moved to California. He had many close encounters with cars in parking lots. The house in Minnesota sold in two days; the garage/estate sale took quite a bit longer. The sticker shock of California real estate was jaw-dropping. We went from a 4,000-square-foot house to a 2,400-square-foot tract home. We paid more for our new tract home in California than we had gotten for our custom one in Minnesota.

We finally left Minnesota after we came to the conclusion that twenty Minnesota winters were twenty too many, and we were done with the bullying. The company we hired to do the moving sale was so efficient that several months later we were still looking for some of the things we asked them not to sell. But none of that mattered; we were off on a new adventure. And Ryan left his history and the bullies behind.

Ryan already had a plan for his new life in California and set out to reinvent himself. Not long after we arrived in June, my son and my husband teamed up to work with a personal trainer. Ryan's metamorphosis began before high school even started. Frank was still in charge of anything physical, but the trainer, Eric Hubscher, added some expertise to the mix. Ryan lost thirty pounds and took up running. He loved the sunny California weather. He happily traded his down jacket and snow boots for shorts and flip-flops. It was almost as if Ryan had always been a California kid. Ryan thought he should wear shorts 24/7, 365 days a year, plus one more in the leap year.

We were careful to plan Ryan's education before we moved. After several trips to observe the high schools in the area, we decided on Westlake High School. We thought the specialized technology program would be perfect for our geeky-techno son who so masterfully wrecked and then repaired our computer. Students had to apply to get in the program. It seemed like the admission process was selective, and it was an honor to be accepted.

Other attractors to this school-within-a-school included a smaller class size of fewer than twenty-five students. Several of his classes would be with the same group of students throughout the day. And there were internships at local technology companies as well as hands-on learning. We painstakingly filled out all the forms with what we thought were the right answers.

We shouldn't have tried so hard, since Ryan would have been accepted no matter what we wrote. We were unaware that the high school was desperately trying to make this new program work and would have accepted Elmer Fudd.

The technology program had trouble enrolling enough students. Those who did enroll were not college-bound and lacked the same enthusiasm Ryan had for learning. The classes, although small, turned out to be more disruptive than the ones with more kids in them. But the director of the program assured us this program was perfect for our son. This wasn't the first time someone talked us into something that wasn't really right for Ryan.

I intervened when there were problems with his technology teacher. She did not like my son and was not shy about letting him know it. I suspected that she was intimidated by his vast computer knowledge, which was clearly more extensive than hers. Frank warned me to not start one of my crusades. I was not allowed to even know the principal or superintendent's names.

At first, Ryan didn't fit again and didn't make many friends. Eventually, we moved Ryan out of the technology program and enrolled him in honors and advanced placement (AP) classes for his junior year. Although California schools ranked almost last for education among the states, Ryan's school was packed with great teachers who truly cared about their students. My son was finally bully free and happy. After he left the technology program behind, his high school experience was so much better.

Ryan said the AP classes packed with thirty-eight students were much more controlled than the smaller twenty-something classes in the technology program. In these AP classes, the students actually wanted to learn. There were rules and discipline at Ryan's new school. It was so different than the highly ranked middle school we left behind. Many of the kids in the AP classes belonged in Nerdsville with Ryan.

Once Ryan was in the right place, he began to blossom.

Ryan relaxed when he didn't have to worry about the bullies anymore. But he still worried too much about getting all A's. It wasn't the only thing my kid thought about but was still at the top of his list.

Ryan also began to participate in activities in school. He joined the track and cross-country teams and the African-American Literature Club. This surprised us because, as I said before, he struggled with sports. You would find Ryan in front of a computer screen rather than on an athletic field. But trying to impress a girl can make a young man do strange things.

Participation in all these new activities resulted from meeting Lamia, a beautiful girl whom he had a crush on. Lamia was black, and we laughed out loud when my fair-skinned son listed the African-American Literature Club as one of his activities on his college applications. Ryan's willingness to join the cross-country and track teams was also her doing.

In the beginning, it was hard to watch Ryan at the track meets. He was the slowest kid on the team. But he never gave up. The coaches provided a supportive environment for all students where everyone strived to improve their own times. They competed against themselves rather than each other. The kids on the team shouted words of encouragement to each other. Lamia cheered him on. Frank and I rooted for him along with the rest of his new friends. Eventually, Ryan was not dead last and only third to last. The coaches saw how hard he worked and recognized him at the awards ceremony as the *Athlete with the Most Heart*. He finally belonged.

When Ryan was younger, we tried team sports like soccer and T-Ball with disastrous results. Not only was he slower and unable to keep up physically, if you consider the multiple things happening on a baseball field all at the same time, Ryan didn't have a chance of succeeding. We didn't do team sports for long because they made Ryan feel awful about himself.

Individual sports like swimming and karate were better suited for him. But we didn't do many sports at all and picked other activities instead. The reason sports worked in high school was because of a combination of things. Ryan was on a team, but his events were individual in nature. He only competed against himself to improve his scores. The encouragement from the rest of the team and coaches didn't hurt, either.

Ryan also joined the Youth & Government program offered through the local YMCA. There, Ryan was definitely in his element. Once again, we used what he loved to motivate him to develop social skills. Ryan loved anything and everything to do with politics. When it was time for us to vote, Ryan researched the entire list of candidates so we didn't have to. He studied every candidate and issue including who should be sewer commissioner. Although he wasn't old enough to cast a ballot, he was diligent in finding out who would best serve our community. Someday he'd love to run for office. He might even be the first president who once had autism.

He made a ton of friends in Youth & Government. Still, no one called him to do things together outside of the time they spent together in the program. And Ryan was still too self-conscious to take that first step. The real reason most of the kids attended this program was not because of a true interest in politics, but for the fun trips and social activities it offered. In contrast, Ryan loved the intrigue of the politics.

Before we left Minnesota, we decided to get rid of one car and travel across the country in the other. Of course, we picked the wrong one, and the minivan died shortly after we arrived in sunny California. We needed another car, and Ryan's hover mother decided he needed another kid-attractor.

My plan went something like this . . .

I started by planting the seed in Frank's head that we needed to buy a *proper* California car. I told my husband a used convertible might be a fun choice. Frank thought I wanted this car to feel the warm California wind on my face. At least, that's what I told him. The real reason was it looked cool, and later Ryan would have a babe magnet. The trampoline we used as a kid-attractor was no longer enough. We needed to up the ante a bit. This was *car therapy*.

I held my breath every time Ryan drove. But I realized it takes two to make a car accident. Surely the other driver would be paying attention and maneuver to miss Ryan.

On the night Ryan passed his driver's test, my husband went into his room to yell at him for talking on the telephone long after he should have been asleep. When Frank came back to our room, he had a huge smile on his face as he asked me, "Who would have believed I'd be yelling at our son to get off the telephone with his friends and he would get his driver's license all in one day?" Ryan was a pretty typical high school kid after he got his license. He stayed up too late, played too many computer games, and liked to instant message with other kids.[44]

Ryan's new driving was a double-edged sword. Back then, Ryan didn't have a clue that some people took advantage of his automotive generosity. My son was more innocent and naive than his peers. It was one of the things I loved most about him, but it also worried me. Some kids weren't really friends, but they used him and his car for their own benefit. They never gave him money for gas or invited him along if they found another ride. I didn't care. At least someone called even if it was only because they needed a ride.

I never worried about Ryan speeding or not following the driving laws. Ryan was a rule follower. He wouldn't start the engine until everyone had seatbelts

---

44 Instant messaging is what kids did before Facebook was invented.

on. Still, I worried whenever he took the car. But it was important that we let him drive, no matter how much it scared me. That was Frank's doing. Ryan's mommy was afraid to let that happen. Frank made me stop being so overprotective. Well, that's not entirely true—he managed to slow me down a little.

I think we had the car in the body shop almost every month of the year. Okay, perhaps I'm exaggerating a bit. In Ryan's defense, he did have to park in a high school parking lot, which was like a very expensive game of pinball. He learned to start every sentence with those three little words: "NOT MY FAULT." The good news was no one got hurt and it gave us a warm feeling to know we helped put our mechanic's daughter through medical school.

Ryan's lack of confidence continued to be an issue. He still waited for friends to call him. Although it happened, it was a rare occurrence. If he wanted to do anything like go to a movie or dinner, he was the one who needed to call and make the arrangements. It was hard for him to get up the courage to do this. Ryan was still afraid of rejection. The scars that resulted from the bullying in middle school never really went away. He still worried too much if people liked him.

Ryan also had severe test anxiety. He worried to excess about having enough time to finish tests. My son, who had once been fascinated with timed situations, now found them tremendously stressful. It was as if he felt he could never find the correct answer in time to win at *Legends of the Hidden Temple*. He was a worrywart as well as a perfectionist. He needed to check things twice to make sure he did everything right on every test as well as homework assignments. I couldn't tell if this was his autism or a gene passed down from Chicken Little (aka me). Eventually, I decided I had to do something if my son were going to get into college. I disclosed Ryan's past to his high school counselor. Mr. Lisowski suggested we put a Section 504 plan in place to give Ryan extra time on tests.

But a 504 meant we needed to inform all his teachers about the reason for the accommodation. I didn't want a repeat of second grade. I didn't want to revisit all those fears and failures. In the end, I trusted the counselor when he told me that the high school teachers were professionals and would never change the way they treated Ryan.

I had to fill out a ton of forms, and I did have to reveal he was once diagnosed with autism. We had a meeting that looked and felt like an IEP meeting, but it wasn't exactly one. Frank was on a trip and couldn't be there. I felt lost in a room full of school personnel without Frank to kick me under the table. I was on my own trying to explain the complexities of my son to people I didn't know. My eyes started to well up, and my voice cracked as I tried to draw the complicated picture that was Ryan. I broke into tears in front of a room full of people I never met before. The 504 was granted, and it did help Ryan with his text anxiety. However, my new worry was that Ryan would use this 504 plan as a crutch.

Some mothers are *never* happy.

The 504 plan was the right thing to do, and only Ryan's Spanish teacher treated him differently after she knew about his autism. She had been Ryan's favorite teacher. Ryan liked her so much he even bought her a new stereo/CD player with his own money after her classroom equipment died. But once she found out about his *difficulties,* she put him down in front of the rest of the class and no longer had time to answer any of his questions.

Ryan still had trouble finding someone to eat with at lunch. Since there was no fear of rejection with the adults around him, he would sometimes spend the lunch hour visiting some of his teachers. The Spanish teacher was the one he loved to visit most. But after the 504, there were no more lunches with her.

Fortunately, Ryan's past issues never mattered to his other teachers. Mr. Baldwin, his AP US History teacher, was impressed by how well Ryan could remember the smallest details about anything having to do with history and government. Mr. Baldwin was never intimidated by my son's knowledge. Even when Ryan questioned something, Mr. Baldwin praised Ryan for getting the facts right. He let Ryan shine and encouraged him.

To practice for the AP exam, Mr. Baldwin divided his class into two competing teams. Then the teams debated and answered questions to earn points. This teacher made his class fun, and his teaching methods made the kids want to study before one of these contests. Ryan's enthusiasm for learning was contagious in the classroom. Mr. Baldwin recognized that. Even though Ryan was not the most popular kid in the class, the other kids would fight to have him on their team! They wanted to win the competition. Ryan's your guy if you are ever

on a game show and need a lifeline. He remembers dates and the most insignificant details about every subject.

Friday night football games were avoided along with dances and many other
social situations. Instead, Ryan chose to stay home or go out to dinner with us.
His dad and I were still his main friends. Weekends were usually spent together
doing the things he liked to do. We went on hikes, to the movies, and had
adventures finding the restaurants he had seen on the Food Network channel.

The exception to this was the one weekend a year when Frank went to the
UCLA/USC game with Megan. Frank didn't want to pay full price for a ticket
since we were already paying full tuition at USC. So Mr. Cheapskate sneaked
into the big game using one of Megan's student tickets.

My husband is a horrible liar, so Megan came up with this big fat whopper if
they happened to get caught. Frank was to say he was a doctoral student studying the long-term psychological effect of parents being forced to send money to
a rival college. Megan required him to wear a Trojan hat to the game and told
him to never talk about UCLA when he sat in the USC student section. This
became a yearly father/daughter tradition for the two of them. But now that
Megan is no longer a student, they have to pay full price for tickets.

Things like USC football made us realize how different Ryan was from most
kids. Megan loved the football games in high school and then later in college.
Ryan wanted nothing to do with the Friday night games that were so important
to the high school social scene. It was more fun for him to stay home and dream
up some new recipe. We stayed home and watched the Food Network together.
I know it is hard to believe, but I even started to like cooking when it was with
Ryan. Once again, his enthusiasm was catching.

Megan was the son Frank never had, and Ryan was at home cooking with
me. Somehow, it worked since they both were happy. But I still worried. My son
was still not quite there socially even though he now had a better handle on
what to do in most social situations. Ryan only went to one dance in high
school, and that was only because the group he went with included Lamia. He
refused to ask a girl to his prom after Lamia moved away.

If I Knew Then What I Know Now

Throughout Ryan's school career, I struggled and re-struggled with the issue of disclosure versus nondisclosure. Sometimes I didn't even disclose things to my own husband. I know Frank would have thought I was certifiable if he knew the real reason for the "babe-mobile." I needed it to help Ryan's future social life. I finally admitted my true motivation to my husband for buying the convertible, which never did attract any babes. Frank being Frank didn't get mad after I revealed the truth.

Disclosure was always a difficult decision when it involved Ryan and school. I worried that if I disclosed that Ryan was once severely affected by autism, his teachers might treat him differently. I also worried that if I didn't mention his autism, he would be academically and socially disadvantaged.

I wanted him to be a regular student in a regular classroom with no accommodations with only his hover mother as his backup. To my son's credit, he survived this decision. But with the SAT and ACT exams looming, I thought I needed to reconsider my nondisclosure decision. This was a forever balancing act.

CHAPTER 36

APPLYING TO COLLEGE—COULD THEY MAKE IT ANY HARDER?

I believe that we parents must encourage our children to become educated, so they can get into a good college that we cannot afford.

—Dave Barry

I HAD NO idea what Ryan should do for college. I should have been grateful that my previously autistic son, who was supposed to be on the fast track to a group home, had a chance at going to college at all. After years of medical treatment he was so much better, but he still had a long way to go socially.

I wasn't grateful so much as on a new mission. I *needed* to get Ryan into college.

For a kid Ryan's age, a normal life was about going to college, so that became my new focus. Although this chapter is about the process we used to help Ryan get to college, it is by no means the only way to get a child to college (or maybe not even the right way).

And not all kids should go to college, and some may not be ready for this big step immediately after high school. Some kids never finish college and still seem to land on their feet. Bill Gates, Oprah Winfrey, Michael Dell, Ellen DeGeneres, David Geffen, and Mark Zuckerberg didn't do so badly without a college degree. These are the choices our family made. Some were good and some not so good. Ultimately, we were successful, but we were not always knowledgeable.

We just tried to make the best decision with the information at the time. Frank kept me from looking back or second-guessing our decisions. The train always needed to move forward.

The college admissions process reminds me more of a beauty pageant than an academic competition. It seems like it's not enough to be smart, you have to have a great song and dance act, as well. Kids need to participate in academic and community activities that make them more desirable to those mysterious admission officers whom you hope are in a good mood at the moment they read your child's application.

What I didn't realize at the time was how important each of these activities would be to further Ryan's personal development and growth. They did so much more than simply make him look good on his college resume. Although he did these academic and socially compassionate activities for all the wrong reasons, these activities helped my son become more accomplished.

First, there was *GEEK camp*. Ryan attended a ten-day technology leadership conference in the San Francisco Bay Area prior to starting his college application process. The reason to attend was solely to make him look good on paper. Ryan had never been to summer camp and, other than a couple of YMCA Youth & Government trips, he had never been away from me for even a sleepover. I was afraid to let him go and worried he wasn't ready. Sometimes, I wasn't sure who was more attached at the hip—him or me.

But he survived, and so did I.

Frank and I picked him up after he finished camp and headed off for lunch with our niece who worked nearby at Google. Heather gave us the complete tour. Fortified by a wonderful free meal provided by Google, my son instantly decided he wanted to work there, too. Who wouldn't? At Google, they feed you free gourmet meals, and you can have as many of them as you want. You can wear jeans to work, and your dog can come with you. Heather mentioned Google hired a lot of people from Stanford and a local private Jesuit school, Santa Clara University. Ryan decided at that very moment he should apply to these schools. Google and the food they served became Ryan's motivation.

To put his plan into action, Ryan began his quest to look good on his college applications. He joined the Jewish and Spanish clubs to complement his

African-American Literature Club credit. Apparently, there was no room left in the Irish-Lebanese American Music Appreciation Club. Ryan was extremely busy, but he came out of his room to eat and say "Hi" every now and then.

Next, he turned his attention to the socially compassionate part of his application and started to volunteer at an assisted living facility. Snooper had left us some time ago and Ryan took Buddy, our next dog, along with him. Again, his focus was on looking good on paper and not too much on compassion. Colleges love volunteer activities. But this decision was another life-changing event for Ryan. His volunteer work at the Agoura Hills Senior Retreat was more educational than any of us could have imagined. When he and Buddy first started there, Ryan assumed he was supposed to run games like bingo and help in only the most general sense. It turned out that the activity he most enjoyed was sitting around and talking to the residents. These older, wiser, and sometimes forgotten folks had so much knowledge and wisdom to share with my son. Their experiences taught him about what was most important in life. The bonus was it gave him more practice with small talk.

Ryan still had difficulty making eye contact with anyone he didn't know well. This was still one more road he needed to travel. But with Buddy by his side, he no longer found it difficult to talk with people he hadn't met before. Buddy served as Ryan's security blanket, his canine icebreaker. Buddy was always a warm and loving topic of conversation. Buddy's special gift was that he always knew who needed him most. At Agoura Hills Senior Retreat, everyone needed a Buddy.

When Ryan handed me a copy of his first college application, I was surprised to see that it read better than Megan's. Ryan had a high GPA, loads of extracurricular activities, and lots of volunteer work. It glowed. No one could see Ryan's autism on his college application. That was the problem. I was back to my disclose/not to disclose conundrum. I wasn't sure if keeping Ryan's autism a secret would serve him best in the college application process. I was ready to do anything to level the playing field for this kid who had dealt with so much already.

Ryan was more intelligent than anyone I had ever met, and he had successfully learned how to compensate for so many of his deficits. But he had trouble with the things that seemed easy to anyone else. Stuff like calling friends to go out to dinner and getting to school on time was still hard for him. It took Ryan too much time to complete homework assignments, and he still worried to excess about every-thing.

I worried that Ryan didn't possess the life skills required for independent living at college. How could he handle the academics, remember to take his meds, do laundry, and stay on his nondairy diet? I always handled these details of life for him. All he had to worry about was getting his homework done. He might have appeared to be normal and he'd done well academically, but he still couldn't remember where he put things, had a lack of confidence, and lingering social skills issues. If I had taken a deep breath and paused, then I would have realized that my fears were similar to every parent whose child is about to take this life step.

After going through the college application process with Megan, I knew just how important the high school counselor's letter of recommendation was going to be. Ryan needed an experienced counselor who could help him navigate this new school as well as write impactful letters. I certainly didn't want my son to have the new counselor on the block, and I expected to get my way. My bending of the rules had always worked for me in the past, but not this time. California was a little different than Minnesota. In Minnesota, my reputation preceded me. All I had to do was ask the principal for something, and it usually happened. The school staff didn't want to mess with Ryan's mother. I rarely had to *get loud*. It didn't work that way in California.

Mr. Lisowski was Ryan's assigned counselor because he had all the H-M last names. He was new to the high school, just like we were. What I didn't realize was that he wasn't new to being a counselor. Even though we had never met the man, I asked if we could switch to Ms. Arnez who had the reputation for being the BEST counselor. Instead of getting upset by my actions, Mr. L. announced at our first meeting, "I'm going to *prove* to you that I'm here to help Ryan." And he did. It didn't take long for him to win me over and show me that *he* was the BEST counselor ever!

When I confided in Mr. L. about Ryan's autism and test anxiety, he listened carefully, Mr. Lisowski recommended we institute a Section 504 plan so we could get Ryan extra time on his SAT and ACT entrance exams. This counselor waded through mountains of paperwork needed to get Ryan the extra time.

I asked Mr. L. if we should let the colleges know about Ryan's autism. Would it give him a leg up or hurt his chances for being accepted? Together, we made the decision that the colleges didn't need to know about Ryan's autism. He said it was not necessary to mention anything about Ryan being in the A-Club on his application or in his interviews since Ryan didn't need any special accommodations in college.

Today, things are different, and the Americans with Disabilities Act makes it illegal for any university receiving federal funding to discriminate against students with disabilities. In reality, stating a disability and working with the Office of Disability Services during the application process can significantly help a student gain admission. Still, I'm not sure we would have done things differently. The decision to disclose/not to disclose depends on your child's needs. If Ryan needed extra help after he was in, he could always contact the disabilities office then. This was the decision we made for Ryan. It is by no means a decision that applies to every child on the spectrum.

Further, there are now public and private universities, such as the University of Scranton and UCLA, that offer specific programs for students with a diagnosis of autism. Whatever route is chosen, be prepared to open and use that tub of documents you have been collecting over the years.

Mr. L. helped us decide what size school was best for Ryan and where he should apply. I worried my son would get lost if he went to a big school. I hated UCLA and didn't thrive in the big-school atmosphere. But for Frank, UCLA was the right choice. My instincts told me Ryan was more like me and needed a more personal education. We listened to my gut and the research that says children with autism do better in smaller settings. A smaller school probably would have worked better for me, but I never would have met Frank if that had been the case.

After completing endless college essays and applications, Ryan and I weren't sure we had any words left. It seemed like Ryan and his mother only knew how to write in 500-700 word segments, and most of what we wrote about in his college essays sounded too good to be true. Getting into college was not only essays and applications; Ryan had to do personal interviews. That worried me. What if he did not make eye contact with the admissions officer? He still avoided eye contact with people who were unfamiliar. But now Ryan knew what he had to do to get in, so he did it.

He was late making the appointment to interview for the engineering slots and scholarships at USC. He still hated making phone calls. When he did finally call, all the interview times in Los Angeles were already taken. That's when our airline travel passes came in handy. Ryan and I jumped on a flight and went to Seattle where there were still interview times available. How crazy is that? We lived an hour away from USC, but we had to go all the way to Seattle for an interview. Ryan must have remembered about the importance of making eye contact during his interviews because he was accepted to six prestigious engineering schools. Three of them offered him scholarships.

He wasn't accepted at Harvey Mudd College or Stanford University. After our visit to Harvey Mudd, we decided it was too small, anyway, even for Ryan. And everyone knows no one gets into Stanford unless you are someone's famous kid, a published author, a star athlete, or invented something the world can't live without. I warned Ryan about that. But he insisted on testing the theory, and I think that was his motivation for applying there (besides the Google factor).

Ryan was awarded merit scholarships to USC, Santa Clara University, and Loyola Marymount University. For a short time, Ryan considered Cal Poly and USC. However, they were both enormous and probably not the right fit for him. Ryan instinctively knew that.

But this was Ryan's life and his decision. We were just happy to make it to this point with a kid who was never supposed to make it at all. Ryan was going to any school he wanted, no matter what bank we had to rob to make it happen. This was still America where you are free to go into major debt to pay for your kid's college. We decided we would just take out more loans if we couldn't afford the school Ryan wanted since the banks already owned us for Megan's college.

Ryan narrowed the choices to Loyola Marymount University in Los Angeles and Santa Clara University in San Jose. Both are Catholic Jesuit schools—perfect for my nice half-Jewish boy. Both offered him a generous scholarship. The schools were medium-sized. Not too big and not too small. Each offered a more personal education. Both guaranteed that your child could finish in four years. Both had classes primarily taught by professors rather than teaching assistants. The big difference between the schools was that Loyola was *forty* miles away and Santa Clara was *three hundred and forty* miles away.

We were afraid if Ryan decided on Loyola, he would spend every weekend in the safety of our house, cooking gourmet meals with me to avoid making friends. Yet Santa Clara felt too far away from the same nest we were trying to push him out of. Could Ryan make it without our support that far from home? Could he manage dorm life, remember to take his meds, manage everything without me, and still do his own laundry? Did he even know how to do laundry?

We were about to find out because Ryan chose Santa Clara.

CHAPTER 37

THE MOST IMPORTANT THING RYAN LEARNED IN COLLEGE WAS NOT ENGINEERING

I have never let schooling interfere with my education.

—Mark Twain

RYAN THOUGHT HE went to college to earn a degree in engineering. He excelled in all his courses, but he gained so much more than just a diploma. He graduated with a degree in *life*. College taught Ryan how to be Ryan.

However, college was not without issues. Moving to college meant more than finding the space in his dorm room for his new clothes and new textbooks. Ryan also needed to find a place for all the old emotional and social baggage he brought from middle school and, to a much lesser extent, high school. Going to college is not so much starting a new chapter in your life as it is the continuation of your life. And Ryan learned to negotiate life—without his hover mother standing right next to him.

Ryan's freshman year was spent living in a dorm suite with seven other guys. He had a rocky start with the social dynamics. One roommate was dealing drugs. He shared a room with another who often invited girls to spend the night. Ryan was sometimes *sexisled* (his term) from his room. He ended up on the couch and didn't get enough sleep before classes or exams. Any kid would have trouble dealing with these complicated social issues. Much to my surprise,

Ryan figured out what to do all on his own. The roommate stopped dealing, and the other entertained only on weekends when Ryan would visit his aunt and uncle; and they all seemed to get along.

But was I done hovering? No. Freshmen were not allowed to bring cars to campus because there were not enough parking spaces. His hover mother got special permission for Ryan to have a car on campus. Once again, I changed the rules to help my son succeed. I bent the truth when I told the school he needed to be able to drive home to see his doctor. This time, he took the "babe-mobile" with him. Since no other freshmen had wheels to get anywhere, Ryan was inundated with requests for rides.

The car was his new kid-attractor, and it worked amazingly well!

When anyone in his dorm wanted a ride, they approached Ryan. He drove everyone everywhere, and gas was our only expense for this valuable social education in courses like "group body piercing" and "midnight pizza runs." As the man with the keys, Ryan never had to initiate friendships or make the first move to meet anyone. They found him, and the social benefits to Ryan far outweighed the cost for gas.

Initially, Justin needed to get places, too. Justin was a friend to everyone, and everyone wanted to be his friend. As one of the most popular kids in his dorm, Justin could have been friends with anyone, but he chose to take Ryan under his wing, and they became genuine friends. Since Justin accepted and included Ryan, everyone else did, too. Justin taught Ryan all the things I couldn't. He became his best friend and dragged him everywhere.

Ryan made up for all the things he missed when he was younger and still affected by autism. Every summer vacation, Ryan took several trips from Los Angeles to San Diego to stay with his college friends. He even went with a group of guys to Hawaii for surfing and fun in the sun. I am happy to report this kid drank beer and went to fraternity parties. I know it is kind of weird and backwards for a mom to want their kid to be part of the drinking scene in college, but this is what college kids do.

Our kids make us view life a little differently.

Ryan even tried the girlfriend thing for three months. He was ecstatically happy, but all good college flings come to an end. Heartbreak is just another part of life. Ryan is now a little gun-shy about trying again. He tells me women are too complicated and he'd rather have a dog. My husband agrees with him. I sometimes wondered if they were talking about me. And should I be insulted by their comments? I know my son will try again. Or maybe some smart girl will make the first move, so he won't have to.

In time, his transformation into becoming a social animal was complete. Ryan's sense of humor is now almost as awful and quick as his father's. There isn't much lacking in his social skills now. Sometimes, he still hesitates to make the first move and waits for friends to call him instead of just picking up the phone. But don't we all?

It was no longer necessary for Ryan's mother to hover. But I just couldn't seem to help myself. I still hovered. Ryan eventually contacted the disabilities office to get extra time for tests, and again we used documentation from the tub that doubled as our file cabinet. This minor accommodation really helped his stress level at school. I don't really believe he actually needed the extra time. But this helped him relax more when taking tests.

Ryan was still overly focused on getting good grades all through college. Once again, I was not the typical college parent. I told him he needed to have more fun instead of having a perfect GPA. I tried to reassure him that B's were okay, and he needed to stop pushing himself so hard. When the pressure got to him, my brother and his wife were his safety net. Dean and Debbie's house was a safe haven when dorm life and school got to be too much. Debbie, the sister I never had, listened with a sympathetic ear and fed him a good meal when he needed to escape for a weekend.

Ryan's fears and insecurities surfaced at the start of every academic year, as predictable as the Minnesota cold he hated so much. He would call home in a panic, worried if he could manage. He did this multiple times during his last grueling year of school. After a series of "I can't do this anymore, and my grades are in the toilet" telephone calls, he still managed a near-perfect GPA.

Sometimes Frank or I had to talk him down from the ledge when he called in a panic. Although the calls mostly came to me, Frank was usually better at helping him than I was. Sometimes, I just wanted him to stop complaining and be grateful for all he had accomplished.

When I got sick of his complaints, I would tell him sternly, "You are almost done, and you *can* do this!" Sometimes, we would argue when he felt it was all too much. He would complain about the same things over and over, trying to vent. I knew that at these times, I was once again the safe harbor where he could say anything that popped in his head. The thing I tell both my kids when they are stressing about completing a goal or taking one of life's big tests is, "I will always love you, *no matter what.*" He knew that I would always love him even if he failed. When he was overwhelmed and reacted by saying he wanted to quit school, I wasn't as patient as I could have been. Here is one of the emails he sent after one of our telephone calls degenerated into yelling:

From: Ryan Hinds
Sent: Tuesday, March 01, 2011 7:36 PM
Subject: My point of view
Mom,

I love you, but I want you to understand my point of view. You tell me that I need to fix my own problems, but my hands are tied. I am not allowed to opt out of the NASA scholarship. And quitting the fraternity is not an option because you want me to have that social experience. The only social experience I have is in the chapter meetings, which ruins my Sunday so I have one less day to go surfing.

I have too many things to do and can't seem to eliminate anything from my obligations. With the amount of homework from all my classes, I have no social life (besides working on homework with friends). Yesterday, I spent upwards of five hours doing homework for only one engineering class, and I couldn't even finish the assignment. This week, I have two other homework assignments, a lab report, and finals I need to start studying for. I just had a phone appointment with Dr. Harvey, and I will try my best to improve my diet, but I honestly do not know what to eat or cook. Everything I like seems to be off-limits, and the cafeteria only has very few healthy, non-dairy choices which provide protein.

I am not going to make any life-changing decisions like quitting something when I feel like this, but everything is on the table. Thank you for understanding.

Love,
Me

Frank was the one to answer his email. He was such a good dad that day. Once again, I hit overload and couldn't do it anymore. I had run out of patience.

From: Frank Hinds
Sent: Wednesday, March 02, 2011 7:37 AM
Subject: I'm proud of you and you can find the solutions
Ryan,

That was a very well-written email. Maybe it's better if you and Mom communicate this way because when you two talk on the phone, it always degenerates into yelling. Anyway, here's the deal. In my opinion, you allow yourself to become paralyzed by your problems instead of looking for solutions. You say you lost your skateboard, but you call Mom to find out what to do about it when the solution is obvious. When your backpack breaks, you call Mom and expect her to figure out what to do about it. When you're having trouble figuring out what to eat, you write Mom and complain about it.

Do you really need Mom to tell you to find someone to help you get into the classroom where you think you left your skateboard? Do you really need Mom to tell you where to go to buy another backpack? Do you really need Mom to tell you what to eat? Mom and I are here for you, but we are here to help you with issues you cannot solve on your own. You know what you need to eat: meat, vegetables, and fruit. Do you think I would be upset if I see on the American Express bill that you are going to decent restaurants and eating proper food? If you think that, you're wrong.

It is your job to find a way to make your life work. If that means not going to a fraternity chapter meeting because you need some time to yourself to do something fun, don't ask us for permission. There are certain times in life that you're just stuck with unpleasant circumstances. Mom hated college. She also wanted to quit. She didn't. I kept getting airsick in flight school. Do you know what it's like going to work, knowing you're probably going to be puking all over yourself? Still, I wouldn't allow myself to quit.

The difference between people who succeed and those who don't is just one thing. Those who succeed keep getting up and trying again after they are knocked down. I've seen you overcome things that most people couldn't. You've just gotten used to Mom coming to your rescue. It's time to get off the Mom-welfare.

So, attack your problems aggressively. Look for ways to solve them. Look at each of your difficulties knowing that you can overcome every issue even though it may take some time. Don't allow yourself to become mired down in them. Don't expect others to solve the problems you can take care of yourself. This does not mean you don't get help. But use the assets you have (professors, graduate students, administrative staff, and the school counselors) to help you find solutions.

I know sometimes you think you can't do this. I know that you can. You just need to start believing that you can, too.

I love you,
Dad

If I Knew Then What I Know Now

My son likes his time alone probably more than most people. The solidarity of the ocean and surfing is another way he escapes the stress of life. Ryan loves anything having to do with the ocean. He and Megan still watch *Shark Week* on the Discovery Channel together. First it was sharks, next came Jacques Cousteau, then scuba lessons. Now, it's surfing.

Ryan traded the chick magnet convertible for our old beat-up Honda because the Honda could hold a roof rack for his surfboard. He gets together with the surfing buddies he met online at various beaches, looking for that perfect wave. I demanded that Ryan attach a plastic laminated card with emergency contact information to his wetsuit just in case of shark attack. Frank tells me this won't really protect our son and is not sure why the sharks wouldn't just eat the laminated card while they're busy munching on Ryan. He said that's what the sharks do on the Discovery Channel.

Over the years, I learned not to place a limit on what our kids can do. I never even considered college when Ryan was still in middle school. I barely considered high school. Back then, all I hoped for was that someday he could hold a job at McDonald's and live independently. I still wasn't even sure he was ready for college when I helped him move into the dorm. However, Ryan always seemed to step up when I threw him in. Never rule anything out.

When Ryan was in high school, I still helped him start every research and English paper. I probably should have made him do more by himself, but he couldn't seem to come up with a single paragraph on his own. His progress was one step at a time and way too slow for my liking. In college, he became an excellent writer when his hover mother was no longer there to help him write his papers. However, I still did a little editing by email for the first part of his freshman year. Now, he writes articles for a political website that blow me away. I wish my writing skills were as advanced as his. Kids will only accomplish as much as you think they can do. And I should have had higher expectations in the writing skills area sooner.

Ryan is no longer someone I can hover over. For me, the hardest part was to stop holding his hand and let him fail. Hover mothers have that problem. Thank goodness for my husband who would make me put him in situations I never would have considered. The thing our children need to learn is that we all fall at times, but the important part we have to help them understand is that they must always get back up and try again.

Ryan's Thoughts About Autism, College, and His Mother

As you have seen in the previous chapters, my mother is a little stubborn. This is not a criticism, but rather a fact that shouldn't really surprise anyone who has read this book. I'm not bothered by this personality trait. It was because of her tenacity that I got better. Sometimes her pushiness can be a little annoying, but there is no one in the world I love or appreciate more.

It is because of this almost perfect yet obsessive mother that I live a pretty normal life, and I am grateful for that. My mom and I fight sometimes, but at times it is kind of fun to mess with her. When she wanted to know every detail about my girlfriend, it was quite bothersome. There are just some things you don't tell your mother. My sister and I decided a long time ago that we love to torment her by *not sharing* information about anyone special in our lives. Some people call that *passive-aggressive* behavior. We think of it as *entertainment*.

I worry I will disappoint my mom if I decide not to get married or have a family. I might want a house full of dogs instead. They are much easier than women. My dad agrees with me. And my mom is a little insulted because she believes she isn't that difficult. Marcia already has a closet full of clothes for the grandchildren who aren't born yet.

The one thing that still bothers me about being on the spectrum is that I'm still dependent on medications to make my immune system work properly. I long for the day when someone invents the thing the world can't live without—a cure for autism.

When I forget to take my medicine or don't watch my diet carefully enough, I must battle to suppress my old behaviors like talking to myself, weird noises, and obsessive touching. They are almost like volcanoes—dormant, though able to erupt at any time. I am no longer considered to be on the autism spectrum medically or socially. I'm just a little nerdy.

The good news is that *nerdy is in*, and in the engineering field, smart and nerdy is almost *expected*. One of my bosses recently told me I have "great people skills." My mom and I had a good laugh over that one. But I guess in comparison to some of the engineers I work with, maybe I do.

Like any other human being, I accept some limitations for my normal life. I am not supposed to have much dairy; I must have good health insurance (my medicine is expensive, even though I am very healthy overall); and last but not least, I have to hear my crazy mother talk about autism nonstop to other parents.

It is very understandable why my mom does this constantly. She has a good heart and just wants to help kids get better. She just wants the same life I now have for everyone who struggles with this painful illness. She wants to save the world from autism and the problems it caused for me and for the rest of my family in the past. And she just might do it.

You don't tell Marcia she can't do something! It will just make her want to do it more and prove you wrong. My mom loves telling anyone who will listen about my *coming out* story. My mom and I didn't share that I was ever diagnosed with autism with many people. She believed sharing was my decision. I guess this book might change that. I won't bore you or tell the *coming out* story the way she does, which includes every little detail. So briefly, here's what happened:

I belong to a fraternity. When my mom and dad came up for parents' weekend, there was a fraternity dinner for all my brothers and their parents. One of my fraternity brothers usually followed me around a little like a lost puppy. It was no different at this dinner. My frat brother should have been nominated as a not-so-obvious member of our A-Club. My mom immediately picked up on what was going on, and we exchanged a knowing glance from across the dinner table that communicated that he was *touched*. That is our own term for someone in the A-Club.

Later, I explained to my mom that this guy always wants to be my friend and follow me around. Before I even finished my sentence, my mom got a little agitated as she revved up into high gear. Next, she almost reprimanded me as she said in a serious tone, "You better be his friend because you remember what it was like not to have any."

I quickly assured her that I'm always nice to this guy and a friend to him. Before she could get any more worked up, I went on to share that just last week I defended him in front of the entire fraternity—about fifty guys or so. My friend was not at this particular meeting, and the rest of the guys were complaining about him and his *strange* behaviors. A few of the fraternity guys became very vocal about not wanting him around and how he made the rest of us look *uncool*. They had no idea he suffered from autism or that that was the reason he acted strange.

I stood up in front of the fraternity and tried to explain to them why he did these annoying things. I had kept my autism hidden for years and this was my *coming out* party. It was almost a relief to talk about what I had kept secret all my life.

I explained to them how our fraternity brother was ill. His immune system didn't work right, and the result was autism. I helped them understand the difficulties he had to face on a daily basis and how he needed us to help him. Next, I told them about my own autism story and how hard it was to be rejected by others. I said that I hoped they would show him compassion. He can't stop doing those strange things. I finished with how, as his fraternity brothers, we must help him and not allow anyone to leave him out.

As I told my mom this story, her eyes misted up. Next she said it was never my grades or academic accomplishments that were important. As the tears ran down her face, she said it was the times like this and what I did for my fraternity brother that made her most proud. She went on to say what I did was the measure of a real man. Next, my mom said she thought I was the best kid ever!

I turned her tears to laughter when I reminded her about James Hopkins. In middle school, he seemed to be the perfect kid. He was popular, smart, and one of the best athletes. James was even the fourth fastest runner in the third grade. During those difficult middle school years, my mother once told me that I should be more like him. That one hurt, and I know she is truly sorry for ever saying that. But that doesn't mean I will ever stop teasing her about it. After I had her laughing through her tears my mom said,

"James Hopkins doesn't even come close to being as wonderful as you are, and I wouldn't want anyone else to be my son."

After I came out, I was asked to speak to a group of around three hundred Santa Clara students and faculty. My parents drove more than five hours to see me speak about my experience with autism. First up was an administrator from a rehab/group home. This dedicated professional talked about what they do there and how it helps their residents. Next, I got up and told my story. I was a bit nervous, but my mom said that's what made it even more amazing because I continued in spite of that. My mom said she could tell I was nervous, but she didn't think anyone else knew. The last scheduled speaker was a dad who was a judge in the area. He spoke about his twenty-four-year-old son, who was not recovered. The judge talked about how hard life is with autism. It has affected the entire family and his *typical* daughter is still suffering with psychological issues as a result. Neither speaker mentioned anything about the medical treatment for autism. They were both so educated, very nice, and yet so wrong about autism. They still defined it as a *life-long developmental* disorder. It makes me sad that so many people still don't get it.

Of course, Marcia, being Marcia, felt compelled to get up and give another point of view. She said she was Ryan's mom and asked if she could say a few words. She spoke about how autism results from a medical condition. After my mom told me what a great job I did, she asked me if what she said was okay. I think she expected me to say she was funny and entertaining, but I didn't. I told her she did well, but I thought she was a bit too *strident.* My mom didn't know what that word meant, so she asked me to explain. I said she came off a bit too strong. At first, I was afraid I hurt her feelings, but she just started to laugh. Next she said, "You know, Ryan, you are really something. My son who was supposed to be autistic is filling in the holes in my vocabulary and teaching me about how to act in public."

I have learned from all my experiences. Middle school had the worst and most lasting impact on my life. Kids in middle school can be very mean, and it didn't make it easier that I was different. I was afraid to tell my mom about the bullying because I thought she would blame me. I was never the same after the other kid they tormented committed suicide. I received so many awful phone calls from the bullies that sometimes I still take a deep breath before I answer the phone. Old fears take time to go away. I also do not have as much faith in people as I should because of what happened to me, and I am very selective in choosing the people I spend time with.

My past experiences have led me to avoid some social situations even when they seem perfectly safe. I am not a big drinker, which made it harder to fit in at college. Don't get me wrong, I enjoy being with others (I hated my internship job at NASA, where I was isolated), but I would rather have a couple of close friends than a lot of average acquaintances. Contrary to my mom's wishes, I don't know if I will ever get married because I fear that I won't be able to find anyone who can understand me. Even so, I have had a good life that most parents would love for their children.

Part 6

Can a Family Survive Autism?

CHAPTER 38

WILL OUR MARRIAGE MAKE IT?

Sometimes we are too busy mopping the floor to turn off the faucet.

—Author Unknown

ALTHOUGH I WOULD not have said this at the beginning of our autism nightmare, our biggest problem was not Ryan. Our biggest problem was autism. *Life on Autism Island* put immense, unending strain on my marriage and on my family. Autism is tough on the child, and it's tough on the rest of us dealing with the child.

It's probably more correct to say, "We *hate* autism, but we *love* the kid."

However, when you are in the throes of yet another screaming match—only this time it's with your husband—no one is thinking clearly, and everyone is way too emotional. At those times, we blame our kid followed by a nice big dose of blaming your spouse and/or his family for being the cause of this entire disaster that has become your life. Stress is the reason why many of the marriages with our kind of kids end in divorce.[45]

---

45   For an article discussing divorce in families with autism, Abbott, Alysia. "Love In The Time Of Autism." *Psychology Today* Volume 46, Number 4 July/August Edition 2013, pp. 60-67. For an abridged version, search the internet for, "Love In The Time Of Autism." Another article on this subject is called "After the Diagnosis: Staying Together as a Couple" http://maryromaniec.com/pdf/afterthediagnosis.pdf and is by Mary Romaniec who also wrote *Victory Over Autism*.

I answer questions for families struggling with autism. Some find me on Facebook and others contact me through my website. Parents don't have to explain anything to me, because I've been there. I just want all kids to have what Ryan now has and I never charge to help. The following is a shortened version of an email from a mom. It exemplifies the problems and daily frustrations created by living with a child with autism.[46]

Marcia,

Tommy knocked over his dresser last night, and my husband lost it. He called our son an "idiot" and a "retard," and he said he hated him. He said we can't have a normal life with him around. My husband said, "All Tommy can do is eat and poop. He can't even have a normal conversation." I know you understand. I hope your husband is supportive. Thanks for listening to me.
  Signed Frustrated Mom

This is how I answered her:

Dear Frustrated Mom,

I get it. There were many similar scenes in our house. Our children with autism put a tremendous stress on a marriage. We all lose it at times. We all react differently to the stress and frustration this diagnosis brings. As women, we want to talk about things over and over again. As moms, that is how we cope. Men are different. Our husbands often just want to solve the problem but can't. So, some disengage and are in denial. But more often since there is no easy fix, men sometimes exhibit what I refer to as Autism Road Rage or ARR. ARR is not exclusive to fathers; moms get it, too. But when I lost it, I knew I still loved my son. However, when my husband lost it, I sometimes wondered if Frank loved Ryan at all. Sometimes I had to protect my son from his own father. There were

---

46   The names were changed to protect the family's privacy.

times when my frustrated husband went after Ryan physically when he was at a loss as to what else to do. I'm embarrassed to say I sometimes did that, too. Neither of us even considered using physical punishment with our other child. But nothing worked with Ryan. Ryan wanted what he wanted, when he wanted it. He was often angry, stubborn, and totally unmanageable.

Ryan didn't have the language to express his needs, so he screamed and had meltdowns. Back then, I was a frustrated mom, too. I tried anything, even grabbing him in a way that mothers shouldn't or smacking him on the butt when he wouldn't listen. It wasn't the right thing to do, and I'm humiliated to admit I actually did that. This was before we knew how to use ABA to address inappropriate behavior.

Frank and I were usually at our best when we had a plan on how to do things. Sometimes, it was the wrong plan, but even so, having a plan helped. But eventually, the plan would go out the window, and we would have a scene like you described. We almost didn't make it through this autism HELL. Try not to hate your husband too much after these awful times (easier said than done). If you both survive this, your marriage will be strong enough to withstand anything.

Your husband is hurting as much as you are, and he probably feels he has to protect you at the same time. Most men don't talk about their fears. And we can't talk about our fears to our husbands because they just get upset and try to fix something that is unfixable. What a big mess our special needs children create.

Best,
Marcia

Another dad described how his marriage ended in divorce because of the stress autism put on the family. This dedicated father put his life on hold to help his son. He was responsible for all his son's medical, behavioral, and educational interventions and only worked from home when he could. His wife was the main breadwinner and traveled a lot.

According to him, she didn't know anything about what was going on with their son. He was resentful because he was doing everything alone. His wife was also resentful because she worked and thought her husband should earn more income for the family.

The sad part is that they both loved their son, and this divorce should never have happened. Now, they have an increased financial burden as they try to support two households while they continue to pay for their son's expensive medical care. They have almost no chance to successfully maintain the consistency and discipline their son needs as he travels back and forth between two residences.

Marriage is tough enough without our kids putting more stress on it. Living with Ryan minus a husband to bring in the bacon would have made his recovery impossible. I can't imagine accomplishing what we did if I had to work and Frank was not around to help me. There were times I hated Frank for his behavior toward Ryan. There were times I couldn't talk to him about anything. The bottom line is that Ryan never would have gotten better without Frank doing all he did.

Even when I blamed Frank or Ryan for our awful circumstances, I somehow held it together and never said out loud what I was actually thinking. I used to tell Ryan that it was okay NOT to share everything that is on your mind. That goes for everyone else in the world, too. Not all truth needs to be spoken. As a matter of fact, to maintain a relationship that is under siege by autism, it is sometimes imperative to have a marital filter. To Frank's credit, no matter how bitchy I got, he wouldn't let me give up on our son, our family, or our marriage.

Parents are different in what they bring to a marriage and a family. I was a mom that slowly lead my children into the wading pool one toe at a time. Frank was the kind of father that made his kids sink or swim. I usually put my arms around our kids and tried to protect them from everyone and everything. I constantly worried about their feelings and tried to keep our kids safe from the rest of the world. Frank had a different approach. He prepared our children to make it on their own and pushed them out of the nest. Children need a little of each in order to succeed.

Although I was too overprotective, Ryan knew I was always there to pick him up when he fell—and I mean that literally and metaphorically. In the beginning, Ryan couldn't do anything for himself, including walk down the street, without me tightly holding his wrist. I had to hold onto him because if he tripped, he would never use his hands to break his fall. He would have landed flat on his face. I often protected him too much from life, even from the situations that provided learning opportunities and natural consequences.

Ryan never would have progressed as far as he did without Frank constantly making me stop acting like his overprotective mommy. Frank insisted that Ryan participate in activities that scared the crap out of me. He played T-Ball, did gymnastics and karate, and joined the track team in high school. I never would have made Ryan do half the things Frank did because I didn't want his feelings hurt when he was, yet again, the worst one on the team.

Fortunately, my son had a strong father in the picture. Frank was instrumental in helping Ryan grow up to be more capable. That's what his dad did. I tried to shield my son from the world because I knew he did not have the same physical capabilities as other kids. That's what his mom did. Our children need someone to protect them and tell them it will be okay as well as someone to encourage and push them into trying new things. More importantly, our children need to learn from both parents how to get back up when they fall.

It was a mistake to constantly argue with my husband about Ryan. Instead, I should have encouraged Frank when he did even the slightest thing right with Ryan. I could have shaped Frank's behavior at the same time I was working on Ryan's. I was so overwhelmed that I forgot *ABA works on husbands, too*. Just like our kids everyone needs encouragement when we see them doing something right. Inappropriate behavior should be ignored as much as possible.

Sadly, most times I didn't have anything left to give Frank. I needed to treat my husband with respect and affection like I did when he was my boyfriend and I was still trying to impress him. Listening and giving credence to his ideas was the best way to get Frank's assistance and support. Instead, I made the mistake of being critical and pointing out what he was doing wrong. I sometimes forgot that Frank loved Ryan, too.

If I Knew Then What I Know Now

It wasn't like we were this wonderful family that always agreed on how to help Ryan. Frank and I fought constantly about how we should do things and what our son needed. I felt alone in the bottomless pit of autism. I never seemed to have time for my husband or anything else. Ryan and our entire family would have benefitted from less fighting.

We were lucky our marriage survived at all; we almost didn't make it.

In hindsight, I have come to the conclusion that when Ryan was at his worst, I held the key to making our home less stressful. I was the one who had the power in the relationship to get what I needed for both my son and our family. What I now know about autism and fathers would have been extremely helpful when Ryan's autism was at its worst.

Remember my *"If You Don't Feel It, Fake It"* therapy for autism? You need a similar tactic for those rough times with your spouse. It's important to treat your partner in the same way you would like to be treated . . . maybe the way you did before you were married and were still trying to impress him or her. By changing my behavior and by making Frank a part of the solution to Ryan's autism, I could have made him an ally instead of just another person standing in my way.

As parents, we are so overwhelmed by all we need to do. Sometimes we make the mistake of relegating our spouse's importance to the equivalence of a piece of furniture. My husband has told me that dads he has spoken with compliment their wives on being great mothers, but most expressed considerable pain over not being shown love, affection, or any sexual interest. I was one of those moms. Fortunately, Frank didn't give up on me or our kids.

If I had known all this way back then, I wouldn't have argued so much with Frank. The fighting interferes with what needs to be done. All parents want to move heaven and earth for their child. They don't want to fight about how to proceed.

The bottom line is that our fighting interfered with what needed to be done to help Ryan. Instead, every family needs to adopt a "we are in this together as equals" approach to survive the tough issues that an autism diagnosis brings to a family.

CHAPTER 39

WHY COULDN'T I JUST BE A DAD?— BY RYAN'S FATHER, FRANK

Being a great father is like shaving. No matter how good you shaved today, you have to do it again tomorrow.

—Reed Markham

I'VE NEVER BEEN an emotional person. I'm a linear, logical, place-for-everything-and-everything-in-its-place kind of guy. That served me well throughout Navy ROTC, flight school, and commercial aviation. Yet to say I was ill-equipped to deal with Ryan's autism may be the understatement of my life.

Dealing with autism is not as simple as dealing with the loss of your dreams. Of course, every dad sees his newborn son and can't help but think in terms of stereotypes. I thought about his first day playing little league, going camping together, his high school football games, and his college graduation. Then you are told you need to start thinking in terms of group homes. The shockwave this sends through you runs so deep that your initial dreams just disappear. You learn to take life in much smaller bites and not look too far into the future. You're soon surprised by the joy you can find in little things. Suddenly you are playing baseball with your daughter and your wife is cooking with your son. The stereotypes are no longer important. Instead the focus becomes that my son talked to a kid at school, he was invited to a birthday party, and he learned how to jump rope. Next thing you know, you're dreaming again. Maybe it's not for the Heisman Trophy; maybe it's only that he plays in the marching band. You can't keep going without dreams, no matter how what they are.

Even after you begin climbing out of the abyss, it is not a constant, steady climb. Two steps forward, one step back. Sometimes two steps forward, three steps back. That experience is both frustrating and frightening. But as long as there is a forward step, there is hope. And as long as there is hope, there are possibilities. Throughout middle school, high school, and even college, Ryan had an occasional meltdown. But we kept going because we had hope and mostly because giving up wasn't an acceptable alternative. Many days, I had to really struggle to see any forward movement.

I remember being angry at the doctor who diagnosed Ryan. I remember wanting to prove her wrong. I thought at the time that this would involve some work on our part but that I'd get control of this like I had gotten control of everything else in my life. I'd power through this: develop a plan, put it in place, and fix the kid. How dumb was I?

The worst part for me was this loss of control. There were times when I became overwhelmed and angry at the thought that this was going to be my life forever. Sometimes I was teased into temporary feelings of joy when Ryan would have a good day—no crying and no hitting. Inevitably, the next day we were all dragged down into autism hell again, Ryan screaming, Marcia and I fighting, and Megan running to her room so that she didn't have to listen to any of it.

But life was most difficult when I didn't have a plan. Not having a plan happens with all kids, but when you have a child with autism, you deal with it constantly. What should we try next? Auditory training, occupational therapy, prism glasses? We bounced around from doctor to doctor, feeling that life was completely out of control. I got pretty angry during these no plan/no control times. When we had no direction, my daughter was not getting the attention she deserved, and I was angry at Ryan because of it. I smacked him when he misbehaved, and I see now I was just trying to get control of a situation over which I had no control. My progress out of this was much like Ryan's: steps forward and backward.

We visited a family in the Bay Area that Marcia had been helping. They were us twenty years ago: older daughter, younger autistic son, and a dad who still had all of his hair. I could see the shell-shocked look on the father's face, the desperate need to be normal, and the nagging realization that there's a good chance it's not going to happen. He showed me all the stuff his son could do—letters, numbers, words, and puzzles. I had done the same thing when Ryan was younger: If I get Ryan to do enough parlor tricks, maybe people will think he's normal and that I'm not a failure.

I think he may have been the first dad I've talked face-to-face at length about what it was like to have a child on the spectrum. He admitted that I was his first too. Why was that? Marcia spends hours conversing with moms via online autism groups, email, and phone. Occasionally, I've spoken briefly to a dad or two and sometimes a mom I needed to convince that her husband was probably not insane.

Men usually think about the situation differently. It's probably a combination of things. First of all, we're men. Men don't always share—food, toys, feelings, etc. Second, to admit to another guy that you are seriously floundering is an admission of failure, and we tend not to do that either.

But with this dad, I decided to break all the rules. We discovered that, in many cases, we had similar thoughts. We were angry about what life had handed us. We agreed that there were times when we felt that it might be necessary to get our sons out of the house. Not that we didn't love them—but as dads, it was our duty to preserve the family unit. Any threats to the stability of the family must be dealt with. And our sons with autism were a definite threat: They caused us to fight with our wives. They made our daughters cry. They put our families into a constant state of chaos.

We also agreed that it was never going to happen for many reasons, one of which was that our wives were running this show, and their instinct was to protect the cubs. We assured ourselves that, as far as our spouses were concerned, if anyone was going to be shown the door, it would be us. But that didn't stop me from leaving military school websites on the computer desktop after a bad day with Ryan.

When Ryan was younger, I think I took his autism much more personally than Marcia. I was easily embarrassed by his behavior and angrier that things weren't working out according to my plan. I would alternately resent Ryan for what he had done to our lives and then feel guilty for resenting this lost and innocent child who was completely overwhelmed by the world around him. I took my anger out on everyone. I am ashamed of myself for that. Thank God Marcia was better at this than I was. When the latest cure du jour turned out not to be one, Marcia would stay up all night reading and come up with our next move. While I was getting over the previous misstep, she would be marching off in a new direction. It was hard to keep up.

If I learned one thing in the Navy, it is someone has to be in charge. Wait, I actually learned two things. The other thing I learned was that the person in charge was not me. I relegated myself to a sup-porting role. Marcia came up with the plan—of course, she bounced ideas off me—and I would figure out the logistics of the plan. It was my responsibility to figure out how to pay for it, book an airline, and reserve the hotel. The details were left to me.

This is not to say that I was only involved in the administration of Marcia's many grand plans for Ryan. I played many roles. When we would set up teaching scenarios, I got to be the bad kid. Ryan and I would go to hardware stores together, ride the elevators at hotels, and read books. I was in charge of the bedtime routine: First was his bath. Then we read a book. And every night we cuddled as I told him his bedtime story. I think that this bedtime routine was what I enjoyed the most, probably because I craved things that allowed me to just be a dad. Feeling normal for just a little while was important to me.

At some point, we decided to get Ryan involved in sports. I had coached Megan in softball and football and had fun doing it. But Megan would have been okay with any coach. In Ryan's case, it was essential that I was the coach. No one else understood what worked with him or got what to do with him. They would not see how easily he was overwhelmed with team sports. If you think about how many things are happening on a baseball or soccer field at the same time, Ryan didn't have a chance. We tried one season each of baseball and basketball and a couple seasons of soccer before we realized it was time to go another direction.

We were much more successful at swimming and karate. It was much easier to focus on getting from one end of the pool to the other or memorizing punches and kicks than the multiple steps of "whom do I throw to if it's a ground ball, a fly ball, with one or two outs, runners on base or not." Ryan was always a fish in water, but he was apprehensive about karate. So, we took karate together and tested for our belts together—it was great.

What we learned was that team sports did not work for Ryan. Sports that were more individual in nature while still having a team aspect were so much better. In karate, Ryan had his own stuff to learn, but he had to help the younger students as well as practice with his peers. When Ryan was in high school, a girl talked him into running on the cross-country and track teams. Again, it was an individual sport where he still had to train with and cheer on his teammates. Today, Ryan still runs and scuba dives, and he is an avid surfer. He is part of a surf group. Perfect.

There were a few things we did right. First, we realized early on that our family had to start working as a team and that working together was the only way Ryan was going to have a shot at succeeding. We also tried to make sure that Marcia and I were not both ready to jump off the ledge at the same time. Somebody had to have enough hope at the moment to talk the other one down. Finally, even though there were plenty of raised voices along the way, I think it helped that Marcia and I always had a similar vision of what we wanted to accomplish. We wanted Ryan to be a part of the world in which he lived. We were not going to be able to change the world to adapt it to Ryan. He was going to have to learn to play to his strengths by using his amazing intelligence, perseverance, and determination.

At the same time, Ryan needed to make up for his weaknesses. He needed to hide his discomfort when he met new people and was put in new situations. As long as we kept his weaknesses somewhere in the middle of the bell-shaped curve, we'd be okay. Ryan had his quirks; he just needed to learn that everyone has their quirks, too. And they just don't put them out on display for the world to see.

Our vision also evolved to include the idea that Ryan has a responsibility to help others. Ryan has, at times, tried to run from his association with autism as fast and far as he could. Can you blame him? This was a kid who was rarely invited to a birthday party, had few friends, and was severely bullied in school. Who wouldn't try to distance himself from that? But Ryan has found a balance.

He doesn't wear an A-for-Autism patch on his sleeve, but he doesn't hide from it either. When a young man was excluded from Ryan's fraternity because he was a little different, Ryan stepped up and told his brothers how he had grown up on the spectrum and had been left out of a lot of things. He wasn't going to sit by and just watch this discrimination happen. I can't imagine the number of touchdowns Ryan would have to score to make me prouder.

I guess what I'm saying is that if you let the loss of your dreams and hope, the lack of control, the resentment, and guilt over the resentment take over your life, you cannot make it out of this. Life becomes that series of small bites, small successes, and, hopefully, only small setbacks. When you come out the other side of this, your family is better for it. My daughter is a more generous, giving, and tolerant person for having helped take care of my son. My wife will help anyone, anytime, with anything. As for me, I'm just lucky to have them.

CHAPTER 40

THERE'S NEVER ENOUGH OF ME TO GO AROUND!

That's what people do who love you. They put their arms around you and love you when you're not so lovable.

—Deb Caletti

SO MUCH OF my time went to Ryan, and yet it still wasn't enough. My life and our family's life were Ryan, Ryan, and more Ryan. Ryan was over-parented, and Megan was under-parented. At the same time, it was Megan's quiet love for her brother and thoughtful suggestions that sometimes held our family together.

As a young child herself, Megan didn't understand Ryan's preferences for playing with objects rather than playing with her. She selflessly gave him any of her toys that he showed an interest in. As he got older, the object he loved best was an orange and yellow Little Tikes car. Ryan lived in that car and drove it all over the house. He would only get out of it when he'd arrive at the large plastic gas pump he used to fill his gas tank.

One day, when Megan was still a little girl, she and I were having a conversation about how young kids don't really know how to share. Megan immediately came to Ryan's defense and announced, "Well, Ryan knows how to share!"

I answered sarcastically, "Really? And what does he share?"

Megan promptly said, "His car." That's when I reminded her it really wasn't Ryan's car—it was hers.

Megan simply answered, "It is his car because he is the one who uses it all the time." Megan came up with the new rule that in our family something belongs to the one who uses it the most.

Megan was usually very patient and loving with Ryan. Even though Ryan pinched Megan, squeezed her arms, and pulled her hair until she cried, she still loved him. When she'd ask me if she could hit him back, my reply was, "When he gets better, you can hit him." Of course, I had no knowledge that he would ever get better and my response amounted to a life sentence of sibling bullying for Megan. My message was that Ryan's autism entitled him to be excused for hitting and biting her and it also carried an implicit rule that Megan was required to behave appropriately around Ryan, no matter how he acted. What I should have done is require Ryan to act appropriately around Megan.

Today, this awful example of *parenting on the edge* continues to be a big joke between my children. Most siblings don't hit each other when they are adults, but my kids may be the exception. Megan holds me to my word. Ryan is better, so she slugs him when he is a smart ass or does something she doesn't like. They share a look of understanding and then laugh. It doesn't matter that he towers over her. She will always be the big sister and he will never hit her back.

Megan carried a heavy burden of expectation. When Megan was only seven, we included her as part of Ryan's educational team. She was one of his most effective therapists. Meg was in charge of teaching Ryan how to play. Back then, he lined up toys and obsessed over certain mechanical things. He didn't yet know how to play with people.

Megan was part of our team—*a big part.*

Megan taught Ryan how to pretend better than any of the adults who had forgotten how to long ago. She was a great therapist, and helping Ryan made her not resent him for taking so much of our time.

Megan and I also had our *special time* every Saturday night. No matter what happened during the week, she knew on Saturday night, it would be just Mommy and her. She didn't have to share me with anyone.

We would plan for our Saturday nights all week long. We'd secretly buy candy and treats that Ryan wasn't allowed to eat. We'd whisper about the things we planned to do on our special night and stash goodies in secret hiding places around the house. After the boys left for their own adventure, Megan and I would cuddle on the couch and watch her favorite TV show, *Dr. Quinn, Medicine Woman*. We ate masses of junk food until our stomachs hurt. We ate all the things we couldn't eat in front of Ryan. Those Saturday nights together were wonderful memories for both of us. After Meg was married and had a dog of her own, she named her Dr. Quinn Medicine Woman (Quinnie for short).

Middle school years were a tough time for Megan. They are for most kids, but her brother made it worse. Ryan's odd behavior embarrassed her. I wanted to shield Megan from the problems, outbursts, and embarrassment Ryan created at home and at school, but that just wasn't possible. Kids that age are mortified by the things their parents do—let alone a brother who acts strangely. At the same time, she felt she needed to protect him from the many kids who were intentionally mean. Sometimes, their meanness toward Ryan spread into meanness toward Megan.

During Megan's middle school years, watching our show together evolved into Saturday nights with her friends. Our new *special time* together became walking Snooper (our dog) around Bredesen Park after school. Sometimes, Ryan was included. If Frank was on a trip, Ryan had to tag along because we couldn't leave him unmonitored in the house. But it was almost like he wasn't there because he never joined in our conversations, anyway.

We talked about everything on those walks. Back then, before everyone had a cell phone, all we could do on these walks was talk. We shared Megan's dreams for the future, and we gossiped about things that happened in school. That's when I tried to casually slip in the important values she needed to learn without sounding like that was what I was doing.

Some days after our walk, we'd watch *Sally Jessy Raphael*. This horrible program that paraded all the bottom feeders in our society was a milder precursor to the reality television shows of today. The guests exhibited every life mistake people shouldn't make. Most parents probably wouldn't let their impressionable teen watch this show, but this program was a great avenue to teach Megan about my own values of right and wrong, without seeming preachy. Sally's show often led us to some very constructive discussions.

Megan's new role during Ryan's high school years included becoming the brother he never had. She answered all his questions on how social events and relationships work with peers, sexual topics, and even how to ask a girl to a dance. She was the fashion police and made sure he looked cool. Ryan had to fit in if he wanted to join in, and Megan knew that wasn't going to happen if I was Ryan's fashion guru. I wore tie-dye shirts and sweatpants—not exactly her idea of high fashion.

Our days revolved around Ryan's needs, his schedule, and all the people coming into our house to provide different therapies. One of my fears for Megan centered on the lack of time and attention she received as a result of Ryan's problems. Were Frank and I a big enough part of her life? How would all this autism chaos affect Megan later in life? Our reason to have a second child was so Megan would have family after Frank and I were no longer here. After Ryan was diagnosed, I worried he could become an endless burden for his sister later. I hoped Megan was getting enough from her parents and that I wasn't messing her up in the process of trying to save Ryan.[47] But what else could we do?

When those thoughts snuck into my head, I remembered my late-night thoughts before Ryan was born when I would sit quietly in the rocking chair and look at his crib. My fear had been a real one. There really weren't enough hours in a day or enough of me to go around.

If I Knew Then What I Know Now

I shouldn't have worried as much as I did about Megan getting enough time and attention. Megan is a better person because of Ryan's autism. Not all siblings have that same happy ending. A family's battle with autism affects every sibling differently. Siblings are at a higher risk for all sorts of psychological issues.

---

47   Green, Laura. "The Well-being Of Siblings Of Individuals With Autism." www.hindawi.com, 2013. Common issues (as excerpted from this article) are: Embarrassment around peers. Jealousy regarding amount of time parents spend with their brother/sister. Frustration over not being able to engage or get a response from their brother/sister. Being the target of aggressive behaviors. Trying to make up for the deficits of their brother/sister. Concern regarding parental stress and grief. Concern over their role in future caregiving.

The challenges of being Ryan's sister helped Megan grow. Ryan's autism forged a more giving and compassionate person who stands up for those who can't protect themselves. Megan was an old, wise soul hidden in a child's body. She had to do too many things for herself at a young age. And when she was done with her needs, she had to help me with Ryan.

As a result of all she dealt with, Megan became one of the most responsible and together people I have ever known. She graduated from the University of Southern California (USC) in three years. After graduation, she immediately had a job in the entertainment industry and supported herself. Within a few years, she went back to school to get a master's degree, so she could work with children on the spectrum. She is a wonderful person with a great work ethic and even better values. That was because we did a few things right. We included Megan as an important member of the team while at the same time made sure she got the individual attention and time she needed.

Megan worked two jobs while going to school to earn her master's in counseling, with an emphasis in ABA. Her supervisors and classroom professors commented on what a gift she has as a behavior analyst. What they didn't realize is that she had her first ABA training session at the young age of seven. She grew up with ABA being part of our everyday lives, so it comes naturally to her. When she passed the test to get her certification as a Board-Certified Behavior Analyst (BCBA), we celebrated that, too. Out of all she has accomplished, it is the way she helps children with autism that makes me the proudest. Still, I sometimes wonder what her life would look like if our house had been autism-free.

On Being Ryan's Sister
by Meg Hinds

I was sixteen and threw a punch at a football player who was twice my size. Matt had announced to my entire group of friends how weird my brother was. I don't know what came over me. I made fun of my brother all the time, but no one else was allowed to do that. So, what did I do? I kept punching Matt until two of my friends pulled me off him. No matter how much he annoyed me, I still had to protect Ryan. The good news was Matt was too shocked by my actions to realize that he could have stopped me without much effort.

In a way, I think it would have been easier if Ryan had a disease like Down syndrome. People know what Down syndrome is, and it's obvious from the moment you meet a person afflicted. Kids don't make fun of those type of kids because they are obviously handicapped. But you can't tell someone has autism by looking at them. Most people thought Ryan was just spoiled and capable of controlling his behavior but choosing not to. They didn't know he was ill, and I certainly wasn't allowed to tell them. My mom thought it was important not to tell anyone because of the stigma attached to the A-word.

Our home was pretty tense growing up. My parents fought constantly about the best way to deal with Ryan. As long as I can remember, our lives revolved around controlling his outbursts and making him better. I recall one incident where I told my mom I wished I could sit behind her—Ryan always had to sit behind my mom in the car. She assured me that I could on the way home. When we walked out of Jerry's market, I got in the seat behind her. Ryan screamed bloody murder and began to pinch and hit me. I got up to move (this was so *not* worth it), and my mom told me to stay put. Ryan wasn't getting his way this time. I smiled the whole ride home—despite the blood-curdling screams in my ear and the fingernails digging into my arm. My mom finally took control from Ryan.

When you're fifteen-years-old and inviting a boy over for the first time, it's nerve-wracking enough making sure your hair is perfect, without worrying about the things your unpredictable brother might do. Adam was my first boyfriend, and I wanted it to go well when we had him over for dinner. What I didn't count on was Ryan. He picked his nose right in front of Adam at the dinner table. It didn't matter that we had told Ryan millions of times not to do that. He knew it was private behavior, but he did it anyway. *I wanted to kill him.* I was so tired of having to apologize or explain

Ryan's embarrassing behavior. But right after that, Ryan made all of us laugh hysterically with his unusual talent of putting both his elbows behind his head. He was such a weird—yet funny—kid.

Since Ryan was always messing up, there was a lot of pressure on me growing up. I felt like I had to be extra perfect. There were no B's—only A's, no detentions, and never even a call home through my entire school career. Trust me, I'm not that smart and definitely not someone who does everything right. I knew how many dreams my parents gave up for Ryan, and I couldn't let them give up on me, too. This was an impossible standard to live up to.

But at the end of the day, Ryan changed me for the better. Because of Ryan, I'm independent. I had to be. As much as my parents loved me, there were only so many hours in the day, and Ryan took up most of them. Ryan taught me that everyone needs a chance and a family who will not give up on him. My friends constantly make fun of me for "taking in the strays" by looking out for people who are a little different and who have no one else. Being a part of Ryan's recovery taught me anything is possible. I am so proud of my little brother.

CHAPTER 41

WHY COULDN'T I JUST BE A MOM?

A mother's love is the fuel that enables a normal human being to do the impossible.

—Marion C. Garretty

THIS BOOK IS the story of Ryan's recovery from autism. It is also the journey of our family's recovery from Ryan's autism. Anyone reading this book can't help tripping over our family's recurring stress, isolation, frustration, misery, and hopelessness. Frank felt this way at times; I felt this way often. Megan hid in her room behind her closed door when she had these feelings. We tried to protect her from the worst of these emotional storms, but that wasn't really possible.

It wasn't only Ryan's behavior that was extreme. At times, my behavior was worse. The thought of our family always living this awful existence, the personal and family energy needed to work relentlessly on Ryan's behavior day and night, and the frustration of seeing only very gradual changes often sent me to the brink of a very dangerous place. Some days, I struggled with dark thoughts of killing Ryan and myself. I cringe now when I think of how often I seriously considered doing this.

Thoughts of what would happen to him in a future of institutions and anonymous group homes tormented me the most. How could I leave him in a group home *all alone*? Megan would be his only visitor. Ryan would interfere with her life, and she would feel guilty if she wasn't there for him. My mind was cluttered with horrible images of my son calling out for me after I was gone.

It was only one thought that stopped me from following through with my delusional plan—how could I leave Megan to grow up without a mother? It was usually during my premenstrual phase that these feelings surfaced. My out-of-control PMS behavior greatly affected Ryan and everyone else who lived with me. When I was not running on all cylinders, he was off, too.

One day, a day I am sure Frank chose by my calendar very carefully, Frank said, "When you're crazy during PMS, the whole house is crazy, and Ryan is uncontrollable." He was right. I knew something had to change if I was to hold it together.

Sometimes help comes in an unexpected way.

Mine came during an appointment with my dental hygienist. Teri did all the talking, and I did all the listening. I was her captive audience since I couldn't talk with her hands in my mouth. Teri shared that she took antidepressants (or SSRIs). Back then, I thought people who relied on those kinds of drugs were weak at best and probably stark-raving lunatics.

Teri, not even embarrassed that she practiced better living through chemistry, revealed that these pills never changed who she was. The SSRIs just made her feel more like herself on a good day. Her revelation thoroughly surprised me because she was one of the most pleasant, together people I had ever met. Teri was kind and a good person. I realized she said these things because she just wanted to help me. She might have shared this about her personal life because she recognized my symptoms and knew I needed help. It takes one to know one.

After starting an SSRI, I became better equipped to deal with all the stress in my life. It didn't take long to see that Frank was correct. If I wasn't okay, then I was incapable of doing anything for Ryan or anyone else in the family. Anyone under the kind of stress I dealt with daily would have difficulty coping. What my family was going through was awful and reason enough to become depressed and anxious. My reaction was what any mom would feel.

A pharmaceutically adjusted Marcia was much more pleasant to be around. And it became much more pleasant to be me. My invention of the *"If You Don't Feel It, Fake It"* self-therapy worked even better with an SSRI assist. Frank, who never even took an aspirin or drank coffee, used to lovingly place my little blue pill on the counter every morning to make sure I never forgot to take it.

If I Knew Then What I Know Now

The SSRI helped me help Ryan. One of the many roles I played as Ryan's Mom was chief interpreter of life. It was my job to explain the world to Ryan when he was still stuck on Autism Island. Every day, I translated for Ryan all the events that occurred and people he encountered that seemed confusing and hard to understand. As a result, my attitude greatly affected his behavior. Ryan's behavior improved when I had a positive attitude instead of one filled with gloom and doom. The keys to making Ryan's world safer and predictable were my attitude and presence.

I also realized to stereotype children with autism as emotionless, as unable to perceive emotion in others, and as intellectually void is both incorrect and demeaning. These children have feelings and perceive the emotional state of others. Remember Tommy from the letter and how his father thought his son was "retarded"? He incorrectly assumed Tommy's intelligence was somehow tied to Tommy's behavior. Children with autism feel things at least the same or maybe even more strongly than the rest of us. What they cannot do is effectively communicate what it is they are thinking and, so very often, intensely feeling.

Part 7

Are We There Yet?

CHAPTER 42

ARE WE EVER DONE WITH OUR KIDS? NO!

Here is the test to find whether your mission on earth is finished. If you're alive, it isn't.

—Richard Bach

MY HUSBAND SAYS he is going to inscribe on my tombstone, *"She was finally DONE."* I long for life to be easy, but it never really is. I'm not sure an uncomplicated life is actually possible for anyone. Anyone looking at my family would think I have it all. My son is fully recovered, and anyone who meets him would never know he was once severely affected by autism. He now works as an engineer for a major aerospace company, and what I wanted most for him actually happened. He is happy, has friends, and is leading a typical life. Ryan recently bought a condo and lives close to the beach.

And yet . . . I'm not done.

I'm always monitoring his health and looking for the next new thing that might correct the issues with his immune system permanently, so he would no longer be dependent on medications. I'm way too involved in his and Megan's lives. I will never be done being Ryan and Megan's mom even though they might like me to just butt out. I know I will have that job until the day I take my last breath.

Once, now long ago, my job was physically exhausting and psychologically debilitating. I was miserable—almost as miserable as Ryan. Today, being Ryan's mom means dealing with normal, usual, ordinary stuff. Now, it is mostly fun. For most parents who live on Autism Island, this usually doesn't happen. They must maintain a controlling role, forever coping with their children's difficult behaviors and continuing to teach the most basic of social and other skills.

Even with Megan, I am never really done. My fiercely independent daughter doesn't let me help much, but I am allowed to babysit her two dogs when she goes out of town. Sometimes, her hectic schedule makes it necessary for me to help her juggle the details of life. And when Megan decided to work with kids who have autism, I encouraged her to make the change. After all the years she put in at USC studying film and the job experience she gained in the movie industry, she really needed to consider the consequences of changing professions. I am so proud that she has chosen such an important calling. She has a gift and changes lives daily.

I will never be done being Ryan and Megan's mom. Although no one can look at Ryan and tell he ever had autism, I know there are still situations where Ryan is unsure of himself. When it comes to matters of character or right and wrong, Ryan always has strong convictions. He is a strong and determined man. Before, Ryan called me to help him with even the smallest decisions that he should have made on his own. I couldn't understand why he spent so much time perseverating about these unimportant things. I always attributed this lack of confidence to the horrible bullying he had to endure in middle school. That was partly true, but some of the reason for his lack of confidence was *me*. I created the problem. It took me years to figure this out, and it happened only after I talked with Barb, my friend, neighbor, and unofficial shrink.

Barb lives across the street and is not really a psychologist at all—not licensed anyway. One day, when Ryan was still in college, I was standing in the middle of the street with my friend sharing my frustration concerning my son. Ryan was so accomplished, yet he still lacked the confidence he should have. Barb gently helped me realize that my overprotective, hover-mother behavior was the real source of Ryan's confidence problem.

Barb said sometimes we do too much for our kids. By handling all their problems, we give them the impression that they can't do things for themselves. She was supportive and kind, but it was almost as if she hit me over the head. Ryan wasn't the problem at all. His lack of self-confidence resulted from *my* actions. While in the past my intervention and hover-mother tendencies were needed, now it was my interference that kept Ryan from succeeding.

By trying to prevent him from falling on his face, I made him feel like he wasn't capable. When he was little, I didn't have a choice; I had to do the things he couldn't do for himself. But this caused me to develop a lifetime habit of taking care of the details in his life for him.

I forgot to let him breathe on his own.

Whenever I did this with his older sister, she bluntly and quickly stopped me from bulldozing in and taking over. Megan just didn't allow it. If I became too pushy or strident (Ryan's wonderful new word for me), she would announce, "Mom, you need to *calm* down—I got this!" That is her signal for me to butt out. Megan started using that phase when I started to edit her college essays without her permission.

The dynamics of my relationship with Ryan changed forever after that conversation with Barb. The next time Ryan called for help, I reassured him that he didn't need me anymore because he was very capable and could handle anything. I went on to say that I was surrendering the "pink slip" to his life. That single comment changed everything. Since then, Ryan has been in charge. He knows I won't be doing things for him anymore; so, he takes care of every detail himself.

After he started to take charge of his life, he didn't look back. That was the summer he traveled to Washington, DC, by himself to make a presentation for NASA.[48] He was picked out of hundreds to make a presentation. Ryan made all of his own plane, hotel, and travel arrangements without any input. He filled

---

48   A video of Ryan making this presentation at NASA can be seen on YouTube. Just put "Ryan Hinds At NASA HQ" in the search engine or go to https://www.youtube. com/watch?v=4-10o3frU1A

out the paperwork to get reimbursed from NASA and spent his time in
Washington exploring the sites. My butting out changed everything.

He was just fine breathing on his own.

CHAPTER 43

IF YOU DON'T KNOW WHERE TO START, START HERE

The way to get started is to quit talking and begin doing.

—Walt Disney

HEARING THAT YOUR child is on the spectrum is frightening and overwhelming. I was once where you are now—devastated by my son's diagnosis and scared out of my mind for my child's future. When we first started to help Ryan, there was no internet or much information to help us. Now we have the opposite problem: there is too much information, and no one agrees on much of anything. Which professionals should we believe, and what information is credible? We can't accept the myths that come with an autism diagnosis. Unfortunately, most children will not get better on their own. The first step toward recovery is deciding that you are no longer willing to stay where you are.

Ryan's story demonstrates that recovery from autism is possible when you combine medical, behavioral, and educational therapies. Some parents make the mistake of only doing behavioral intervention because "experts" have told them that is the only proven treatment for autism. Parents, behaviorists, educators, and medical professionals must all work together as a team. Each of us has a piece of the puzzle.

Please forgive me if I mention things in this section that I have already talked about in the book. This is the short version of the information you need to know that was most important for helping my son. We did things scientifically.

Although I wanted to fire everything at Ryan's broken immune system, we did things one at a time. That was the only way to know what was effective and which medications made a difference.

We started Ryan on a dairy-free diet. Next came the antifungal and antiviral drugs, an SSRI, and Leucovorin to counteract his MTHFR gene mutation. My son never took the long list of supplements that many of the autism specialists prescribe, but Ryan does take iron, vitamin D-3, and fish oil. My son has been on these prescription medications continuously without stopping.

If you don't know where to begin, a good first step is by changing your child's diet. This can be done immediately even before you find the right doctor to help repair your child's immune system. At first, I was *not* convinced eliminating dairy from Ryan's diet would change anything. We were the kind of family that had pizza at least once a week and ate a lot of junk food. The old National Dairy Council's advertisement proclaimed, "Milk is Good for Every Body." I used to believe that, but that just isn't true for our ASD kids.

One of my personal heroes, the late Dr. Bernie Rimland, founder of the Autism Research Institute (ARI), suggested I take Ryan off dairy products for a week. He told me that at the end of the week I should give Ryan a glass of milk to see what happened. At first, I wondered what a cow could possibly have to do with helping my son? But because I was desperate and didn't know what else to do, we changed his diet.

We eliminated all foods that had dairy in the ingredient list. This included cow's milk, cheese, yogurt, casein, and lactalbumin. The change in Ryan's behavior was astounding. Ryan became more tuned-in and more responsive. His weird noises, screaming, biting, and pinching lessened in frequency and intensity. I never did give him that glass of milk at the end of the week.

Still, I worried the rest of our family would all be deprived because Ryan could not have milk products. I had no clue as to what foods I could substitute for dairy in recipes. I spent hours in the grocery store reading labels. I wrongly convinced myself that to help my child, I would have to be chained to the kitchen counter, make two different menus for every meal, and cook from scratch. It took some time to figure out that wasn't true. Our family learned how to eat at restaurants, have prepackaged foods, and have fast food while at the same time eliminating dairy from Ryan's diet.

When we first started life without milk, my son melted down whenever he accidently ate something that contained even the smallest amount of dairy. If I unknowingly gave him something that contained dairy, a more thorough reading of the food label confirmed what I already knew from observing the change in Ryan's behavior. Most times, his ears turned red, his strange noises increased, and he was much harder to deal with.

I learned that when Ryan ate an offending food, when I increased his exercise and water intake, the effects of the foods did not last as long. When a child has an allergic reaction and is taken to the emergency room, they are given adrenalin to speed up and rid their systems of the substance that affected their immune response. When we increased the exercise and water, there was a similar effect.

Daily exercise is still essential for Ryan for his immune system to work better. When he was younger, Ryan rode his bike, jumped on the trampoline, went to the playground, took walks, or did something physical every day. When he accidentally got something he reacted to, we went swimming. I don't know why swimming worked so well for my son. Maybe it increased his metabolism and we didn't worry about the chemicals in the pool. The swimming helped more than any effect from the chemicals.

On Ryan's first allergy test, he reacted to everything. What I didn't understand back then was that the real problem was my son's broken immune system. It was easy for Ryan to fall over when he didn't have two feet firmly planted on the ground. As time went on and his immune system improved, that changed. After two years of helping him regain his health, we repeated the same allergy test. It showed that not many foods still caused a reaction. It showed that only thing he needed to continue to avoid was dairy.

For every meal, our entire family drank water. This saved us a fortune at restaurants over the years. We limited the amount of sugar and fruit juice Ryan consumed (sugars feed *Candida* [aka yeast]). The overgrowth of *Candida* was the reason Ryan stimmed, acted silly, and exhibited that drunk-like behavior.

At times he was hyper, and other times he had no energy at all. He was only allowed two fruits per day in order to limit his sugar intake. *Candida* is a yeast-like fungus that is present in everyone's body. A healthy immune system normally keeps *Candida* from being a problem, but that isn't true for our kids.

Many individuals with compromised immune systems react to gluten. Ryan was never gluten free. Gluten can always be removed later if necessary. But doing both at the same time (casein and gluten) can be overwhelming.

It is important to note whole wheat and whole grains aren't tolerated well by kids with a compromised immune system. Ryan's doctor told me more processed bread would be easier for Ryan to digest. He said to buy the cheapest dairy/casein-free white bread I could find. This seemed confusing because it went against everything I knew about eating right. Suddenly, almost all the rules about nutrition *didn't* apply anymore—at least not to my kid. Whole grains were out. And foods from health food stores were no longer okay for Ryan.

Individuals with autism each have different medical issues and need medical treatment specifically tailored to them. It was not one thing that helped Ryan recover. It was a combination of many little things that caused his immune system to function better. The majority of our doctors have been taught autism is a developmental or psychiatric disorder. Don't be surprised if a physician thinks you're crazy when you ask about medical treatment. Even though they are dedicated and caring doctors, they never got Autism 101 in medical school. Maybe if we stopped calling it "autism" and called it what it is—a messed up immune system—more kids would get the medical treatment they need and deserve.

The doctor who changed Ryan's life was not an autism specialist; he was a physician who understood how the immune system works. In the blog section of my website (www.autism-and-treatment.com), there is a post called *HOW TO FIND THE RIGHT DOCTOR TO BEAT AUTISM.* In it are websites that list doctors by location and zip code. It also has my contact info if you need help coming up with a plan.

Although we are desperate to help our kids, we must think with our heads instead of our hearts. All doctors are not created equal. We must avoid any physicians who aren't doing this for the right reasons. Anyone who promises a miracle cure or instant fix is not the expert you want. And if a treatment sounds too good to be true, it probably is.

Almost all individuals improve with medical treatment. So, don't give up too soon. Our kids have been ill for a long time, and it takes time to get better. Although Ryan is now typical, his recovery from autism was S-L-O-W. "Miracles" can happen for many children by reducing the total load on the immune system. Our loved ones can regain their health, but that is a long process and only happens with hard work and sweat equity.

Doctors who know how to treat autism medically understand that once the body works, the brain follows. Remember, Google is your friend. Type in the kind of doctor (e.g., immunologist, Lyme specialist, PANDAS, functional medicine, integrative medicine, or autism) and list some cities that are near you. Some of the best physicians are hard to find. They try to stay below the radar since they often use interventions that are not yet considered mainstream medical practice. Once you find the right doctor and treat your child's autism medically, the symptoms diminish in intensity. But if you don't see significant improvement in six months, it is time to start the search again.

When picking a doctor, remember you are the expert on your child. If I had listened to everything Ryan's doctor told me to do or ordered me not to do, it would have delayed his progress. **It is important to learn to trust your instincts**. That doesn't happen right away. Once I realized that I knew my son best and needed to be the final decision maker when it came to medical intervention, things started to improve. **With experience, it became easier to know what was science, what made sense, and what we should try or avoid.**

I used to be one of those parents who only wanted to use supplements and natural remedies. But we must use whatever works best to help our kids. I tend to steer clear of the doctors who prescribe a lot of supplements. Their protocols are often impossible to continue, especially when you have a younger child who doesn't yet know how to swallow pills. We can only get so many medicines in our kids and must do the things that have the biggest impact. That being said, many families have recovered kids by only using supplements.

To save time and to rule out physicians who don't do what your child needs, call the doctor's office and ask questions. One question that will immediately eliminate many doctors is this: "Will the doctor prescribe antivirals and anti-fungal medications when warranted?" Some doctors only use these meds for a short time. They think all our kids need is a month or two on the medications. That is usually not the case, and many kids need to be on them continuously and indefinitely. Some individuals are able to stop the medications when their immune system kicks in, but my son has not been one of them.

Ryan's bloodwork showed he had HHV-6 (a Herpes simplex virus). HHV6 is an acute infection generally involving the frontal and/or temporal cortex and the limbic system. It is the leading cause of encephalitis in children and adults in the United States. His labs also showed the presence of the Epstein Barr virus. Viral infections can alter a body's immune function. The antiviral medications can help with this.

Another important question to ask the doctor's office is how often blood tests are done to make sure there are no adverse effects from the medications. (We did them every two-three months.) The reason God made blood tests is to make sure the medications have no long-term ill effects to the liver or kidneys. Ryan is now an adult and has been on these meds continuously since he was about four. He has never had a blood test with an abnormal kidney or liver reading. Reactions to these medications are rare, but if it happens, you can stop any medication that causes an issue.

Sometimes, you have to go to many doctors before you find the one to help your child. One parent told me they went to multiple doctors without much success or improvement. But after they found the right doctor, her son went from only saying "yes" and "no" to speaking three-word sentences and making other huge gains. Another mom went to the same pediatrician as we did. Unfortunately, they did not have the same life-changing results we did. Although her son improved with our doctor's protocol, it wasn't enough and did not address the root cause of her son's autism. This warrior mother didn't find the right doc until her son was sixteen years old. But she never gave up and went to four more doctors until she found the one who knew how to treat the Lyme disease and parasites that were holding her son back. Now her son is in school for the first time. He is getting all A's in mainstream high school classes. He has an aide to help him learn how school works, because he was only homeschooled before. This is a great example of why we should NEVER GIVE UP until we find the answers to help our children.

Ryan is still dependent on medications to keep his immune system working. I think of all the things we did to help Ryan's immune system function better as a treatment and not a cure. When my son builds up a tolerance to a medication, he has to switch to another. For him this seems to happen yearly, and we know it is time to make a change when the autism symptoms start to creep back in. Ryan tried to stop the antifungal medication as an adult. He said he felt tired and felt the compulsion to talk to himself out loud. After he decided to go back on the meds, things shortly returned to his normal baseline.

Even if I could have instantly corrected all of Ryan's medical issues with a magic wand, he still needed to be taught what he couldn't learn before. I used to think that all our problems would be solved if Ryan just learned to talk more. What I didn't understand is that kids on the spectrum don't start speaking in full sentences as soon as their immune systems start to function again. Don't use speech as the indicator of whether a medical protocol is working. Improvements in speech take time, and the results are not immediately apparent. Please consider that it takes at least three years for most neurotypical kids to acquire functional speech.

It is really hard to keep talking to a kid who doesn't respond. All I got was that blank stare. Ryan gave me nothing—not a look and not a smile. The lights were on, but nobody was home. But I continued to talk to Ryan anyway. I didn't realize until after he improved that he had learned so much from our one-sided conversations.

Ryan's bizarre behaviors often overshadowed the fact that we truly were making progress. I *never* missed it when Ryan did something wrong! I couldn't notice his improvement in speech because I was too busy with his tantrums in the mall.

Sometimes, parents mistakenly perceive actual development as a new behavior issue. They think their kids are getting worse. No matter what their chronological age, children pick up where they stalled out and must go through the same developmental stages. If a child was two when typical development stopped, they resume at age two. And two-year-old behavior doesn't look so good in a seven-year-old body. An older child who is two years old developmentally is much harder to deal with than a zonedout kid who doesn't care about anything. An increase in behavior problems can actually be a good sign.

Our kids need a focused rehabilitation program until they start to learn like other kids. So, choose the program you like (e.g., ABA, Floortime, RDI, Son-Rise, TEACCH), and stick with it. They all work once their immune systems start to function better.

When my son was forced to comply after we started ABA, his behaviors got really bad. He began hitting, biting, and pinching us. Once he realized we weren't giving up no matter how hard he tried to make us, things improved. **Reward the behaviors you want to increase, and try to ignore (whenever possible) the negative behaviors you need to eliminate. Look for those rare moments when your kid does something right.**

Concentrate on changing one behavior at a time. If you try to correct too many behaviors at once, our kids get the message they can't do anything right and shut down. So, pick the behavior that drives you crazy, and only work on eliminating that one. Then, pick the next one you need to address. Ryan's inappropriate behavior changed gradually despite the fact that I wanted it to change immediately. As Ryan became healthier, we were able to we move away from a strict ABA stimulus-response model toward a more natural way of teaching. But **nothing worked before we helped Ryan's immune system function better—** not even ABA.

How much ABA is enough ABA? We did about ten hours a week of someone formally working with Ryan. However, since we were all trained in ABA, we used these techniques throughout his waking hours. ABA was implemented in the most natural settings using games and Ryan's interests to keep him focused and working. If you count up the ABA hours in Ryan's day, we probably did more than the recommended forty hours per week. Yet it didn't seem that way to Ryan or us because we were *playing*. We taught him each skill as soon as we saw a need. When he didn't know how to do something, school was immediately in session. We just did what parents should do naturally with kids but with a little ABA thrown in. Most times, Ryan had no idea we were teaching him or that we did everything with specific goals in mind.

The room where Ryan slept was always the cleanest in the house. I changed his sheets at least once a week. We also changed the filter on the heater once a month instead of every three. Sometimes, I put the pillows he slept on and his favorite stuffed animals in the freezer for a couple of hours (that kills dust mites). We only used paper cups in the bathrooms. I also threw the toothbrushes and toothbrush holders in the dishwasher once a week. For laundry, I used a liquid detergent with no dyes or perfumes. I don't know if these small things eliminated immune triggers. But they are easy to do and not expensive.

Most people don't understand how difficult our lives are. Some relatives believe our kids are spoiled; they think the real problem is our parenting. But if you are a parent in the A-Club, I don't have to explain that to you. Still, part of me thought my relatives might be right when they said I created Ryan's issues. And remember parenting by the regular rules doesn't apply when you have a kid on the spectrum. It took time for me to realize: AUTISM IS NOT MY FAULT! Some of us have to repeat that phrase over and over until we actually start to believe it.

I couldn't look too far ahead because I might have given up. When I didn't have a plan and had no idea of what to do next, I just kept putting one foot in front of the other. Recovery takes time and a never-give-up attitude. Some people call this perseverance; I call it being more stubborn than our kids.

The hardest part of this diagnosis is to live with the fear for our children's future. Will my child ever be able to live independently? Who will take care of him after my husband and I are gone? My son's life would have been very different if we had accepted his autism or believed what the so-called experts said.

It angers me when I hear someone say we need to accept autism. Autism *is never* a gift. Our children *are* the only gift. Treating the symptoms of autism doesn't change the wonderful things about our children. It just allows them to be who they were supposed to be before autism came into our lives.

When Ryan was still in middle school, my dream was that someday he could hold a job at McDonald's and live independently. Yet, I wasn't sure that was even possible back then. I know many families who worked as hard as we did without the same results. But there are new treatments coming every day, and the only way to know if something can help your kid is to try.

Don't look too far ahead because this autism stuff can be overwhelming. I made many mistakes along the way. But the one thing I did right was to keep going no matter how bad things got. Don't worry if you don't get it right on the first try; U-turns are allowed. Recovery is the hardest thing you will ever do, but it is so worth it! And God help anyone who gets in our way!

WE MUST WIN THIS WAR!

Remember, if you're headed in the wrong direction, God allows U-turns!

—Allison Gappa Bottke

IMPROVED HEALTH AND even recovery are possible for many children when they are treated medically in conjunction with focused educational and behavioral rehabilitation. Sadly, and for reasons no one fully understands, complete recovery may not be possible for all children. Our family's triumph over autism should never impart the idea that those who did not achieve a similar outcome did not care enough or work hard enough. Each child with autism travels on a different path and has different medical issues. But every individual improves with proper medical intervention.

Children are recovering from autism, and yet the general public and many doctors don't realize this is possible. That is what must change! An autism diagnosis no longer has to mean "game over." And parents no longer have to stand by to helplessly watch their children slip away.

I hope in the near future that Ryan's story becomes the norm, rather than the exception. There are some stories of full recovery from autism—but not enough of them. I've met a few of these delightful young adults. However, I am haunted by the fact that some parents who did all the right things and worked just as hard as I did still have kids who didn't fully recover.

I have survivor's guilt.

Over the years, I have wondered why Ryan was so fortunate. I came to the conclusion that some children may have immune systems that are too broken or compromised to fix with the current interventions. And then there is the luck and timing piece. Were these kids who are still struggling in the right place at the right time to get the proper medical, behavioral, and educational interventions? Were the medical interventions done long enough, at the right dosages, and in the right order? Did their ABA people do the rehabilitation correctly? Were these children lucky enough to get the right teachers who had high expectations? There were so many life-changing events for my son that resulted simply from luck and circumstance.

Hard work made things happen, but Ryan's recovery involved so much more. I want more children to recover. There are too many kids not getting what they need. Valuable time is lost when parents have to wade through massive amounts of information and misinformation to help their child. And it is difficult to go against the ideas of our trusted, well-meaning doctors. It has taken way too much time to change minds and shift the paradigm from a psychiatric disorder a *treatable medical condition*.

Also families who have recovered children seldom tell their stories or *come out*. This is because of the ignorance and negative stigma associated with autism. They escaped from Autism Island and are never going back. Most don't want to remember those difficult times. And those who do speak about recovery soon realize no one believes them anyway. The disbelievers say that our now-typical children must have been misdiagnosed. I suspect the same comments will be made about Ryan from some people who read this book. But I have the videos to prove it.

Although my son is now leading a full and productive life, he is not cured. Ryan is still dependent on medications to help his immune system work optimally. It is hard to keep up with what's new in research. It is very time-consuming to keep sifting through which interventions may be legitimate and which ones are not. I have trouble determining which new treatments will make a difference and should be investigated and possibly pursued. But, as Ryan's mom, I must keep searching for that final fix that could right his immune system *permanently*. As parents, we are never done.

I have spent several chapters relating our family's experience with the medical interventions Dr. Harvey used. Ryan continues to be guided by his protocol to this day. However, I do not want to give the impression that *this kind of medical intervention* is the take-home message for recovering *all* children from autism. That was simply the best medical option available for my son at the time. There are so many more choices, as new research has come along.

I know many families that went down a different path and still got the job done. Check out Jennifer Giustra Kozek's book called *Healing without Hurting: Treating ADHD, Apraxia and Autism Spectrum Disorders Naturally and Effectively without Harmful Medications*. Or Mary Romaniec's book called *Victory Over Autism*. These are only two of the numerous success stories out there.

I used to be one of those parents who only wanted to use supplements and natural remedies. But I changed my mind. Maybe because I couldn't get my son to take them all, as there were just too many. Who knows if we would have had the same outcome if we had only used supplements? For the type of autism Ryan had, the medical treatment we used, and our modified ABA program, worked. I am thrilled for those who have recovered their kids by only using supplements, but that didn't work for us.

Now I think we should use whatever works. MDs or DOs who use both supplements and prescriptions are the best kind of doctors. That's why I tell the families I help to look for a functional medicine doctor or an immunologist for medical treatment. The doctor who helped my son most was not an autism specialist, but a pediatrician who understood how to correct the problems with his immune system. Finding the right doctor still remains one of our biggest challenges. And even the visionary doctor who helped us most didn't have all the answers to help my son. Sometimes to help our kids we have to use multiple doctors.

For my son, removing dairy had a huge impact, but, at first, that just seemed strange. It was hard to understand what cows could have to do with the treatment of autism. And for Ryan, the medications that had the biggest impact were antifungals, antivirals, leucovorin, and an SSRI. He had to take iron because he had low ferritin stores and used Zyrtec® and Beconase Aq nasal spray during allergy season. We treated each of Ryan's medical issues one at a time.

Some children are able to stop the prescription medications when their immune system starts working again. But as of yet, my son isn't one of them. Ryan has been on an antifungal prescription continuously since he was about five and an antiviral since he was ten. The good news is he never had an irregular reading on his blood tests when it came to kidney and liver function.

When Ryan tried to stop the antifungal medication a few years back, he called me within a couple weeks and said he didn't feel well. When I asked him what he was feeling, my son said he felt very tired and felt a compulsion to talk to himself out loud. So he went back on them. Ryan alternates between several medicines to make sure they remain effective. When he builds up a tolerance to a medication and it stops working, he switches to another. (He needs to alternate medications about once a year.)

Medical treatment alone would not have been enough. ABA alone would not have been enough. It was this combination that made it possible for him to completely recover and learn what he couldn't learn before.

The medical piece is the hardest part for me to understand. I am not a doctor. All I ever wanted to be was my children's mom. When I come across new medical research, *I ask the people I trust*, who are much more knowledgeable than I. Deciding whether to leap into something new or stick with the current plan often leads me to revisit old insecurities. Insecure or not, sometimes we have to take that leap of faith.

My latest leap has been into the world of genes and autism. Researchers have identified specific genes whose cellular pathways and function may directly contribute to the behaviors we now label as autism. Medical interventions can counteract the effects of these genetic abnormalities. In the future, the study of genes may provide the flow chart needed to know which treatments will be effective with which kids.

Recently, we learned from blood test results that Ryan has a single methylenetetrahydrofolate reductase (MTHFR)[49] gene polymorphism. Many well-credentialed scientists agree that even with a genetic predisposition to being environmentally sensitive, an environmental trigger is necessary for autism to occur. But the take-home message is that even with an underlying gene mutation, Ryan was able to make **remarkable progress with targeted medical intervention**.[50]

Ryan was prescribed a specific form of folate based on the results of this MTHFR gene test.[51] According to neurologist Richard Frye, MD, PhD, and my MTHFR guru, the prescription medication Leucovorin helps remedy the

---

49 Methylenetetrahydrofolate reductase (MTHFR) polymorphism of genes 677 and 1298 and catechol-O-methyltransferase (COMT) are of current interest. 5,10-methylenetetrahydrofolate reductase (NADPH) makes the enzyme methylenetetrahydrofolate reductase and enables homocysteine (an amino acid) to make methionine. MTHFR 677C>T (rs1801133) and 1298A>C (rs1801131) reduce enzymatic activity. MTHFR and COMT mutations can cause compromised detoxification pathways and decrease glutathione. Supplementation is specific to the individual's genetic expression.

50 Engel, Stephanie & Daniels, Julie. "On The Complex Relationship Between Genes And Environment In The Etiology Of Autism." *Epidemiology* Volume 22, Issue 4, July 2011: pp. 486-488. This article provides information on higher than expected rates of MTHFR mutations in parents of a child with autism. There is currently substantial interest in identifying specific genes and alleles whose cellular pathways and functioning status may directly contribute to the behaviors we now label as "autistic." Dr. Richard Frye's work in this area can provide the reader with easily accessible information they may wish to discuss with their doctor. Some children have made substantial progress when the medication leucovorin was added to their treatment. That medication worked to cause a behavioral change when the MTHFR gene and single nucleotide polymorphism (SNP) profiles were involved. Some children with autism have specific allele and SNP combinations that made remarkable progress with supplementation based on the results of their specific gene tests.

51 Individuals with different Allele/SNP results require different prescription formulation.

effects of this gene mutation.[52] This was the same medication I secretly kept in place many years ago after Dr. Harvey told us to stop everything else we were doing. Leucovorin was instrumental in developing my son's speech way back then. But we stopped seeing the doctor who originally prescribed it, and eventually we ran out.

Ryan started taking leucovorin again after college. Just when I thought my kid couldn't get any better physically, he did. But as is often the case, my son didn't respond to the new medication with an immediate or positive response. Initially, Ryan was more tired than usual and had no energy. His doctor told him to hang on for a few weeks.

Two to three weeks after he started leucovorin, Ryan was no longer tired at the end of the workday and was soon running on all cylinders. He became the go-to guy at work. When he was away from his desk, giving a tour, his boss couldn't wait for him to return to solve a problem she encountered in his absence.

Maybe MTHFR status will be a game changer for your child, and maybe it won't. If your child does not have this gene polymorphism, then you need to keep searching. We have certainly chased our share of medical dead ends. There have been many things that have looked promising but did not pan out. But there is always hope because there is always something new coming down the road.

Unfortunately, the reason the autism puzzle is so difficult to solve is because each child has different medical issues that need to be addressed. Autism is complex. We all want that magic bullet. Yet we need to use what is out there *now* to help our children as long as it is biologically plausible and can be done safely under appropriate medical supervision. If I had waited for the mainstream medical establishment to research Dr. Harvey's protocol and validate it as a

---

52   Dr. Frye did a study to document his hypothesis about leucovorin, but the time it takes to be accepted by the rest of the medical community is way too long. See the blog post on my website called "What the Heck Is The MTHFR and What Does It Have To Do With Autism?" for the latest info. For more info on Dr. Frye and his work go to: https://recoveringkids. com/2017/11/06/conference/?fbclid=IwAR133JG61qk9x5xxM81zhvCfXb7plfZ WgisBVK7TM9T971MGXi8jZtDquiA

proven treatment for autism, God only knows where Ryan could have ended up. He definitely wouldn't be where he is today.

That being said, all medical treatments must be under a doctor's care. And as I said before, all doctors are not created equal. Trust your gut when assessing if something new is safe and should be tried to help your child.

And for those of you who have tried it all, we still can never give up because every day new treatments are being developed.

The research into mitochondria and interventions at the cellular level looks promising for a subset of autism. Current research linked ASD to dysfunctions in the mitochondria.

Mitochondria are bean-shaped tiny parts of the cell responsible for producing energy and are the powerhouses of the cells. Mitochondria turn fat, sugar, and protein into energy. "Ultimately, understanding the energetic aspects of neurodevelopmental disorders may lead to entirely new kinds of treatments, and preventive strategies that would target mitochondria," according to Zhenglong Gu a research scientist at Cornell University. We must also learn more about the potential use of rituximab and peptides.

Dr. James Adams and Dr. Frye are doing trials for microbiota transfer therapy (MTT) for both children and adults on the spectrum. Their research is showing great promise. Treatment simply involves swallowing a liquid medication to repair the issues with gut health. One parent in the trials told me that after only two weeks, her seven-year-old gained fifty words and was potty trained for the first time. And the gains for her son have remained. Another parent whose son was in the adult trials told me her son was no longer in pain and is now having typical bowel movements for the first time in his life. And when the gut is healed, then the kids begin to progress. This microbiota therapy didn't have to be repeated like so many treatments do. When microbiota transplants finally become approved to treat autism, Ryan wants one. Our hope is that with this therapy, Ryan may no longer have to be dependent on the antifungal meds.[53]

---

53 For more info on the microbiota trials, go to http://autism.asu.edu. When I spoke to Dr. Adams and asked him if Ryan could be in his microbiota transplant study he said he couldn't because Ryan is no longer considered to have autism. I also asked Dr.

We also need to gain a deeper understanding of how the immune dysfunction affects our children. For some children, IVIG infusions have made all the difference. And stem cells have changed outcomes. But we need to know more. But I have great hope for their future use and pray with time they will provide answers for more people and bring permanent gains.

Genetic testing may help us learn which treatments are most effective for which individuals. As parents, it is up to us to work with our doctors to improve how our children's immune systems function.

We must also set the tone for everyone to work as a team. That is the best way to minimize the chaos this disease creates in families. We must partner with our doctors, behaviorists, teachers, and anyone else who could possibly help our children.

Try not to be as crazy as I was and worry about every possible thing that could go wrong. I used to believe if I didn't get it right on the first try, Ryan would not get better. That just wasn't true. I made many mistakes along the way, but the one mistake we must never make is to give up before we find the answers to help our children.

I long for the day when someone gives the world a "cure" for autism. But for now, we just manage it. It helps me to think in terms of "treatments" and not "cures." I compare it to the way a diabetic needs insulin to make their body work properly.

The medical treatment only makes it possible for our children to learn. Often we think all our issues will be solved if our children just gain speech. But it is important to remember speech is not a good indicator that a medical treatment is bringing improvements. It takes typical kids without any health issues almost three years to learn language. We can't assume the medical treatment isn't working if our children don't immediately start talking in full sentences.

Adams what may benefit our kids in the near future. He said his protocol has helped many (you can find it at www.autismNRC.com). Dr. Adams believes fish oil, when given at the right dose can also be of benefit. He would like to see more research on antifungal meds and how to keep the candida from returning.

In addition, an intensive rehab program is needed to catch our children up on all they missed. Any program you chose works when the medical issues have been addressed. When medical treatment is combined with rehab, that makes the rehab programs work faster and recovery is possible for those who couldn't recover before.

Autism is never easy. Just keep putting one foot in front of the other. Don't look back or spend time thinking about the mistakes. We must always move the dream forward. And don't give up when you are exhausted. You can give up when you are done.

We must never give up until we find the answers for all children. That is the only way to win the war against autism. And we must win this one because there are too many kids not getting better.

ALONE there is little we can do about autism...
TOGETHER we will be unstoppable.

Part 8

Appendices and More Info

APPENDIX I

FRANK'S LETTER TO THE DOCTOR WHO DIAGNOSED RYAN

ONE OF MY favorite things Ryan's dad did through the years was a little vengeful, and maybe even a little mean. Whenever Ryan did anything extraordinary, my husband sent an email to the psychiatrist who diagnosed my son. He'd inform her of the new and wonderful thing Ryan just accomplished, which she said could never happen. Frank has written several emails to her over the years. I included one of them below. She never answers, but that doesn't stop him from sending them. These emails continue to be very therapeutic and part of our family's healing. But more important than that, we want this *expert* to learn that kids can recover before she pronounces another *life sentence* on a family. I can't wait until Frank sends her a copy of this book.

From: Frank Hinds
Sent: Friday, May 4, 2007
Subject: My son, Ryan
Dear Dr. Goodman:

This is an update on my son Ryan's progress. You diagnosed Ryan with PDD-NOS at the age of four. You told my wife and me that he would need special schools, be unable to deal with people, and had a good chance of ending up in *an institution or group home. You said if we were lucky, someday he might get to work in the basement of some company where he wouldn't have to talk to anyone.*

Ryan is now eighteen and a senior in high school. Ryan was one of seven students from his high school out of a class of 560 selected for this Celebration of Excellence honor. (If you do the math, that puts him in the 98.75th percentile.) The award was not for running a computer or memorizing inane facts (as YOU might have predicted), it was for SOCIAL SCIENCE.

I'm taking time out of my day to write you, not because I have a lot of time on my hands. You see, next week we get to go to Ryan's end of season track banquet where he will receive a letter in track for running the 800- and 1600-meter runs. This award will go well with the letters he earned in Cross Country and Track from last year. The week after that, we attend a dinner at the Reagan Library, where Ryan has been selected as a Ronald Reagan Library Scholar. In the middle of this, Ryan is taking four AP exams. Of course, that is not unusual for him, having taken three exams last year, scoring two 4s and a 5 (out of 5 possible).

He graduates in June and his schedule doesn't let up. Ryan will continue helping out at a local nursing home and start a summer job to earn money for college. Oh, I forgot to mention that Ryan was accepted at Santa Clara University, the University of Southern California, Loyola Marymount University (with Honors), California Polytechnic University (San Luis Obispo), and the University of California, both Irvine and Santa Barbara campuses.

Ryan chose Santa Clara University both because of the outstanding engineering program and the fact that they along with Loyola offered him the most scholarship money of the THREE schools that offered him MERIT-based scholarships. Did I mention that Ryan had to interview for these scholarships with university alumni and staff (you know, the kind of people he shouldn't be able to talk to)? He'll miss his best friend (surprise, Ryan has friends) who'll be attending UCSB, but he's already met some great kids at Santa Clara University.

Have I left anything out? Oh, yeah, my wife and I would like to thank you once again for making us so angry with your diagnosis/prognosis that we were determined to prove you wrong. I assume you won't respond to this email just as you have failed to respond to all of the others.

Thanks again,
Frank Hinds

AUTISM—THE REAL STORY NEEDS TO BE TOLD

Please share this article with anyone it might help. It is available to share from my website (www.autism-and-treatment.com). You have my permission to reprint it and share it everywhere.

Imagine a world . . . where children with recurring fevers, unexplained seizures, and chronic rashes are denied medical treatment.

Imagine a world . . . where increasing numbers of children show up in our schools without speech, lost in their own worlds, and have no hope for the future.

Imagine a world . . . where children with severe sleep disorders, limited speech, nutritional deficiencies, stomach problems, and severe allergies are sent to psychologists and psychiatrists.

When you have a child with autism, you don't have to imagine any of this. If your child has been diagnosed with autism, this is the world you live in. How can we just stand by and let this happen?

Some say the increase in autism is due to better diagnostic tools and awareness. Don't believe it! The increase in autism is REAL! No one can miss a child with autism. They have epic meltdowns in the grocery store and they throw award-winning tantrums in restaurants. They do and say strange things. Some never say anything at all, including, "I love you."

Still there is hope. The solution to the autism crisis seems complicated, but in reality, it is simple if you know the truth about autism. Autism is a complex medical condition caused (in most part) by an immune system that is not working properly.

My son, Ryan, was diagnosed with autism at age four. I was told there was nothing I could do. A psychiatrist, who was a leading authority on autism, told me that my son would probably need to be institutionalized. She was wrong.

Ryan's recovery helped me realize autism is a treatable and changeable condition. Treating him medically took time; the road was long and difficult. It felt as if it would last forever! Our family made many sacrifices and many mistakes along the way. Some days we were barely hanging on by our fingernails. But, the only institution Ryan ever ended up in was the university where he graduated Magna Cum Laude. NASA paid for most of his master's degree after he completed a paid internship with them. Today, he works as an engineer at a major aerospace company when he is not surfing or going out with friends.

We need to stop looking at autism backwards. Autism is not the cause of the many medical conditions our children suffer from. In reality, it is the other way around. The dysregulation of their immune systems results in the symptoms we call autism. Autism needs to be taken out of the psychiatric journals and put into the medical books where it belongs. Physicians who know how to treat autism medically understand that once the body works, the brain follows.

Unfortunately, there is no easy fix or magic bullet to heal our children. It takes time to repair a child's compromised immune system. And each child has different medical issues. Once the body has healed, a child still needs focused educational and behavioral interventions to catch up on what was missed when they were too sick to develop normally.

Even though our children are often said to have low intelligence, don't believe it. The book Carly's Voice demonstrates just how smart our kids really are. Carly lacked speech and couldn't communicate with her parents until she learned how to type at age ten. She still hasn't gained the ability to speak but after reading her story no one would ever question just how intelligent and capable she is. Carly is a great example of why we can't give up and why we need to solve the autism problem. We need to put an end to this disease that is taking our children and robbing them of happy and productive lives.

Even if you don't have a child on the autism spectrum, you probably have one in your child's classroom. When a child is ill with autism, they rarely recover completely without medical treatment no matter how much money is spent on their education. Our educational funds are limited and sometimes used ineffectively. The autism epidemic takes away from all of our children, including the healthy ones.

Autism awareness is no longer enough. We need a doctor on every corner who says, "I know what this is, and I know how to treat it." The world needs to realize our children are not broken—they are sick! They can get better with proper medical treatment combined with focused rehabilitation. Many children have already made the long, difficult journey to recovery. If these children can be healed, more can be helped. We no longer have to sit and watch helplessly while our children slip away.

Don't believe all you've been told about autism. You know that your child is ill. You've caught a glimpse, however brief, of the loving, vibrant child who is hidden behind the veil of autism. You know they are in there. We must join together to give our children a future. We can agree that this is a medical and treatable condition. This must be our message; unwavering, unapologetic and most of all, unified. The infighting among different groups about what causes autism and how to fix it must stop. That is the only way we will win the war against autism. We must never give up until we find the answers for our children.

AUTISM GROUPS, ANOTHER WAY OFF THE ISLAND

Parents of children with autism are warriors and quick to learn about the latest research that helps our children. As a result, there are many autism discussion groups on the internet and Facebook that are extremely current with the research about what we can do to help our children get healthier.

I belong to several groups and try to help parents start down the complex road to recovery. These groups cover everything from new medical research to questions posed by parents on how to deal with schools and other everyday issues associated with autism. I have learned so much from the informed people in these groups. There is a lot of sound medical information disseminated along with a lot of garbage, too. *Read thoughtfully.*

These online discussion groups serve as support for those of us who live on Autism Island. We talk to each other about everything. I consider these people to be my best friends, because we have shared so many intimate details of our lives over the years.

Strange as it sounds, I would not recognize most of these people if I walked past them on the street. They live all over the world and they know things about me that I would never admit to anyone else. It is bizarre how this A-Club can make us instant friends and confidants. My friends in these groups get it. They understand what it is like to have a kid with autism. It is so comforting to not have to explain our frustrations or feelings. We would die for our kids and love them more than anything, but at the same time hate them for creating this craziness and difficulty in our lives. On my website there is a lot of information to help you. And I'm constantly updating it because *I am never done*!

REFERENCES

There are many good books, websites, apps, and videos about autism. I've included a few here, but there is so much more.

I found the cheapest and most effective way to teach my son was by using technology. I bought every computer program I could by the *Edmark Company* because their programs were linguistically based. When my son was playing *Millie's Math House*, he was also learning language. My favorite game is still *Thinkin' Things One*. These programs are still available today, because they have stood the test of time. They are also inexpensive because they are older.

I wish we had a computer tablet or smartphone when we were trying to teach Ryan all the things he didn't know. Our kids love technology. As a result, autism apps are extremely helpful for managing your child's daily routines and providing the motivation to learn. For individuals who are nonverbal or have limited verbal ability, these apps can be essential to help them communicate.

When I was looking for educational materials to use with my son, I used to hang out at the teacher supply stores. Our kids love workbooks because they are predictable. I liked everything Frank Schaffer did, but there are hundreds more. And the inexpensive workbooks you can buy at drug stores or other retail stores work too.

Your child's speech teacher and other parents are also great resources. I got a lot of ideas on how to teach conversation from watching Ryan's speech teacher. Steal the stuff that works and do more of it at home. Borrow materials and remember to make it fun for your child. Don't forget to use what your kids love or obsess about to teach them.

There are a multitude of websites and blogs that make recommendations about which apps are best to teach conversation skills, friendship, interaction skills, emotional awareness, and behavior management. There are no correct answers when it comes to choosing the right applications. You know your kid best and what motivates him/her.

YouTube is a great tool for teaching many things your child needs to learn. It is also effective for teaching ABA techniques. The Listening Program (TLP), Fast Forward, vision therapy, and Brainjogging are also great resources. In addition, the website for this book, www.autism-and-treatment.com is constantly being updated. Email me there and I will do my best to answer your questions and help your family any way I can. I want all kids to have what Ryan now has.

Other Resources:

Maurice, Catherine. *Let Me Hear Your Voice: A Family's Triumph Over Autism.* New York: Knopf, 1993.

Maurice, Catherine; Green, Gina; & Luce, Stephen. *Behavioral Intervention for Young Children with Autism: A Manual for Parents and Professionals.* Austin: Pro-Ed., 1996.

Barbera, Mary: *The Verbal Behavior Approach: How to Teach Children with Autism and Related Disorders.* Jessica Kingsley Publishers 2007.

Freeman, Sabrina; & Dake, Lorelei. *Teach Me Language: A Language Manual for Children with Autism, Asperger's Syndrome and Related Developmental Disorders.* Langley: SKF Books, 1997.

Gladysz, Dominka. *Immune Abnormalities in Autism Spectrum Disorder—Could They Hold Promise for Causative Treatment?* Molecular Neurobiology Abstract January 2018

Hughes, Heather. *Immune Dysfunction and Autoimmunity as Pathological Mechanisms in Autism Spectrum Disorders.* Frontiers in Cellular Neuroscience. November 13, 2018

Mannix, Darlene. *Social Skills Activities for Special Children.* San Francisco: Jossey-Bass, 2008.

Mannix, Darlene. *Life Skills Activities for Special Children.* San Francisco: Jossey-Bass, 2009.

Mannix, Darlene. *Social Skills Activities for Secondary Students with Special Needs.* San Francisco: Jossey-Bass, 2009.

Michelle, Lonnie. *How Kids Make Friends*. Freedom Publishing Company. 2000.
(This inexpensive paperback was not written especially for families dealing with autism but has very important information all kids need to know to make friends.)

Sharma, Melinda. *A Parent's Guide to the Common Immune System Issues in Autism Spectrum Disorder*. Published 2016.
(This book has important information for you and your doctor. It includes the tests you may want to ask your doctor to order.)

Sheridan, Kate. *Could an Antibiotic Treat Autism? Medication to Reduce Brain Cell Inflammation Could Treat Widespread Disorder*. Newsweek Tech and Science. February 9, 2018

BIBLIOGRAPHY

Abbott, Alysia, "Love in the Time of Autism." *Psychology Today* Volume 46, Number 4 July/August 2013: pp. 60–67.

Ablow, Dr. Keith, "Deplin: A 'Medical Food' That Treats Depression." FoxNews.com, June 18, 2013.

Canfield, Jack and Hansen, Mark and McNamara, Heather and Simmons, Karen. *Chicken Soup for the Soul: Children with Special Needs.* Deerfield Beach, Florida: HCI, 2006.

Conniff, Richard, "The Body Eclectic." Smithsonian. Volume 44, Number 2, May 2013: pp. 40-47.

Engel, Stephanie and Daniels, Julie, "On the Complex Relationship Between Genes and Environment in the Etiology of Autism." *Epidemiology* Volume 22, Issue 4, July 2011: pp. 476-485.

Faber, Adele, and Mazlish, Elaine. *How to Talk So Kids Will Listen & Listen So Kids Will Talk.* New York: Avon, 1982.

Faber, Adele, and Mazlish, Elaine. *Siblings Without Rivalry.* New York: W.W. Norton & Company, 1987.

Frost, Lori and Bondy, Andy. *The Picture Exchange Communication System Training Manual, 2nd Edition.* Newark, DE: Pyramid Educational Consultants, 2002.

Goldberg, Michael and Goldberg, Elyse. *The Myth of Autism: How a Misunderstood Epidemic is Destroying Our Children.* New York: Skyhorse Publishing, 2011.

Goldberg, Michael and Mena, Ismael and Miller, Bruce, "Frontal and Temporal Lobe Dysfunction in Autism and Other Related Disorders: ADHD and OCD." alasbimnjournal.net, July 1, 1999.

Green, Laura. "The Well-being of Siblings of Individuals with Autism." *International Scholarly Research Notices*, Volume 2013, Article ID 417194, February 18, 2013.

Hacker, Bonnie, "Early Referrals for Speech and Language Challenges On the Rise." *Emerge a Child's Place*, April 2012.

Hacker, Bonnie, "Mothers Found to Overestimate Children's Language Development." *Emerge a Child's Place*, September 2011.

Hacker, Bonnie, "Mounting Evidence that Mothers Overestimate Language Development." *Emerge a Child's Place*, April 2013.

Helt, Molly, et al., "Can Children With Autism Recover? If So, How?" *Neuropsychological Review* Volume 18, 2008: pp. 339-366.

Herbert, Martha and Weintraub, Karen. *The Autism Revolution: Whole-body Strategies for Making Life All It Can Be.* New York: Ballantine Books, 2012.

Irlen, Helen. *Reading by the Colors: Overcoming Dyslexia and Other Reading Disabilities Through the Irlen Method.* Garden City Park: Avery Publishing Group, 1991.

Landalf, Helen and Rimland, Mark. *The Secret Night World of Cats.* Hanover: Smith and Kraus, 1997.

Kopp, Katherine, "Infants' Gaze Shifting May Predict Autism." *Carolina Parent*, May 2013 p. 29.

Maurice, Catherine. *Let Me Hear Your Voice: A Family's Triumph Over Autism.* New York: Knopf, 1993.

Michelle, Lonnie. *How Kids Make Friends.* Evanston: Freedom, 1995.

Nathe, Margarite, "Signal to Noise." *Endeavors* Volume XXVIII, Number 2, Winter 2012, pp. 14-19.

Rapp, Doris. *Allergies and the Hyperactive Child.* New York: Simon & Schuster, 1979.

Rapp, Doris. *Is This Your Child?* New York: William Morrow & Company, 1986.

Rapp, Doris. *Is This Your Child's World?* New York: Bantam, 1996.

Rapp, Doris. *The Impossible Child in School, At Home: A Guide for Caring Teachers and Parents.* Aylesbury: Allergy Research Foundation, 1989.

Center for Disease Control and Prevention. *"Learn the Signs. Act Early."* cdc. gov, March 27, 2014.

Diagnostic and Statistic Manual of Mental Disorders, Fourth Edition (TR), 2000, American Psychiatric Publishing.

Diagnostic and Statistic Manual of Mental Disorders, Fifth Edition, 2013, American Psychiatric Publishing.

Procedural Safeguards: *Handbook On Parents' Rights, Public Schools of North Carolina,* Revised April 2009.

Treating Autism and Autism Treatment Trust, *"Medical Comorbidities in Autism Spectrum Disorders."* autismtreatmenttrust.org, March 2013.

ACKNOWLEDGMENTS

I want to thank everyone who helped tell Ryan's story. A special thanks to Tony Lyons, Caroline Russomanno, and Mark Gompertz from Skyhorse Publishing for all your help making this book possible and sharing our story. And to my agents Leslie Garson and Michael Wright, because of your hard work more families will know autism is medical, treatable, and outcomes will change.

Dean Abramson was indispensable in making this book happen. Dean had my back when I needed him most, and all it cost me was a few home-cooked meals and some very fattening desserts.

Teri Arranga, the grammar queen editor, drove me crazy making sure everything in this book was absolutely correct. She held my hand, encouraged me, and kicked my butt when I needed that too.

Sian McLean helped with the direction of the book. Without her, I might still be talking about this book instead of having written it.

And to my dear friend Dr. Melinda Sharma, thank you for your relentless commitment to helping children, knowledge about immunology/autism, and attention to detail. She ensured I got my facts right.

To Pam Smith, Gena McElwain, and Mindi Fischer Polenz, you helped develop and implement Ryan's modified Applied Behavior Analysis (ABA) program. Without your help and guidance, our family never would have made it. You were our sanity in the darkest time of our lives.

Bryce Miler wrote the letter to the editor that led us to the medical care that changed Ryan's life. Catherine Maurice's book, *Let Me Hear Your Voice*, provided my first inkling that our children can get better. Catherine's story gave me hope and continues to be relevant today. It was the first book I read that offered real solutions.

Dr. Bernie Rimland and Dr. Sidney Baker were the first to show us there might be a way out of this hell. I am forever grateful for all the researchers and physicians who treat autism as a medical condition. They are changing the paradigm and showing the rest of the world that autism is medical and treatable.

The advances from Dr. James Adam's and his research team have changed outcomes. Micobiota Tranfer Therapy (MTT) will be a game changer for our kids. And the advances with stem cells have given us hope for the future. As a result of the dedication of these pioneers, some of our children will live full, happy, productive lives.

Ed and Teri Arranga improve lives daily with their AutismOne nonprofit. Dr. Steve Edelson of the Autism Research Institute (ARI), Ann Millan, and all the others who are totally committed to making a difference for individuals with autism. There are too many of you to mention but for each of you, this is all about hope, helping others, and creating possibilities for our children.

And to all of Ryan's teachers, and the other professionals who helped Ryan and our family escape from Autism Island. You helped us through the rough times and made my son feel loved and cherished when he was still different and so alone. It took so many of you to help one little kid make it.

A special thanks to both my tech divas, Diana Lee and Lisa Orsic, your encouragement and skills helped this technology impaired mom more than you will ever know.

And, to Barb Weisel, my friend, neighbor, and unofficial shrink, you keep me on track in life, and continue to remind me to butt out of Ryan and Megan's lives.

And finally, to all the parents who shared your personal stories, your experiences, and heartaches. Your words will encourage others to continue the fight. We will never give up!

ABOUT THE AUTHOR

Marcia Hinds has more than fifteen years' experience as an educational and behavioral consultant. She works with children on the autism spectrum and advocates for their families. Marcia holds a bachelor's in Psychology and Sociology from the University of California at Los Angeles (UCLA). She is a credentialed K-12 teacher. Ironically, Marcia, along with her husband Frank, worked in the UCLA Young Autism Project under Dr. Ivar Lovass as undergraduates at UCLA. As therapists they used Applied Behavior Analysis (ABA) before all the research was in about the effectiveness of ABA. Thirteen years later, that training came in handy when Ryan came along and their lives changed forever.

Marcia's most impressive credential for writing this book is that she is Ryan's and Megan's mother and her family survived their war against autism. As a result of combining medical, behavioral, and educational interventions, Ryan recovered. Ryan now works as an aerospace systems engineer for a major company. But more important than that . . . Ryan has friends, a social life, and is happy. In short, he is living the life all parents want for their children. He does everything the "experts" said would never happen. Ryan's inspirational story brings hope to families in the trenches still struggling to help their children.